Alternative Medicine Guide to

Heart Disease

BURTON GOLDBERG

and the Editors of

ALTERNATIVE MEDICINE DIGEST

 FUTURE MEDICINE PUBLISHING

TIBURON, CALIFORNIA

Future Medicine Publishing, Inc.
1640 Tiburon Blvd., Suite 2
Tiburon, CA 94920

Editor: Richard Leviton
Senior Editor: Stephanie Marohn
Assistant Editor: Nina Giglio
Research Editor: John Anderson
Art Director: Janine White
Cover and book design: Amparo Del Rio Design
Indicated images: LifeART Images Copyright©1989-1997
by TechPool Studios, Inc. USA

Manufactured in the United States of America.

10 9 8 7 6 5 4 3 2 1

Library of Congress Cataloging-in-Publication Data

Goldberg, Burton, 1926-
    Alternative Medicine Guide to Heart Disease /
Burton Goldberg and the Editors of Alternative
Medicine Digest.
    Includes bibliographical references and index.
    ISBN 1-887299-10-6 (trade paper)
    1. Heart—Diseases—Alternative treatment. I. Title
RC684.A48G65   1997
616.1'206—dc21   97-39816
                                          CIP

Portions of this book were previously published,
in a different form, in *Alternative Medicine: The
Definitive Guide* and *Alternative Medicine Digest*.

Important Information

BURTON GOLDBERG and the editors of *Alternative Medicine Digest* are proud of the public and professional praise accorded Future Medicine Publishing's series of books. This latest book continues the groundbreaking tradition of its predecessors.

The health of you and your loved ones is important. Treat this book as an educational tool that will enable you to better understand, assess, and choose the best course of treatment when heart disease strikes, and how to prevent heart disease from striking in the first place. It could save your life.

Remember that this book on heart disease is different. It is not another catalog of mainstream medicine's conventional treatments and drugs used to treat heart disease. This book is about *alternative* approaches to heart disease–approaches generally not understood and, at this time, not endorsed by the medical establishment. We urge you to discuss the treatments described in this book with your doctor. If your doctor is open-minded, you may actually educate him or her. We have been gratified to learn that many of our readers have found their physicians to be open to new ideas.

Use this book wisely. Because many of the treatments described in this book are, by definition, alternative, they have not been investigated, approved or endorsed by any government or regulatory agency. National, state, and local laws may vary regarding the use and application of many of the treatments that are discussed. Accordingly, this book should not be substituted for the advice and care of a physician or other licensed health care professional. Pregnant women, in particular, are especially urged to consult with a physician before commencing any therapy. Ultimately, you, the reader, must take responsibility for your health and how you use the information in this book.

Future Medicine Publishing and the authors have no financial interest in any of the products or services discussed in this book, other than the citations to Future Medicine's other publications. All of the factual information in this book has been drawn from the scientific literature.

Contents

PART TWO—High Blood Pressure (Hypertension)

PART THREE—Stroke

You Don't Have to Die of Heart Disease

HEART DISEASE is a disease of the 20th century. Atherosclerosis, the hardening, thickening, and clogging of the arteries, was virtually unknown in 1900. Today, it is a major killer of Americans. This book will show you why heart disease is rampant, how to reverse it using natural, alternative modalities, and how to prevent it from returning or occuring in the first place. This book will explain—and give you the proof—why heart disease is a function of nutrient deficiency and toxicity, and how you can avoid bypass, angioplasty, heart transplants, and other highly invasive cardiac procedures.

Today, an estimated 57.4 million Americans have one or more types of heart disease. Heart disease is responsible for half of all deaths in the United States. In addition to the huge cost in human suffering, the medical costs of treating this epidemic are astronomical. As you will learn in this book, conventional medicine is making little progress in stemming the tide of this epidemic. This is because, for the most part, it only offers assistance when an individual's heart disease has become a serious problem. And that assistance fails as a solution because it does not address the underlying causes of heart disease.

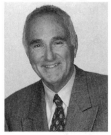

Cholesterol-lowering drugs, high blood pressure medication, angioplasty to clean out the arteries, and coronary artery bypass surgery—the most common "solutions"—may temporarily relieve the symptoms. Often, however, they don't even accomplish that, but instead introduce dangerous side effects and further complications in the patient's condition. For example, cholesterol-lowering drugs have been found to actually increase your risk of heart attack and stroke. Channel blockers, the drug of choice for high blood pressure, increase your risk of developing cancer.

As you will learn in this book, invasive medical procedures such as angioplasty and coronary artery bypass surgery are frequently unnecessary and produce no benefit to the patient at all. Some people endure multiple operations (one patient whose case is discussed in this book underwent 14 angioplasties) without result or their condition returns later. In addition, bypass surgery is dangerous, many people suffering strokes or other damage to their brain as a result of the operation.

Much of this is needless suffering because heart disease is one of the most preventable chronic degenerative diseases. This is both the good news and the bad news; bad news because many of the nearly one million annual deaths from heart disease didn't need to happen, but good news because the epidemic can be brought to a halt. Alternative medicine has practical solutions for reversing and preventing heart disease. The message is: you don't have to die from or even be sick with heart disease.

The doctors in this book have years of experience treating heart disease and will show you how you can keep your heart healthy and, if you already have heart disease, how you can reverse it. They don't use just one therapy, but draw on a range of alternative medicine approaches. As heart disease is not caused by one factor alone, the best treatment will involve multiple methods to remove each contributing cause. The doctors in this book know that in order to permanently reverse any health condition, you must find and remove the multiple factors that created it. This is a basic principle of alternative medicine and the reason why it succeeds where conventional medicine often fails in the treatment of chronic disease.

The first place many alternative physicians begin is with diet, exercise, and lifestyle habits. Sometimes, reversing heart disease is as simple as making changes in these areas. In other cases, supplements are needed to address specific nutritional deficiencies which have contributed to the patient's condition. Therapies which have proven

Much of this is needless suffering because heart disease is one of the most preventable chronic degenerative diseases. This is both the good news and the bad news; bad news because many of the nearly one million annual deaths from heart disease didn't need to happen, but good news because the epidemic can be brought to a halt.

particularly invaluable in the treatment of heart disease include chelation and hyperbaric oxygen. Chelation therapy is a highly effective and noninvasive method of clearing the arteries and reversing atherosclerosis (clogging of the arteries due to plaque, or buildup, on the arterial walls), the main cause of heart disease. Hyperbaric oxygen therapy has been remarkably successful in reversing the damage caused by stroke, even years afterward, by getting oxygen to oxygen-deprived brain tissues.

You may well ask—Why haven't I heard about these treatments? The answer is: politics and greed. The U.S. medical monopoly, comprised of the major pharmaceutical companies, physicians' trade groups, insurance companies, and government bodies such as the National Institutes of Health and the Food and Drug Administration, have a literal investment in keeping nonpatentable and inexpensive treatments from the public. Widespread use of chelation and hyperbaric oxygen therapies would cut deeply into the conventional medical profit pie—because these therapies work and by using them people can avoid very costly (and highly profitable) medical procedures such as coronary artery bypass surgery and angioplasty, not to mention years of taking expensive heart medications.

You don't need to take my word for it. In this book, you will learn how some of the best treatments have been suppressed. Consider the case of David A. Steenblock, D.O., a specialist in hyperbaric oxygen therapy, who was driven into bankruptcy by state medical authorities to the detriment of his many patients (see Chapter 16, pp. 244-249). Or look at what happened to heart researcher Kilmer S. McCully, M.D., when he published an article in a prestigious scientific journal on his discovery that it was homocysteine, not high cholesterol, that was really behind atherosclerosis. If this idea were to gain widespread acceptance, where would that leave the huge industry devoted to lowering cholesterol? Dr. McCully was fired from his job at Harvard University after the article was published (see Chapter 1, pp. 33-37).

It is important for you, the reader, to understand what is going on in the U.S. regarding health care because you are being denied access to medical treatment that can save your life. You have the right to these treatments and I am doing everything possible to see that you get them. One way I can do that is by publishing this book. The more information you have about your options, the more you can make informed choices and then demand the medical care you deserve, because you don't have to live with heart disease—and you certainly don't have to die from it. God bless.

—Burton Goldberg

You may well ask—Why haven't I
heard about these treatments? The
answer is: politics and greed. Widespread
use of chelation and hyperbaric
oxygen therapies would cut deeply into the
conventional medical profit pie—because
these therapies work and
by using them people can avoid very
costly (and highly profitable) medical
procedures such as coronary artery bypass
surgery and angioplasty, not
to mention years of taking expensive
heart medications.

User's Guide

One of the features of this book is that it is interactive, thanks to the following 11 icons:

Here we refer you to our book, *An Alternative Medicine Definitive Guide to Cancer,* for more information on a particular topic.

This means you can turn to the listed pages elsewhere in this book for more information on the topic. For example, if you are reading about toxicity as a contributing cause for cancer in Chapter 25, this icon directs you to Chapter 33 for practical information on detoxification protocols; it also guides you to those cancer doctors in Part One who have detailed programs for detoxification.

This tells you where to contact a physician, group, or publication, or how to obtain substances mentioned in the text. This is an editorial service to our readers. Most importantly, the use of this icon empowers you right now, by giving you a source to acquire something vital to your health, quickly and easily. Whenever possible, we give you complete contact information for all substances mentioned in the text. All items are based on recommendations from the clinical practice of physicians in this book. The publisher has no financial interest in any clinic, physician, or product discussed in this book.

Many times the text mentions a medical term that requires explanation. We don't want to interrupt the text, so instead we put the explanation in the margins under this icon. This gives you the option of proceeding with the text or taking a moment to learn more about an important term. You will find some of the key definitions repeated at different places in the book so you don't have to search for the definition.

 This sign tells you there may be some risks, uncertainties, side effects, or special contraindications regarding a procedure or substance. **Pay close attention to these icons.**

 Here we refer you to our best-selling book, *Alternative Medicine: The Definitive Guide*, for more information on a particular topic.

 This icon will alert you to an article published in our bimonthly magazine, *Alternative Medicine Digest*, that is relevant to the topic under discussion.

 This icon asks you to give a particular point special attention in your thinking. It is important to the overall discussion at hand.

 This icon highlights a particularly noteworthy point and bids you to remember it.

 In many cases, alternative medicine is far less expensive than conventional treatments. This icon means that the widespread acceptance of the therapy or substance under discussion could save considerable health-care money.

 More research on this topic would be valuable and should be encouraged to further substantiate or clinically prove a promising possibility of benefit to many.

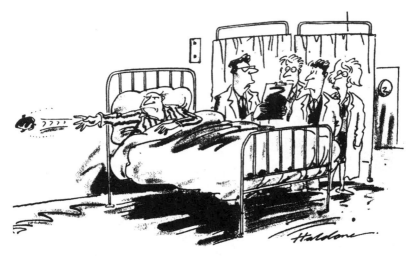

"It looks as though Mr. Markham has rejected his new heart."

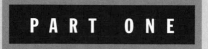

PART ONE

Heart
Disease

What Causes Heart Disease?

THE UNITED STATES leads the world in death rates from cardiovascular disease (pertaining to the heart and blood vessels). More loosely called heart disease, it is the leading killer of Americans, now causing half of all U.S. deaths.[1]

Among the conditions included in the category of cardiovascular disease (CVD) are coronary heart disease (decreased blood flow to the heart usually caused by atherosclerosis), congestive heart failure (cardiomyopathy), heart attack (myocardial infarction), stroke, chest pain (angina pectoris), high blood pressure (hypertension), arrhythmia (irregular heartbeat), rheumatic heart disease, and hardening of the arteries (arteriosclerosis, of which atherosclerosis, involving fatty arterial wall deposits, is the most common).

There are an estimated 1,500,000 new and recurrent cases of heart attack every year. The majority occur with no warning. This makes it vital to practice good heart health.

According to the American Heart Association (AHA), every 33 seconds an American dies of CVD—that's about 954,000 deaths annually or about 42% of all mortalities. Every 20 seconds, an American suffers a heart attack, and every 60 seconds, somebody dies from one, reports AHA. Among deaths attributed to CVD, 52.3% are women and 47.7% are men. African Americans suffer CVD at much higher rates than whites: the rate of death from CVD among black males is 47.4% higher and among black females it's 69.1% higher.

Before we look more specifically at heart disease and what causes it, here's a preview of the alternative medicine techniques we cover in this book to help you on your way to a healthy heart. In the following section, **James R. Privitera, M.D.**, of Covina, California, explains a revolutionary technology to detect a heart attack in the making and outlines a program to reduce your risk.

Preventing a Heart Attack

Heart attacks are a particularly lethal outcome of cardiovascular disease. In 1994 alone, 487,490 people died from heart attacks and there are an estimated 1,500,000 new and recurrent cases every year.[2] The majority of heart attacks occur with no warning, making it vital to practice good heart health.

If you think you're prone to a heart attack or have health factors suggesting the possibility of one, there is a simple, inexpensive way to "ask" your body if conditions exist to make a heart attack possible. Even better, once you know your level of risk, it's easy to take preventive steps, using nutrition, to keep it from ever happening.

This simple, inexpensive technique is called darkfield live blood microscopy. We draw a drop of your blood from your fingertip and place it on a microscope slide. Then a special lens inside the microscope projects an intimate view of your living blood onto a television or computer screen by way of a video camera. A Polaroid camera is hooked up to the device enabling us to take photographs of a patient's blood condition before and after treatment. The result is a *living* picture of the cellular you.

What Silent Clots Can Do Without Warning

The advantage of using a darkfield microscope instead of the more conventional brightfield is that we can see much more detail, such as the contours and shapes of red blood cells and platelets. In a cubic centimeter of blood from a

A "silent" heart attack can be prevented through a darkfield examination of your blood, followed by a precise nutritional prescription to reduce platelet clustering.

healthy individual, there are usually close to 300,000 platelets, which are disc-shaped elements essential for blood clotting.

In most cases, clotting is good because it stops uncontrolled bleeding; but if excess clotting happens in a blood vessel, it can cause a heart attack. When platelets start clustering (aggregating) and sticking together in the blood, they form a clot, which can block the flow of blood through that vessel. Then, if the platelet aggregation is three to four times larger than a red blood cell (which is often the case), it will block the movement of the red blood cells through a capillary (a tiny tributary blood vessel) and stop them from releasing oxygen to the tissues, producing a lower oxygen concentration. This clinical condition, characterized by a shortage of blood flow to the heart, is called ischemia (iss-KEY-mee-uh).

The biggest problem about blood clotting inside your blood vessels is that you probably will have no idea it's happening. When patients come to the office with chest pains (a strong indication of risk), I immediately have a look at their blood. But about 80% of heart attacks are painless, which means the ischemia due to blood clotting

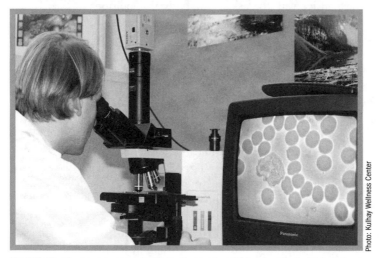

Photo: Kulhay Wellness Center

Darkfield microscopy reveals distortions of red blood cells (which in turn indicate nutritional status), possible undesirable bacterial or fungal life forms, and blood ecology patterns indicative of health or illness.

Dr. Privitera's Program to Reduce the Risk of Heart Attack

- **Kyolic EPA:** EPA (eicosapentaenoic acid, a fatty acid) with garlic and fish oil; 280 mg, 5 times daily
- **Karuna GLA-240:** GLA (gamma-linolenic acid, a fatty acid), containing 1,000 mg of pure borage seed oil and 10 IU of vitamin E; 250 mg, once daily
- **Kyolic Garlic:** 6 capsules daily; 240 mg each
- **CardioSpare:** magnesium and potassium aspartate; 500 mg, 2 capsules after each meal, providing 49 mg of elemental potassium and 33 mg of elemental magnesium
- **Thyroid Chew:** porcine thyroid glandular extract; ¼ g daily
- **Natur Practic Super Enzyme:** containing pancrelipase, pancreatin, pepsin, betaine HCL, papain, amylase, ox bile extract, and others; 2 after each meal
- **Vitamin E:** 1,000 IU daily
- **L-carnitine:** 250 mg, 2 before each meal
- **Raw Heart:** glandular extract from cattle heart, plus added magnesium, manganese, and potassium; 3 times daily
- **Vitamin C:** 5,000 mg daily, divided into 2 doses
- **PhytoPharmica:** aqueous liver glandular extract, containing 100 mcg vitamin B12 and 550 mg liquid liver fractions; 2 times daily
- **Selenium:** 200 mcg, once daily
- **Karuna Maxxum-4:** multivitamin and antioxidant; 2 after each meal

For more information about **Karuna GLA-240** and **Maxxum-4**, contact: Karuna, 42 Digital Drive, Suite 7, Novato, CA 94949; tel: 800-826-7225 or 415-382-0147; fax: 415-382-0142. For **Kyolic EPA** and **Kyolic® Aged Garlic Extract™**, contact: Wakunaga of America Co., Ltd., 23501 Madero, Mission Viejo, CA 92691; tel: 714-855-2776; fax: 714-458-2764. For **CardioSpare**, contact: G, Y, and N Industries, 2407 Grandad Way, Carlsbad, CA 92008; tel: 800-526-3030 or 619-434-6360; fax: 619-434-0816. For **Thyroid Chew**, contact: Merit Pharmaceuticals, 2611 San Fernando Road, Los Angeles, CA 90065; tel: 800-696-3748 or 213-227-4831; fax: 213-227-4833. For **Natur Practic Super Enzyme**, contact: Randal Products, P.O. Box 7328, Santa Rosa, CA 95407; tel: 707-528-1800; fax: 707-528-0924. For **L-carnitine**, contact: DaVinci Laboratories, 20 New England Drive, Essex Junction, VT 05453; tel: 800-325-1776 or 802-878-5508; fax: 802-878-0549. For **Raw Heart**, contact: Licata Enterprises, 5242 Bolsa Avenue, Suite 3, Huntington Beach, CA 92649; tel: 800-926-7455 or 714-893-0017; fax: 714-897-5677. For **PhytoPharmica aqueous liver glandular extract**, contact: PhytoPharmica, P.O. Box 1745, Green Bay, WI 54305; tel: 800-376-4418 (consumer information), 800-553-2370 (licensed healthcare practitioners) or 414-469-9099; fax: 414-469-4418.

produces no pain or gasping and therefore gives you no warning.

You may be driving the car and suddenly slump over the wheel with a silent heart attack. This frightening event may be prevented through a darkfield examination of your blood, followed by a precise nutritional prescription to reduce platelet aggregation. In the darkfield blood pictures (see p. 18), the platelet cluster looks like a blob of oatmeal poured onto a black surface. This is what blood clotting looks like, and it's also the face of a condition that could produce a heart attack.

How Carlon Avoided a Triple-Bypass Surgery

Carlon, 62, came to me with high blood pressure (170/70), chest pains, and a five-year history of serious heart problems, including a moderate heart attack. He had undergone numerous mainstream treatments, which hadn't helped him, and now his conventional physician was urging him to have triple-bypass surgery.

"A total of 14 doctors of the highest degree told me I couldn't live without this surgery, that it was imperative," Carlon reported. "They all agreed that this was the 'only' way they had to keep me alive." They told him if he did not have the surgery in two weeks or less, he would probably die.

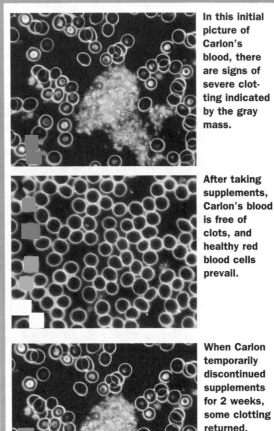

In this initial picture of Carlon's blood, there are signs of severe clotting indicated by the gray mass.

After taking supplements, Carlon's blood is free of clots, and healthy red blood cells prevail.

When Carlon temporarily discontinued supplements for 2 weeks, some clotting returned.

Carlon didn't buy this pessimistic forecast and refused the surgery. He came to me for help. "I believe God built a cage over my heart for a reason. It doesn't need to be messed up with a knife," said Carlon.

I performed a comprehensive mineral analysis from a sample of Carlon's hair and a darkfield examination of his blood. He was seriously low in selenium, magnesium, zinc, chromium, and manganese, and he had some large clots which, incidentally, are asso-

"A total of 14 doctors of the highest degree told me I couldn't live without [bypass] surgery," Carlon reported. It took only three months of chelation and supplementation for his chest pains to disappear. That was five years ago. He bypassed the bypass and is doing well.

ciated with a magnesium deficiency. My treatment program for Carlon had two major aspects: chelation therapy and a nutritional prescription.

First, Carlon started having intravenous chelation twice weekly to improve his circulation and remove heavy metals from his system. Chelation therapy is a clinically proven method of binding up ("chelating") and draining toxins and metabolic wastes from the body while at the same time increasing blood flow and removing arterial plaque. In chelation, a nontoxic substance called EDTA is intravenously infused over a 1½- to 3½-hour period; usually 20-30 treatments are recommended at the rate of one to three sessions per week.

Second, I developed a nutritional supplementation formula for Carlon to help thin his blood and dissolve the clots. Although the nutrients and dosages must be adjusted to the conditions of individual patients, the list (see p. 17) will give the reader a practical idea of how a nutrient program can help prevent heart attacks.

It took Carlon three months of chelation and supplementation for his chest pains to disappear. Even better, at that point he was able to ride his bicycle 25 miles a day with no discomfort. That was five years ago. He bypassed the bypass and is doing well. Carlon follows a reduced dosage maintenance plan for supplements and has chelation about once monthly. "I have skipped the scalpel five times in my life," Carlon told me recently. "I thank God I was stubborn enough to choose my own doctors." ■

To contact the author: NutriScreen, Inc., **James R. Privitera, M.D.**, director, 105 North Grandview, Covina, CA 91723; tel: 818-966-1618; fax: 818-966-7226. Dr. Privitera provides detailed instruction manuals in darkfield microscopic interpretation and nutritional prescribing to licensed healthcare professionals. Dr. Privitera is the author (with Alan Stang, M.A.) of *Silent Clots: Life's Biggest Killers* (1996), The Catacombs Press™ (same address as NutriScreen, Inc.).

For more about **chelation**, see Chapter 3: Scrubbing the Arteries Naturally, pp. 70-92.

The Heart Disease Epidemic

Conventional medicine believes that the answer to fighting heart disease lies in treating certain symptoms such as high blood pressure or in lowering cholesterol with medication. Americans make about 147 million office visits to doctors every year for hypertension and heart

How Your Heart Pumps Blood

The heart is a hollow muscular organ in the chest that contracts rhythmically to circulate blood through the body. The heart sends blood rich with oxygen and nutrients out to the body's tissues and also pumps blood from the rest of the body to the lungs to be re-oxygenated.

The average heart measures 3½" x 4¾" and weighs between 8 and 14 ounces. At rest, the heart normally beats 60 to 80 times per minute (100,000 times per day) and during exercise or stress may beat up to 200 times per minute. The average amount of blood pumped per beat of the heart (at rest) is 2.5 ounces (1,980 gallons per day).

The heart is really two pumps side by side. Each pump consists of two chambers, the *atrium* above and the *ventricle* below. There are left and right atria, and left and right ventricles. These chambers are connected by valves which allow blood flow in one direction only. The rhythm of each heartbeat is regulated by a part of the heart muscle that is connected to the central nervous system; this rhythmic action serves as a natural pace-maker.

Blood flows through the heart on the following course: Blood that has been oxygenated in the lungs flows into the left atrium, then is pumped through the left ventricle out through the aorta to replenish the whole body. Oxygen-depleted blood returns from all parts of the body to the

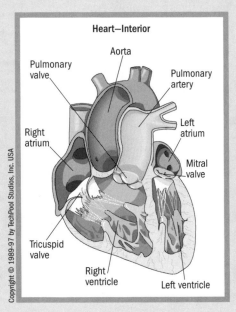

Heart—Interior

Aorta
Pulmonary valve
Pulmonary artery
Left atrium
Right atrium
Mitral valve
Tricuspid valve
Right ventricle
Left ventricle

disease, according to a report in *American Health*. Expensive coronary artery bypass surgeries and angioplasties are performed with increasing regularity, while cholesterol-lowering drugs further fuel the skyrocketing costs associated with heart disease. Coronary artery bypass surgery is called an "overprescribed and unnecessary surgery" by many leading authorities.[3] Complications from such treatments are common and the expense to the health care system is extraordinarily high.

In 1994, an estimated 501,000 bypass surgeries at $44,000 each were performed on Americans, and 47% of these were done on men right atrium, where it is pumped through the right ventricle via the pulmonary artery to the lungs.

Each heartbeat has two phases, diastole (the resting phase) and systole (the contraction). During the diastolic or resting phase, the left atrium fills with oxygenated blood from the lungs and the right atrium fills with oxygen-depleted blood from the body. The contraction begins from the top of the heart as both atria squeeze the blood into the ventricles: the right atrium through the tricuspid valve into the right ventricle, the left atrium through the mitral valve into the left ventricle.

The contraction then continues from the bottom of the heart, squeezing both ventricles upward. The right ventricle moves blood through the pulmonary valve and into the pulmonary artery, then to the lungs. Blood from the left ventricle is pumped through the aortic valve and into the aorta, then out to all parts of the body. The diastolic or resting phase starts again as all valves close and the atria begin to refill.

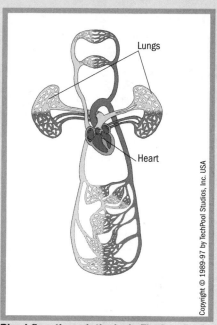

Lungs

Heart

***Blood flow through the body.* The heart pumps blood rich with oxygen (the darker shade) to the tissues of the body through the arteries; blood from the body (the lighter shade) moves through the veins back to the heart and on to the lungs to be re-oxygenated.**

and women under age 65. In the same year, 404,000 angioplasties at $21,000 each were performed (65% on men, 53% on people under age 65). Total costs of cardiovascular disease for 1994, both direct (hospitalization, procedures, and drugs) and indirect (lost working time), were an estimated $259 billion.

Some physicians choose to reduce a patient's risk factors for heart disease by considering preventive measures such as stress reduction, exercise, dietary improvement, weight control, and the elimination of smoking. "Although these methods have resulted in some leveling off

Heart Catheterization Increases Risk of Death

According to a study published in the *Journal of the American Medical Association (JAMA)*, the conventional medical procedure called "right heart catheterization" may increase a patient's risk of death. Performed for information-gathering purposes, the test involves inserting a catheter (tube) through the neck to measure blood pressure inside the heart.

The method has never undergone strict scientific trials and should therefore be considered experimental. However, it is widely used as a diagnostic tool in conventional cardiac treatment. Over 500,000 people are estimated to receive this test every year in the U.S.

Reviewing over 5,000 critically ill heart patients, the *JAMA* study concluded that those who have right heart catheterization may be more likely to die. "If you had 1,000 patients, you would have ended up in our population with about 50 more deaths," states researcher Dr. Joanne Lynn of George Washington University. "That's a substantial number, and we should be very concerned about it." Apply these numbers to the total who have the test and the result is 30,000 more deaths every year. The researchers state that, as people don't die during the test, but later, the cause of the increased risk is unknown at this time and will require further study.[5]

of the rate of heart disease," says Garry F. Gordon, M.D., D.O., (H) M.D., of Payson, Arizona, co-founder of the American College of Advancement in Medicine, "the 'epidemic' of heart disease continues and conventional medicine continues to use drugs and surgery as the primary treatments." Equipped to treat heart disease only when it has reached its most serious and life-threatening stages, conventional medicine is largely failing in its battle against the epidemic.

90% of Patients Receive No Benefit from Bypass Surgery

When it comes to thinking about modern medicine, outrage is a useful attitude, says Lynne McTaggart, editor of the popular and outspoken British medical newsletter *What Doctors Don't Tell You*.

The content of her daily mail frequently makes McTaggart "livid" because her readers tell her about the latest way in which they have been damaged by conventional medicine and the inexcusable failure on the part of physicians to tell their patients the dangers inherent in a drug or procedure. These letters prompted McTaggart to write a book (also entitled *What Doctors Don't Tell You*).[4] She wrote it because, as she states it, "I don't want you to be another statistic."

McTaggart warns the reader that her book is likely to be unsettling, especially in the revelation

The "miracle cure" of beta blockers to lower high blood pressure also evaporates when you look at the outcomes, McTaggart says. A British study of 2,000 patients with high blood pressure showed that in barely 50% of the cases blood pressure dropped to a moderately healthy level as a result of taking hypertension drugs.

that "much of what your doctor tells you isn't true." Her goal is usefully subversive, too: she wants every reader to become an informed medical consumer, able to distinguish between when a doctor is needed and when their advice is best ignored.

To facilitate this radicalization of the medical consumer, McTaggart exposes the "diagnostic excesses" of X rays, MRIs, lab tests, and ultrasounds; she analyzes the shortcomings of medicine's "miracle cures" (antibiotics, steroids, antidepressants, and chemotherapy); and she critiques the routine use of surgery for breast and prostate cancer, hernias, and heart disease, among other topics.

For example, bypass surgery for heart disease, at an average cost of $44,000 per operation, is "one of the most unnecessary operations of all," says McTaggart. Heart surgeons have known since the 1970s that bypass does not improve survival except for patients with severe left ventricle coronary disease, while U.S. government statistics state that about 90% of patients receive no benefit. The "miracle cure" of beta blockers to lower high blood pressure (hypertension) also evaporates when you look at the outcomes, McTaggart says. A British study of 2,000 patients with high blood pressure showed that in barely 50% of the cases blood pressure dropped to a moderately healthy level as a result of taking hypertension drugs.

Study Finds 50% of Bypass Operations Unnecessary

Researchers at the Maine Medical Center found that the number of bypass surgeries and angioplasties performed in a region of the U.S. depends en-tirely upon the amount of diagnostic testing of patients, but not necessarily upon actual medical need, according to the *Journal of the American Medical Association*. The researchers estimated that 80% of all heart testing procedures are inappropriate and that 50% of all bypass operations in the U.S. are unnecessary. The total 1993 cost of Medicare billings of diagnosis and treatment of heart disease was $1 billion.

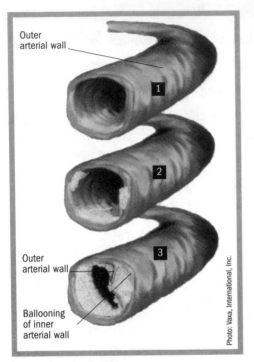

Photo: Vaxa, International, Inc.

How Arteries Thicken
1. A normal, healthy artery with open and clear passages.
2. The beginning of cholesterol plaque buildup within the artery. The inner artery wall is also beginning to weaken and bulge with cholesterol and toxic deposits.
3. Severely restricted artery with cholesterol plaque filling the majority of the passage. Note further breakdown and ballooning of inner artery wall.

In a similar European study of 12,000 patients, only 30% reached their target blood pressure levels with drugs; and in 1993, an American study stated that only 20% of patients on blood pressure drugs experienced the intended results. Further, for hypertension drugs are the major cause of hip fractures among the elderly, while they are linked with an elevenfold increase in diabetes cases, reports McTaggart.

"Our faith in medical science is so ingrained that it has become woven into the warp and woof of our daily routine," says McTaggart. But we may be deeply imperiling our health by putting our faith in a medical approach based on "unscience," she argues. Outcome statistics suggest that in many cases "Western medicine not only won't cure you but may leave you worse off than you were before."

Many treatments we take for granted—for heart disease, breast cancer, and asthma, for example—have been adopted without a single valid scientific study demonstrating their safety or efficacy, says McTaggart. In fact, *New Scientist* estimated that 80% of today's medical procedures have never been properly tested. McTaggart comments: "For all the attempts to cloak medicine in the weighty mantle of science—a good deal of what we regard as standard medical practice today amounts to little more than 20th-century voodoo."

Outer arterial wall

Outer arterial wall

Ballooning of inner arterial wall

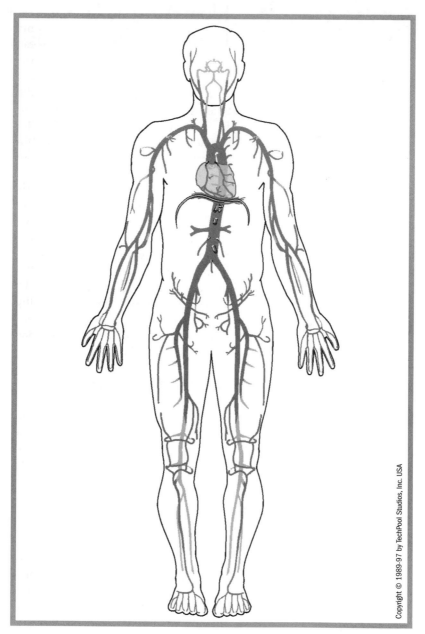

The circulatory system. A network of arteries (shown here) carries oxygenated blood from the heart to all parts of the body. A system of veins carries blood back to the heart.

See Chapter 14: What Causes Stroke?, pp. 230-236.

How Atherosclerosis Leads to Cardiovascular Disease

A common precursor of heart disease is atherosclerosis (thickening of the arterial walls, the most common form of arteriosclerosis). In atherosclerosis, the inner arterial walls harden and thicken due to deposits of fatty substances. These substances form a plaque that, with buildup, causes a narrowing of the arteries.[6] Over time, plaque can block the arteries and interrupt blood flow to the organs they supply, including the heart and brain (see illustration, p. 24).

Atherosclerosis of the coronary arteries (the arteries supplying the muscle of the heart), known as coronary heart disease, is one of the most common forms of heart disease in the United States today. Coronary heart disease can lead to heart attack, coronary occlusion, and angina, while atherosclerosis of the cerebral arteries (the arteries that supply blood to the brain) can precipitate strokes. Coronary occlusion and heart attacks can in turn lead to another heart condition, congestive heart failure.

Heart Attack

When atherosclerosis occurs in the coronary arteries, it can deprive the heart of oxygen-rich blood until the affected area of the heart literally dies, causing a heart attack (myocardial infarction), sometimes leading to cardiac arrest (heartbeat stops) that can result in death. Often, a diminished blood supply to the heart exhibits few symptoms until the blockage is so great that a heart attack results. However, while a heart attack may appear to come on suddenly, it often begins with years of physical neglect, such as a poor diet and lack of exercise. Genetic predisposition can also be a crucial factor.

Coronary Occlusion

In coronary occlusion (blockage of the heart arteries), arteries that course over the surface of and penetrate into the heart muscle become narrowed so that blood flow through them is restricted. The heart muscle stops receiving adequate amounts of oxygen and nutrients and the person develops angina. This means the heart muscle's pumping capacity has been exceeded. Coronary occlusion is commonly caused by atherosclerosis, the buildup of plaque and clogging in the arteries that can lead to heart attacks.

Angina

Angina (discomfort, heaviness, pain, or pressure in the chest or throat) can result when there are lesions in the coronary arteries or in the walls or valves of the heart. These lesions diminish the supply of oxygenated blood to the heart muscle, causing discomfort to radiate from the throat or chest to the shoulder and, in some cases, down the left arm. Angina is a warning sign that there are problems with the heart, but it is not necessarily a precursor of a heart attack if appropriate treatment is initiated.

There is also "silent angina," which means a person may have shortness of breath, numbness in the arm, dizziness, or other vague symptoms that appear when they overexert or become emotionally stressed. About one-half of all people with coronary clogging develop this silent angina form of coronary occlusion. Unfortunately, often the first time they know they have heart disease is when they have a sudden heart attack. That's why coronary disease is such a common killer, because half the people die before they ever reach the hospital.

Congestive Heart Failure

Congestive heart failure (cardiomyopathy) means failure of the heart muscle. The heart becomes literally congested with blood and dangerously weakened. The most common cause of this is coronary occlusion and heart attacks. After you "kill" a large section of your heart muscle through repeated heart attacks, there is not enough heart muscle left to pump blood out of the heart. The pressure and volume of blood inside the heart's pumping chamber build up, putting additional pressure on arteries and veins in the lungs; fluid leaks into the lungs, and the congestive heart failure process begins. A typical sign of congestive heart failure is shortness of breath either with minimal exertion or when lying down at night.

How Plaque Forms in Arteries

Atherosclerosis may be well underway even at birth. In investigating the deaths of newborn babies in Scandinavia from a variety of causes, it was found that nearly 97% had some degree of arterial thickening, the first step in heart disease.[8] Plaque formation in arteries usually follows prior damage to the inner lining of the arteries.

According to William Lee Cowden, M.D., an internist and cardiologist based in Richardson, Texas, deficiencies of nutrients such as vitamin C, vitamin E, and magnesium make this inner lining more susceptible to damage and plaque formation. "Small tears can occur in the lining of the arteries after a sudden very high blood pressure episode brought on by stress," explains Dr. Cowden, who adds that "the vessels cannot always dilate rapidly enough to accommodate the sudden increase in pressure, and tearing occurs."

Dr. Cowden explains how collagen (a protein of the connective tissue), clotting proteins, and other chemical substances are released into the bloodstream to repair the tear. These substances adhere at the site and attract platelets, special blood cells responsible for clotting. "Other cells are attracted to the repair site, including white blood cells laden with oxidized cholesterol which is deposited at the site and initiates soft plaque formation," says Dr. Cowden. "Calcium is then drawn to the site and solid plaques, which are more difficult to remove, are formed."

Matthias Rath, M.D., author of *Eradicating Heart Disease*,[9] calls atherosclerotic desposits the body's "blood vessel repair mechanism" and traces its development back to the Ice Age. According to Dr. Rath, animals don't have heart attacks or strokes because they can manufacture vitamin C and therefore maintain high body levels of this important antioxidant. The human body, on the other hand, lost the ability to manufacture vitamin C thousands of generations ago through what Dr. Rath terms a "genetic accident," the enzymes needed to produce vitamin C becoming defective.

Humans became dependent on diet to supply sufficient vitamin C until the Ice Age when plants were destroyed and people could not get any fruits or vegetables. An epidemic of scurvy (caused by severe vitamin C deficiency) followed. In scurvy, blood vessel walls grow weak and become leaky. A compensation mechanism, atherosclerotic deposits, evolved in the human body, says Dr. Rath. Today, our diet is generally not deficient enough in vitamin C to produce scurvy, but our vitamin C intake is low enough to produce heart disease.

That vitamin C plays a vital role in heart health is supported by a

Despite the evidence to the contrary, dietary cholesterol is regarded by many as the single most important factor in heart disease. This view persists even though a significant percentage of coronary heart disease occurs in people with normal or low cholesterol.

study of more than 11,000 Americans tracked for an average of ten years.[10] Dr. James Enstrom (of the University of California at Los Angeles, School of Public Health) and his colleagues compared the heart disease rate of those eating an average diet (which in our modern world is low in vitamin C) and those supplementing their diet with an average of 300 mg of vitamin C daily. Among men, the supplementation cut their heart disease rate in half. Among women, it was reduced by one-third. Dr. Enstrom's study is one of the largest, and a significant body of research lends weight to the importance of vitamin C in reversing heart disease and maintaining cardiovascular health.

See **Vitamin C,**
Chapter 5: Nutritional
Supplements,
pp. 109-111.

Cholesterol is Not All Bad

Cholesterol, which has long been cast as the villain in heart disease, is a waxy, oily compound vital to the body's health and functioning. Contrary to popular belief, the body, in fact, needs cholesterol. It is an essential component in cell membranes. Your body also needs it to make bile salts which help absorb the fat-soluble vitamins (A, D, E, K) and essential fatty acids from your small intestine. Cholesterol, a steroid, is also involved at the beginning of the pathway that manufactures key male and female sex hormones and steroidal hormones, including pregnenolone, testosterone, estradiol, estrone, progesterone, and cortisol. These are critical for the health of the immune system, the mineral-regulating functions of the kidneys, and the smooth running of the hormonal systems in men and women.

Cholesterol is not only obtained through the diet, but produced by the liver. According to Dr. Cowden, the human liver synthesizes about 3,000 mg of new cholesterol in any 24-hour period, a quantity equivalent to the amount contained in ten eggs. "This new cholesterol is used to repair cells," he says. "In fact, in most people less than 5% of the cholesterol in the bloodstream gets there through diet." Dr. Cowden adds that "when cholesterol levels get too low, depression, lung disease, and even cancer can be the result."

Cholesterol levels in the body are determined by measuring the

Cholesterol's contribution to heart disease appears to depend on the presence of oxidized cholesterol in the bloodstream. LDL cholesterol becomes harmful only after it has been oxidized (the process of a substance combining with oxygen).

Lipoproteins are in two principal forms. Low-density lipoproteins (LDLs) are combination molecules of proteins and fats, particularly cholesterol. LDLs circulate in the blood and act as the primary carriers of cholesterol to the cells of the body.

An elevated level of LDLs, the so-called bad cholesterol, is a contributing factor in causing atherosclerosis (plaque deposits on the inner walls of the arteries). A diet high in saturated fats can lead to an increase in the level of LDLs in the blood. High-density lipoproteins (HDLs) are also fat-protein molecules in the blood, but contain a larger amount of protein and less fat than LDLs.

HDLs are able to absorb cholesterol and related compounds in the blood and transport them to the liver for elimination. HDL, the so-called good cholesterol, may also be able to take cholesterol from plaque deposits on the artery walls, thus helping to reverse the process of atherosclerosis. A higher ratio of HDL to LDL cholesterol in the blood is associated with a reduced risk of cardiovascular disease.

levels of lipoproteins in the blood (proteins that carry fats in the bloodstream). These include high-density lipoproteins (HDLs) and low-density lipoproteins (LDLs). Testing cholesterol levels allows physicians to determine how effectively the body is metabolizing cholesterol and how much remains in the bloodstream. LDL cholesterol is often referred to as "bad" cholesterol because it appears to deposit fats on arterial walls and causes the most arterial damage.[11] HDLs are often called "good" cholesterol because high levels are associated with a reduced risk of heart disease. HDLs may contribute to the removal of "bad" cholesterol from the body.[12]

The Cholesterol Myth

Despite the evidence to the contrary, dietary cholesterol is regarded by many as the single most important factor in heart disease.[13] This mistaken view persists even though a significant percentage of coronary heart disease occurs in people with normal or low cholesterol. It should also be noted that in the first decade of this century consumption of animal fat and cholesterol in the United States was close to mid-century levels. Yet the epidemic spread of atherosclerosis and cornonary heart disease did not appear until the middle of the century. In addition, after coronary heart disease peaked in the 1950s, it slowly declined between 1960 and 1980 even though dietary cholesterol levels rose slightly during those years.

The so-called French paradox further refutes the cholesterol myth. Despite a high intake of total fat, the French have a low incidence of coronary heart disease. It has been suggested that this may be due to the limited presence of hydrogenated fats (damaging trans-fatty acids) in the French diet. Similar "paradoxes" are found in other populations. Eskimos consume huge amounts of dietary cholesterol, have high blood cholesterol and yet low rates of mortality due to coronary heart disease. Northern

Asiatic Indians eat a high percentage of their calories as fat, mostly from butter, yet have an exceptionally low incidence of cardiovascular disease.[14]

Dr. Cowden cites one of many medical examples which refute the notion that all cholesterol is bad and high levels will lead to heart disease. "I have a man in my practice who had a cholesterol count of 300 to 400 for many years," reports Dr. Cowden. "But because he's taking high levels of antioxidant nutrients and avoiding processed foods high in oxidized cholesterol, he's had no plaque formation and has even had plaque regression." Clearly, you would be well advised to consider these facts before turning to a cholesterol-lowering drug as the solution to your heart condition.

Do Cholesterol-Lowering Drugs Even Work?—Since many people with heart disease also have elevated blood cholesterol levels, physicians have traditionally prescribed cholesterol-lowering drugs as part of their treatment program, although new research suggests that it is not the levels of cholesterol but the levels of *oxidized* cholesterol which represent high risk for heart disease.

There is also new information concerning the safety, side effects, and efficacy of cholesterol-lowering drugs. It has been found, for instance, that the drugs used to lower LDL (low-density lipoprotein) cholesterol actually raise it in people who already have the highest levels.[15] In addition, these medications can lead to serious complications. A study conducted in Finland reported that deaths from heart attacks and strokes were 46% higher in those taking cholesterol-lowering drugs.[16]

Newer drugs being touted as safer also have harmful side effects. Studies have shown that Mevacor (lovastatin) lowers the levels of coenzyme Q10, an antioxidant that helps the body resist heart damage, in the bloodstream.[17] A coQ10 deficiency can accelerate congestive heart failure, according to Dr. Cowden. "Studies show that most people with congestive heart failure have a deficiency of coQ10 in their heart muscle," he says. "The lower the levels, the worse the congestive heart failure. But studies also show that patients who were supposed to die 15 years ago from congestive heart failure are still alive, primarily because of taking coenzyme Q10 daily." This may be why many people in Japan use coenzyme Q10 in the place of cardiac drugs.

Trans-fatty acids are found in margarine and other oils which have been hydrogenated (combined with hydrogen) to lengthen shelf-life. Ingredient lists on food labels often designate these oils as "partially hydrogenated," but the partial is a misnomer as far as the body is concerned. When vegetable or animal oils are highly processed and hydrogenated, they are partially converted into an abnormal form called trans. These trans-fatty acids can block the normal digestion pathways of fatty acids. This, in turn, can contribute to the development of heart disease and cancer and interfere with the immune system.

For more about **coenzyme Q10**, see Chapter 5: Nutritional Supplements, pp. 115-119.

Oxysterols can also be generated internally through exposure to environmental pollutants and pesticides such as DDT. Chemicals that oxidize cholesterol include chlorine and fluoride, both of which are ingested from tap water.

Widely used cholesterol-lowering drugs such as Mevacor and gemfibrozil (Lopid) can cause cancer in mice and rats and possibly humans, state researchers at the University of California at San Francisco. Rodent exposure that was carcinogenic was at the same order of magnitude as the maximum dose typically given to humans, reports *Science News*. The researchers noted major discrepancies for carcinogenicity in the listings for these drugs in the 1994 versus 1992 editions of the *Physicians' Desk Reference*, supposedly the standard for accurate drug information.

Sidney M. Wolfe, M.D., advises that drugs should not be the first choice for lowering cholesterol unless other circumstances exist. "A change from animal to vegetable proteins often corrects high cholesterol," says Dr. Wolfe. "Supplementation [of fiber] can significantly lower total cholesterol and LDL cholesterol by absorbing water and softening the stools in your intestine."[18]

The Real Problem is *Oxidized* Cholesterol

Cholesterol's contribution to heart disease appears to depend on the presence of oxidized cholesterol in the bloodstream. LDL cholesterol becomes harmful only after it has been oxidized (the process of a substance combining with oxygen), according to Dr. Cowden. Once oxidized, LDL cholesterol can initiate plaque formation on arterial walls which in turn can lead to atherosclerosis and ultimately to heart attacks and strokes.[19]

Overwhelming evidence shows that the risk of heart attacks and strokes can be greatly decreased through dietary changes, exercise, stress reduction, and nutritional supplementation to help prevent excessive oxidation of cholesterol in the blood. "We've been living on cholesterol phobia for 20 years," says Richard Passwater, Ph.D., of Berlin, Maryland, "but nothing matters unless you prevent the oxidation of cholesterol."

One way oxidized cholesterols (known as oxysterols) enter the bloodstream is from processed foods.[20] According to medical researcher Joseph Hattersley, M.A., of Olympia, Washington, many oxysterols reach people through the air-dried powdered milk and eggs used in processed foods, as well as in fast food products.[21] Lard, kept hot and used repeatedly to cook French fries and potato chips, is loaded with oxysterols, as are gelatin preparations, says Hattersley. "Scrambled eggs and hamburgers are big culprits in the production of oxysterols," states Dr. Privitera. "Oxygen and intense heat from cooking quickly oxidizes unsaturated fats."

Oxysterols can also be generated internally through exposure to environmental pollutants and pesticides such as DDT.[22] Chemicals that oxidize cholesterol include chlorine and fluoride, both of which are ingested from tap water.[23] Chlorine has been shown to have an effect on the arteries, and fluoride lowers thyroid function which in turn allows levels of cholesterol and homocysteine (see the following section) to rise.[24] Chlorine in drinking water also forms trihalomethanes (THMs, carcinogens formed when chlorine interacts with organic chemicals in water) which, according to Hattersley, create oxysterols.[25]

A German study (1991) looked at the coronary arteries of 163 males with chest pain and concluded that the arterial narrowing was due more to blood levels of homocysteine than of cholesterol.

Electromagnetic stress (overexposure to electromagnetic fields emitted by power lines, household appliances, and computers, among other electical devices) is another source of oxysterols. Various stressors such as infections, traumas, and emotional stress can also raise oxysterol levels.[26]

The Homocysteine Connection

There is a significant and growing body of evidence that the biggest culprit responsible for oxidizing cholesterol and producing atherosclerosis, and, therefore, heart disease, is homocysteine, a substance naturally found in the body. In 1969, heart researcher Kilmer S. McCully, M.D., published an unorthodox conclusion in the *American Journal of Pathology* regarding this new possible cause of heart disease. The move soon cost him his job at Harvard University.

Dr. McCully proposed that homocysteine could, when allowed to accumulate to toxic levels, degenerate arteries and produce heart disease. Homocysteine, an amino acid, is a normal by-product of protein metabolism; specifically, of the amino acid methionine,

QUICK DEFINITION

Oxidation-reduction refers to a basic chemical mechanism in the cell by which energy is produced from foods. Electrons (negatively charged particles in an atom) are removed from one atom, resulting in "oxidation" of this first atom, and then are added or transferred to another atom, resulting in "reduction" of this second atom. This continual process of energy metabolism is actually a flow of electrons, or a minute electrical current within in the cell.

33

Elevated homocysteine has the potential of displacing high cholesterol levels as the major dietary factor in heart disease. Dr. Cowden notes that this problem is overlooked, in his view, largely because there is no pharmaceutical drug to "fix" elevated homocysteine levels. "If there was, homocysteine would become just as big a problem as cholesterol."

which is found in red meat, milk, and milk products and which does not create a problem when present in *small* amounts. Methionine is converted in the body to homocysteine, which is normally then converted to cystathionine, a harmless amino acid. But in individuals deficient in the enzyme necessary to convert homocysteine to cystathionine, homocysteine will be abnormally high. Excess homocysteine may generate free radicals which are capable of producing oxysterols.

The conversion in the body of homocysteine to cystathionine requires sufficient levels of vitamin B6, folic acid, and vitamin B12.[27] Also, if sufficient antioxidants are present in the bloodstream (vitamins C and E, and beta-carotene, for example), oxysterols can be neutralized and prevented from damaging the vessel walls. But stress depletes the body of vitamin B6 and vitamin C, and this depletion can lead to a further buildup of homocysteine, which can in turn cause the generation of oxysterols.

Dr. McCully observed that children with elevated levels of homocysteine showed signs of blood vessel degeneration similar to that observed in middle-aged adults with heart disease. He next demonstrated that when rabbits were injected with homocysteine, they developed arterial plaque within three to eight weeks. Homocysteine apparently curtails the ability of blood vessels to expand, keeping them restricted and narrow. It produces this effect by increasing connective tissue growth and by degenerating the elastic tissue in the arterial walls, says Dr. McCully.

Dr. McCully argues that high-protein diets, more than fats and cholesterol, seem to be a prime cause of heart disease. In "honor" of his novel theory, subsequently backed by considerable clinical support, Harvard denied him tenure and effectively fired him.

The Hypothyroidism Connection

An underactive thyroid gland can contribute to heart disease and the propensity to sustain a heart attack, according to Broda O. Barnes, M.D., a Connecticut physician who specialized in identifying and treating the many unsuspected connections between low thyroid activity and numerous health problems. "I am convinced that we are seeing today many more people with low thyroid function than ever before," explained Dr. Barnes in 1976, "and that the rising incidence of heart attacks is related to the rising incidence of hypothyroidism."

Dr. Barnes demonstrated the correlation of low thyroid function and heart disease in a study of 1,569 patients in his practice, grouped according to six categories of age or heart status. As a frame of reference, Dr. Barnes used the statistics reported by the now classic Framingham Heart Study (begun in 1949) which tracked the health status of many thousands of men and women over several decades. Dr. Barnes found that among women 30-59 years old, while there were 7.6 expected coronary cases according to the Framingham results (where no thyroid treatment was given), among his thyroid-treated patients, there were no cases.

Similarly, for those women with high risk (high cholesterol or high blood pressure), Framingham results predicted 7.3 cases, but there were none among Dr. Barnes' patients. For women over 60, Framingham predicted 7.8 cases to zero observed in Dr. Barnes' group; for men 30-59 years old, the ratio was 12.8 (Framingham) to 1 (Barnes); for high-risk males, it was 18.5 to 2; and for men 60 and over, it was 18 to 1. In summary, out of an equivalent patient population, Framingham results expected 72 coronary cases; among Dr. Barnes' thyroid-treated patients, there were only four cases.[28]

The evidence continues to mount in support of Dr. McCully's homocysteine theory. It has been found that men with high homocysteine levels have three times more heart attacks than men with low levels.[29] In 1992, researchers at Harvard University School of Public Health showed that men with homocysteine levels only 12% higher than average had a 3.4 times greater risk of heart attack than those with normal levels. Also that year, a study in the *European Journal of Clinical Investigation* showed that 40% of stroke victims had elevated homocysteine levels compared to only 6% of the controls.

The *Journal of the American Medical Association* (1995) reviewed 209 studies linking homocysteine with heart disease and concluded that the evidence demonstrates that homocysteine represents a strong independent risk

To reach **Kilmer S. McCully, M.D.**, contact: Veterans' Affairs Medical Center, 830 Chalkstone Avenue, PL & M (113), Providence, RI 02908; fax: 401-457-3069.

For more about the **thyroid**, see "The Reason Behind Weight Gain, Fatigue, Muscle Pain, Depression, Food Allergies, Infections...." *Digest* #16, pp. 52-56.

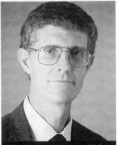

William Lee Cowden, M.D.

A possible dental involvement is another factor to consider. A large percentage of people who have heart disease have some type of abnormal dental process (such as a root canal tooth or previous tooth extraction site) in the mouth.

factor. In 1996, *The Lancet* stated that homocysteine was to be considered an independent risk factor for stroke even after adjustment for other risk factors.

Put simply, the homocysteine theory suggests that heart disease is attributed to "abnormal processing of protein in the body because of deficiencies of B vitamins in the

See **Essential Fatty Acids**, Chapter 5: Nutritional Supplements, p. 119-120.

diet," says Dr. McCully. In short, "protein intoxication" starts damaging the cells and tissues of arteries, "setting in motion the many processes that lead to loss of elasticity, hardening and calcification, narrowing of the lumen and formation of blood clots within arteries."

Elevated homocysteine has the potential of displacing high cholesterol levels as the major dietary factor in heart disease. A German study (1991) looked at the coronary arteries of 163 males with chest pain and concluded that the arterial narrowing was due more to blood levels of homocysteine than of cholesterol. Recently, Dr. McCully declared: "Elevated blood homocysteine is estimated to account for at least 10% of the risk of coronary heart disease in the U.S. population." Dr. Cowden notes that this problem is overlooked, in his view, largely because there is no pharmaceutical drug to "fix" elevated homocysteine levels. "If there was, homocysteine would become just as big a problem as cholesterol."

An effective way to lower homocysteine is through vitamin B6, often combined with folic acid and vitamin B12, Dr. McCully further discovered. Excess levels of homocysteine are correlated with deficiencies in these nutrients which, as mentioned, are required for the conversion of homocysteine into a nontoxic form. Dr. McCully recommends 350-400 mcg daily of folic acid, 3-3.5 mg of vitamin B6, and at least 3 mcg daily of vitamin B12.[30] Dr. Cowden additionally recommends taking betaine hydrochloride (the stomach's principal digestive acid) and vitamin C to lower homocysteine levels in the blood.

According to Mark Nehler, M.D., and colleagues at Oregon

Health Sciences University in Portland, at least 50,000 annual deaths from coronary disease could be prevented by supplementation with oral folate (folic acid), based on their analysis of patient outcomes (and mortalities) of other published studies.[31]

Before we go on to talk about all the ways you can prevent and treat heart disease, here is a look at another doctor's heart treatment protocol to illustrate the *multimodal* approach most alternative physicians use. In the following section, **William Lee Cowden, M.D.**, discusses his comprehensive program to promote heart health.

The Healthy Heart

All the causes of heart failure are reversible, to some degree, using a multifactorial process. There are many people whose heart problems get steadily worse until the only thing conventional medicine can offer is a heart transplant. Yet several patients in my practice who were told this was their last option have never had to have a transplant. Instead, they used natural techniques to improve their heart muscle function to the point where they became active people again. Here's what you need to do.

Your diet needs to move away from standard American fare toward one more plentiful in uncooked vegetables, fruits, and raw grains, seeds, and nuts, but no peanuts. Reduce your intake of dairy products, most animal meats, and refined white flour and sugar. Increase your intake of cold-water fish oil (such as sardine, herring, or mackerel), which is high in an omega-3 fatty acid called EPA (eicosapentaenoic acid). EPA prevents the formation of a clot-forming substance involved in heart disease. Flaxseed contains another omega-3 fatty acid called alpha linolenic acid (ALA) which is normally converted by the body into eicosapentaenoic acid, but stress and nutrient deficiencies block this conversion. For this reason, I recommend that most people living in a city (or an equivalently stressful environment) should take EPA supplements.

Completely avoid all fried foods and hydrogenated vegetable oils because their trans-fatty acids increase atherosclerosis, probably more so than butter. Another nutrient important for reversing heart disease is magnesium, to pre-

QUICK DEFINITION

Omega-3 and omega-6 oils are the two principal types of essential fatty acids, which are unsaturated fats required in the diet. The digits "3" and "6" refer to differences in the oil's chemical structure with respect to its chain of carbon atoms and where they are bonded. A balance of these oils in the diet is required for good health. The primary omega-3 oil is called alpha-linolenic acid (ALA) and is found in flaxseed (58%), canola, pumpkin and walnut, and soybeans. Fish oils, such as salmon, cod, and mackerel, contain the other important omega-3 oils, DHA (docosahexaenoic acid) and EPA (eicosapentaenoic acid). Omega-3 oils help reduce the risk of heart disease. Linoleic acid or cis-linoleic acid is the main omega-6 oil and is found in most plant and vegetable oils, including safflower (73%), corn, peanut, and sesame. The most therapeutic form of omega-6 oil is gamma-linolenic acid (GLA), found in evening primrose, black currant, and borage oils. Once in the body, omega-6 is converted to prostaglandins, hormone-like substances that regulate many metabolic functions, particularly inflammatory processes.

The Thyroid Gland

The **thyroid gland**, one of the body's seven endocrine glands, is located just below the larynx in the throat with interconnecting lobes on either side of the trachea. The thyroid is the body's metabolic thermostat, controlling body temperature, energy use, and, for children, the body's growth rate. The thyroid controls the *rate* at which organs function and the *speed* with which the body uses food; it affects the operation of all body processes and organs. Of the hormones synthesized in and released by the thyroid, T3 (triiodothyronine) represents 7%, and T4 (thyroxine) accounts for almost 93% of the thyroid's hormones active in all of the body's processes. Iodine is essential for forming normal amounts of thyroxine. The secretion of both these hormones is regulated by thyroid-stimulating hormone, or TSH, secreted by the pituitary gland in the brain. The thyroid also secretes calcitonin, a hormone required for calcium metabolism.

Hypothyroidism is a condition of low or underactive thyroid gland function that can produce numerous symptoms. Among the 47 clinically recognized symptoms are: fatigue, depression, lethargy, weakness, weight gain, low body temperature, chills, cold extremities, general inappropriate sensation of cold, infertility, rheumatic pain, menstrual disorders (excessive flow or cramps), repeated infections, colds, upper respiratory infections, skin problems (itching, eczema, psoriasis, acne, dry, coarse, and scaly skin, skin pallor), memory disturbances, concentration difficulties, paranoia, migraines, oversleep, "laziness," muscle aches and weakness, hearing disturbances, burning/prickling sensations, anemia, slow reaction time and mental sluggishness, swelling of the eyelids, constipation, labored and difficult breathing, hoarseness, brittle nails, and poor vision. A resting body temperature (measured in the armpit) *below* 97.8°F indicates hypothyroidism; menstruating women should take the underarm temperature only on the second and third days of menstruation.

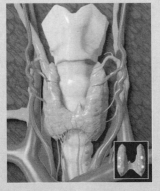

vent the coronary arteries from going into spasm, which can produce a heart attack. Magnesium deficiency is common in the U.S. because magnesium is lost from the kidneys whenever a person is under stress. There is also a relationship between magnesium and EPA levels. If you are deficient in EPA fish oil, you will become deficient in magnesium: this is guaranteed. You can never catch up on a magnesium deficiency

There is also a relationship between magnesium and EPA levels, says Dr. Cowden. If you are deficient in EPA fish oil, you will become deficient in magnesium: this is guaranteed. You can never catch up on a magnesium deficiency if you are EPA-deficient, so make sure you take EPA and magnesium together.

if you are EPA-deficient, so make sure you take EPA and magnesium together.

Selenium deficiency is another common cause for atherosclerotic disease. For heart health, you need about 200 mcg of elemental selenium a day. Other heart-healing nutrients include the antioxidant vitamins E and C, beta carotene, vitamins B3 and B6, bioflavonoids, and sulfur-containing amino acids such as L-taurine, N-acetyl cysteine, or glutathione. Particularly helpful in reversing plaque formation in the arteries are the amino acids L-lysine and L-proline and the antioxidant pycnogenol, from grape seeds or maritime pine bark. The amino acid L-carnitine, which helps to transport other amino acids and fatty acids into the cells, is also useful. People who have congestive heart failure are often deficient in L-carnitine. Keep in mind that all these nutrients work in concert with one another and it's important to develop a total supplement program.

In addition to diet and nutritional supplementation, the alternative medicine techniques of chelation and hyperbaric oxygen therapy can both prevent and treat heart disease by painlessly and noninvasively clearing the arteries.

A possible dental involvement is another factor to consider. A large percentage of people who have heart disease have some type of abnormal dental process (such as a root canal tooth or previous tooth extraction site) in the mouth. Most commonly this is an infection of the jawbone, usually located at the third molar, or wisdom tooth site, in any of the four jaw locations. These infections usually cause an inflammatory response that speeds up the process of artery hardening. Typically, the teeth on the left side of the mouth affect the left side of the heart; those on the right side affect the right side of the heart. If doctors would recognize and treat this, and work with biological dentists, many people who have heart attacks, arrhythmia, or congestive heart failure could see improvement in their conditions.

Often in a case of coronary disease, I recommend that patients have all the mercury amalgams removed from their teeth. Aside from the documented effect that mercury can leach from dental fillings and

William Lee Cowden, M.D. is coauthor of *An Alternative Medicine Definitive Guide to Cancer* (Future Medicine Publishing, 1997). To order, call 800-333-4325. To contact Dr. Cowden: Conservative Medicine Institute, P.O. Box 832087, Richardson, TX 75083-2087; fax: 214-238-0327.

be distributed throughout the body, it can also leak into specific nerve ganglia (stelate, vagus, or cardiac) which regulate heart function, as I've observed in some of my heart patients. Mercury in these ganglia can cause autonomic nervous system (ANS) imbalance and therefore affect heart function. Spasms can occur in blood vessels or the heart itself as a result of an ANS imbalance. As mentioned earlier, this type of spasm can cause a heart attack.

In these patients, the mercury was poisoning those ganglia, which led to heart problems such as impaired blood supply or disturbed heart rhythm. When we got the mercury out of their teeth, then used chelating (binding-up) agents such as DMPS to get the mercury out of their body tissues, the heart problems cleared up and they were able to discontinue using their various heart medications for arrhythmia and angina. Some people who are helped by EDTA chelation (an effective alternative to angioplasty for atherosclerosis) may be benefiting because it pulls heavy metals from the nerve ganglia serving the heart.

One of my patients with a heart rhythm disturbance had considerable mercury distributed in his body, but it was especially concentrated in the submandibular nerve ganglion (below the jaw). In addition, an infection in the third molar socket of the patient's jaw at the site of a previous wisdom tooth extraction was also contributing to the heart problem.

Through the energy lines called meridians in acupuncture, this site was energetically linked with his heart and the jaw infection was harming that organ. When the infection and mercury leakage and poisoning were corrected (including mercury amalgam removal), his heart arrhythmia resolved. ∎

The Mercury Hazard for the Heart

Health researcher H. L. Queen cautions that "the possibilities for involvement of mercury in cardiovascular ailments are so broad" that doctors, from family practitioners to cardiologists, are advised to "routinely address the issue of chronic mercury toxicity (and other heavy metal toxicities) early in the patient's treatment program."

Queen cites Russian research, first reported in 1974, showing that when electrocardiograms were prepared from rabbits exposed to mercury vapor, abnormal changes were apparent in the readings, probably due to an inactivation by mercury of certain heart enzymes necessary for heart muscle contraction. Other research has identified mercury as a contributing factor in arterial disease as well as other problems affecting the heart and arteries; mercury appears to interfere with the normal processing of nutrients that supply arterial smooth muscle, leading to their becoming rigid, Queen says.

Mercury toxicity may also interfere with the processing of cholesterol from arterial cell walls (called Type II hyperlipoproteinemia) and in depositing cholesterol in the liver for removal from the body, says Queen. Further, because it interferes with certain fat-removing enzymes, "mercury may be contributing to the high total serum cholesterol" characteristic of those people vulnerable to arterial disease. In fact, Queen advises that any time there is an unexplained elevated cholesterol level that a physician check for mercury toxicity.

Queen also warns that it can be highly dangerous to suddenly lower a patient's cholesterol (such as with conventional cholesterol-lowering drugs) if they have a preexist-

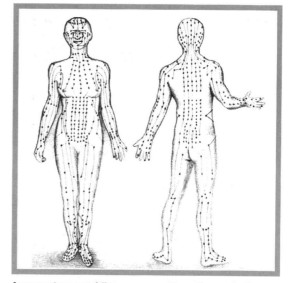

Acupuncture meridians are specific pathways in the human body for the flow of life force or subtle energy, known as *qi* (pronounced CHEE). In most cases, these energy pathways run up and down both sides of the body, and correspond to individual organs or organ systems, designated as Lung, Small Intestine, Heart, and others. There are 12 principal meridians and eight secondary channels. Numerous points of heightened energy, or *qi*, exist on the body's surface along the meridians and are called acupoints. There are more than 1,000 acupoints, each of which is potentially a place for acupuncture treatment.

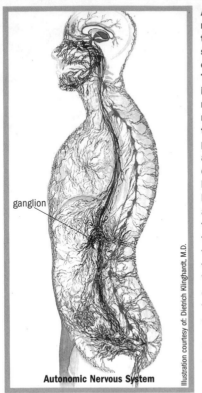

ganglion

Autonomic Nervous System

Illustration courtesy of: Dietrich Klinghardt, M.D.

A *ganglion* is a bundle, knot, or plexus of nerve cell bodies with many interconnections that acts like a sorting and relay station for nerve impulses. There are several dozen ganglia throughout the body. The *autonomic nervous system (ANS)* involves elements of both the central nervous system (CNS) and peripheral nervous system (PNS), is controlled by the brain's hypothalamus gland, and pertains to the automatic regulation of all body processes such as breathing, digestion, and heart rate. It can be likened to the body's automatic pilot, keeping you alive without your being aware of it or participating in its activities. Neural therapy focuses its injections of anesthetics into body structures whose nerve supply is linked with the autonomic nervous system.

Within the ANS, there are two branches—the parasympathetic and sympathetic branches, which are believed to counterbalance each other. The parasympathetic nervous system slows heart rate, inhibits activity, conserves energy, and calms the body, but stimulates gastric secretion and intestinal activity.

See Chapter 3: Scrubbing the Arteries Naturally; Chapter 4: The Dental Connection; Chapter 5: Nutritional Supplements; and Chapter 7: Other Alternatives for Heart Health.

ing but untreated mercury toxicity. "Because mercury has an affinity for lipoproteins and lipoidal tissues, any sudden lowering of cholesterol without a reduction in the body burden of mercury would encourage a transfer of previously circulating mercury to the lipoidal tissues of nerve and brain cells." This in turn could produce behavioral problems including, potentially, violent or impulsive behavior, or other symptoms of chronic mercury toxicity, Queen comments.[32]

An underactive thyroid gland can contribute to heart disease and the propensity to sustain a heart attack, according to Broda O. Barnes, M.D., a Connecticut physician who specialized in identifying and treating the many unsuspected connections between low thyroid activity and numerous health problems. "I am convinced that we are seeing today many more people with low thyroid function than ever before," explained Dr. Barnes, "and that the rising incidence of heart attacks is related to the rising incidence of hypothyroidism."

CHAPTER 2

Caring for Yourself

USE DIET, EXERCISE, AND LIFESTYLE CHANGES TO IMPROVE YOUR HEART

ANY DISCUSSION OF HEART health needs to address diet, exercise, and lifestyle issues such as stress level and emotional well-being. Research has demonstrated the relationship between heart disease prevention and healthy practices in these three areas. For example, eating a vegetarian diet lowers your risk of death from heart disease; exercising just ten minutes daily can significantly reduce the likelihood of heart disease; but anxiety and stress increase the risk of having heart problems.

"The average American lifestyle, combining too little exercise, too much stress, and a diet of highly processed foods often deficient in essential nutrients, has rendered this nation's population especially vulnerable to the ravages of heart ailments," says William Lee Cowden, M.D.

During the teenage and young adult years when bad dietary and exercise habits can most easily be altered, much can be done to protect the body against heart disease. Although initial damage done to the arteries can cause the buildup of plaque, it can be corrected through modifying your diet, building an exercise program into your life, and attending to emotional and psychological concerns.

The Modern Diet and a New Understanding of Nutrition

"Nutrient density is the hallmark of good food," says Paul McTaggart, a nutrition researcher from Ventura, California. Defined

Although initial damage done to the arteries can cause the buildup of plaque, it can be corrected through modifying your diet, building an exercise program into your life, and attending to emotional and psychological concerns.

as the relative ratio of nutrients to calories, foods low in nutrient density are often termed "empty-calorie" or "junk" foods.

The leading nutritional problem in the United States today is "overconsumptive undernutrition," or the eating of too many empty-calorie foods, says Jeffrey Bland, Ph.D., a biochemist and nutrition expert from Gig Harbor, Washington. Although people in the United States consume plenty of food, it is not the right kind of food. Studies have concluded that almost two-thirds of an average American's diet is made up of fats and refined sugars having low to no nutrient density. Consequently, the remaining one-third of the average diet is counted on for the essential nutrients needed to maintain health, which may or may not be from high-nutrient-density food. The result is often nutrient deficiencies which can rob the body of its natural resistance to disease, lead to premature aging, and weaken overall physiological and psychological performance.

The American diet is full of trans-fatty acids which numerous studies have linked to heart-disease risk. These harmful fats are oils which have been hydrogenated to lengthen shelf-life. This altered form is foreign to human metabolism and can block the normal digestion pathways of essential fatty acids, necessary for numerous metabolic functions. Trans-fatty acids are found in margarine and processed, packaged foods such as cakes, cookies, crackers, cereals, donuts, and potato chips, among many other products. Margarine, long promoted as a heart-friendly substitute for butter, has now been proven to be just the opposite. Intake of margarine is significantly associated with risk of heart disease.[1] *Science* reports that hydrogenated fats increase the risk of coronary heart disease.[2]

QUICK DEFINITION

Trans-fatty acids are found in margarine and other oils which have been hydrogenated (combined with hydrogen) to lengthen shelf-life. Ingredient lists on food labels often designate these oils as "partially hydrogenated," but the partial is a misnomer in terms of the effect on the body. When vegetable or animal oils are highly processed and hydrogenated, they are partially converted into an abnormal form called *trans*. These trans-fatty acids can block the normal digestion pathways of fatty acids. This, in turn, can contribute to the development of heart disease and cancer and interfere with the immune system.

Lipoproteins are in two principal forms. *Low-density lipoproteins (LDLs)* are combination molecules of proteins and fats, particularly cholesterol. LDLs circulate in the blood and act as the primary carriers of cholesterol to the cells of the body. An elevated level of LDLs, the so-called bad cholesterol, is a contributing factor in causing atherosclerosis (plaque deposits on the inner walls of the arteries). A diet high in saturated fats can lead to an increase the level of LDLs in the blood. *High-density lipoproteins (HDLs)* are also fat-protein molecules in the blood, but contain a larger amount of protein and less fat than LDLs. HDLs are able to absorb cholesterol and related compounds in the blood and transport them to the liver for elimination. HDL, the so-called good cholesterol, may also be able to take cholesterol from plaque deposits on the artery walls, thus helping to reverse the process of atherosclerosis. A higher ratio of HDL to LDL cholesterol in the blood is associated with a reduced risk of cardiovascular disease.

Studies have found that total fat intake, independent of type, is not strongly associated with coronary heart disease. However, trans-fatty acids raise LDL (low-density lipoprotein) cholesterol and result in reductions of HDL (high-density lipoprotein) cholesterol. In other words, the *type* of fat, not the total fat, is the significant factor.[3]

Dietary management can be highly effective in reversing heart disease. "Ninety percent of heart attacks are caused by blood clots at the site of an atherosclerotic lesion, and 90% of strokes are caused by platelet aggregation [blood clotting]," says James R. Privitera, M.D., noting that dietary changes and nutritional supplements can be used to correct these problems. Dr. Privitera suggests eating foods low in saturated fats (fats from animal products such as butter, milk, and meat) and high in complex carbohydrates, and taking vitamins C, B6, and E, garlic, and the essential fatty acids EPA and DHA.

Soy products can significantly lower cholesterol. Although cholesterol itself may not be the cause of heart disease, the more LDL cholesterol you have in your blood, the more there is available for oxidation, which is where heart problems can begin. By eating three servings a day of any soy product, you can lower your cholesterol level by nine points, according to a report of 38 studies published in the *New England Journal of Medicine*. As a reference point, a tofu burger and a glass of soy milk provide one serving each and one soy protein drink is equal to three servings. The report further stated that the more soy people ate, the more their cholesterol level went down.[4]

Simply eating a lot of fruit and vegetables can help prevent heart problems, according to researchers at the University of Otago in Dunedin, Scotland. "At least ten prospective studies have shown that high intakes of fruits and vegetables confer protection against cancer, cardiovascular disease, and stroke."[5]

Dean Ornish, M.D., assistant clinical professor of medicine at the University of California at San Francisco, used a vegetarian diet, exercise, and stress-reduction techniques to reverse arterial buildup of plaque.[6] His "reversal diet" is almost entirely free of cholesterol, animal fats, and oils. Dr. Ornish found that the condition of those patients who followed the diet improved, while the condition of those who continued eating a diet high in fat got worse.[7]

According to Dr. Cowden, however, the success of Dr. Ornish's diet is due not primarily to low levels of cholesterol and fats but to both low levels of methionine (an amino acid found in red meat, milk, and milk products, and a precursor to homocysteine, a free-radical generator capable of oxidizing cholesterol) and a high intake of vegetables and grains. These foods are rich in the vitamins (B6, C, E, and beta carotene) necessary to act as co-factors for antioxidants and antiatherogenics (substances preventing atherosclerosis).

Dr. Cowden offers the following dietary guidelines to help prevent heart disease:

■ Eat minimally-processed foods (avoid additives and preservatives and foods containing powdered eggs or powdered milk).

■ Buy organic foods (free of pesticides, herbicides, steroids, and antibiotics) whenever possible.

■ Avoid irradiated foods whenever possible.

■ Increase fiber from sources like green leafy vegetables, fresh raw fruits, bran, whole grains, and psyllium.

■ Reduce fat intake, especially fried foods, animal fats, and partially hydrogenated oils. Increase complex carbohydrates such as whole grains, beans, seeds, and potatoes.

■ Use monounsaturated oils (such as cold-pressed olive oil and canola oil), omega-3 oils (from flaxseed or deep ocean fish), and omega-6 oils (from borage, black currant, or evening primrose). Oils must be fresh and cold-pressed—rancid oils can be harmful.

■ Reduce meat, sugar, tobacco, and alcohol consumption—all are sources of free radicals. For example, sugar can cause damage to gallbladder and bowel functions, which can in turn lead to reduced absorption of fat-soluble antioxidant nutrients like vitamin E and

Good News for Chocolate Lovers?

The results of a recent study are a chocolate lover's dream come true. Researchers at the University of California at Davis found that chocolate has high amounts of phenol, a chemical that helps reduce heart disease risk by preventing cholesterol in the bloodstream from oxidizing. It is oxidized cholesterol that clogs the arteries. The phenol in 1.5 ounces of milk chocolate is equal to that in five ounces of red wine, known for its beneficial effects on heart health (to the delight of wine lovers). The study further discovered that chocolate contains a significant amount of antioxidants which also help prevent oxidation.[8]

Unfortunately, chocolate is high in calories and saturated fat along with the heart-enhancing phenol. Since obesity and a diet high in saturated fat increase your chances of heart disease, eating more candy bars as part of your total heart-health program is probably not a good idea.

Margarine, long promoted as a heart-friendly substitute for butter, has now been proven to be just the opposite. Intake of margarine is significantly associated with risk of heart disease.

the increased absorption of free radicals produced by bacterial action in the stagnant colon.

Dr. Cowden also puts many of his heart patients through a detoxification regimen consisting of a vegetarian diet, vegetable juices mixed with garlic, and, in some cases, cayenne, as well as low-temperature saunas. Detoxification in this context means cleansing the internal organs, especially the liver, gall bladder, and intestines, of accumulated toxins. This program helps to cleanse the body of toxins which may be contributing to free radical damage to the artery walls and the buildup of arterial plaque. He also often uses homeopathic remedies to aid in the detoxification.

To reduce the level of oxidized cholesterol in the bloodstream, noted health educator Richard Passwater, Ph.D., suggests combining a dietary regimen (under 30% of daily calories from fat so as not to raise LDL cholesterol levels) with a personalized nutritional supplementation program. "What needs to be done is to first control the LDL cholesterol through diet, then raise the antioxidant level to prevent oxidized cholesterol from doing damage," says Dr. Passwater. Clearly, a healthy diet that limits sources of homocysteine-generating fat, such as red meat and fried food, can keep the body's systems operating more smoothly.

> ## Weight and Longevity
>
> Leaner men live longer, says a Harvard School of Public Health poll of 19,000 men. Those men with the lowest mortality rate had weights 20% below the average for their age while men whose weights were 20% above the ideal body weight had a 2.5 times higher risk for cardiovascular disease.

Eating onions and apples and drinking black tea can also contribute to heart health. These items contain high concentrations of quercetin, a bioflavonoid, and are inversely associated with coronary heart disease mortality rates. In other words, the more onions, apples, and black tea you consume, the lower your risk of dying from heart disease. A bioflavonoid is a pigment within plants and fruits that acts as an antioxidant to protect against damage from free radicals and excess oxygen. In the body, bioflavonoids enhance the beneficial activities of vitamin C and therefore help keep the immune system strong.[9]

A recent study found that men in the highest third of dietary quercetin levels had a 53% lower risk of coronary heart disease than those in the lowest third.[10]

Grapeseed Oil is Good for the Heart

Although there are a number of products that lower total cholesterol, there are few that operate selectively, raising HDL (the "good" cholesterol) while lowering LDL (the "bad" cholesterol that deposits fats on arterial walls). According to both the Helsinki and Framingham Heart Studies performed on thousands of patients over several years, each percentage increase in HDL is correlated with a significant decrease in the incidence of cardiac events.

Grapeseed oil has a high concentration of vitamin E (60-120 mg/100 g), making it a significant source for this nutrient. Grapeseed oil is 76% linoleic acid, an essential fatty acid also known as omega-6, and as the body doesn't produce linoleic acid, it must be acquired through the diet. Linoleic acid is important for producing prostaglandins, hormone-like substances in the body involved in reducing platelet aggregation (blood clotting) and inflammation.

Reducing your intake of saturated fats can help lower your risk of developing heart and circulatory problems. Substituting grapeseed oils for your usual cooking or salad oil can contribute to this healthful goal. Among cooking oils, grapeseed oil has one of the lowest levels of saturated fats at only 9%.

Grapeseed oil is one of the few foods that can simultaneously reduce LDL and increase HDL cholesterol levels; both of these change are beneficial to heart health. In a study published in *Arteriosclerosis* in 1990, researchers at the State University of New York Health Science Center at Syracuse studied the effects of grapeseed oil on 33 men and women with initially low HDL levels. They were tested for cholesterol and triglyceride levels, then instructed to use one ounce of grapeseed oil daily for four weeks. In just this short period, blood tests of the subjects showed a 17.2% reduction in triglycerides and a 10.4% increase in the level of HDL cholesterol.

QUICK DEFINITION

Omega-3 and **omega-6 oils** are the two principal types of essential fatty acids, which are unsaturated fats required in the diet. The digits "3" and "6" refer to differences in the oil's chemical structure with respect to its chain of carbon atoms and where they are bonded. A balance of these oils in the diet is required for good health. The primary omega-3 oil is called alpha-linolenic acid (ALA) and is found in flaxseed (58%), canola, pumpkin and walnut, and soybeans. Fish oils, such as salmon, cod, and mackerel, contain the other important omega-3 oils, DHA (docosahexaenoic acid) and EPA (eicosapentaenoic acid). Omega-3 oils help reduce the risk of heart disease. Linoleic acid or cis-linoleic acid is the main omega-6 oil and is found in most plant and vegetable oils, including safflower (73%), corn, peanut, and sesame. The most therapeutic form of omega-6 oil is gamma-linolenic acid (GLA), found in evening primrose, black currant, and borage oils. Once in the body, omega-6 is converted to prostaglandins, hormone-like substances that regulate many metabolic functions, particularly inflammatory processes.

Detoxification involves a variety of techniques to rid the body of poisons accumulated as a result of a polluted environment (air, water, and food), exposure to toxic chemicals and pesticides, accumulated stress, faulty dietary practices, and chronic constipation or poor elimination, among other factors. Detoxification methods include fasting, intestinal cleansing, enemas and colonics, lymph drainage procedures, chelation, biological dentistry, water and heat therapies, therapeutic massage, and bodywork techniques.

Grapeseed oil is one of the few foods that can simultaneously reduce LDL and increase HDL cholesterol levels; both of these changes are beneficial to heart health.

For a source of grape-seed oil, contact: Salute Santé! Grapeseed Oil, Food & Vine, Inc., 301 Poplar Avenue, Suite 6, Mill Valley, CA 94941; tel: 415-388-7792; fax: 415-388-9933. Napa Valley Grapeseed Oil Co., P.O. Box 561, Rutherford, CA 94573; tel: 707-963-0544; fax: 707-963-3150.

Another study by the same team again showed the beneficial effect of grapeseed oil on cholesterol levels. This study (*Journal of the American College of Cardiology*, 1993) involved 56 men and women with initially low HDL levels. The subjects were instructed to substitute in their daily diet up to 45 ml of grapeseed oil for the oil they normally used for cooking and salads. Blood tests were taken at the beginning of the study and after three weeks. At the end of the test period, the subjects showed no significant changes in total cholesterol levels or weight. However, there was a 7% reduction in the level of LDL ("bad") cholesterol and a 13% increase in HDL (the "good" cholesterol) levels. "The use of grapeseed oil in a daily diet appears to improve both HDL and LDL levels in weight-stable subjects with initially low HDL levels," concluded David T. Nash, M.D., lead researcher on the study.

Raising the amount of HDL in your blood is important because there seems to be a strong correlation between HDL level and the risk of both heart disease and impotence. The effect on cardiovascular health was shown in a long-term study of heart disease called the Helsinki Heart Study. This study called thousands of volunteers to assess their risk of heart disease based on cholesterol levels. The study followed 4,081 men, 40 to 55 years old, over a five-year period. Cholesterol levels were artificially altered (LDL level lowered, HDL level raised) using a drug called gemfibrozil. Every three months, the subjects were examined and tested for signs of heart disease.

The results showed that LDL/HDL levels in the blood are an important indicator of health. Over the five-year period of the study, there were 34% fewer incidents of heart disease in the treated group compared to the placebo group and also fewer deaths (14 vs. 19). During the fifth year of the study, the treated group had 65% fewer heart attacks than the placebo group.

A low level of HDL (and corresponding higher level of LDL) is a major danger sign for the development of heart problems, according to the study, more so than overall cholesterol level. "The increase in the concentration of serum HDL cholesterol and the fall in that of LDL cholesterol were both associated with reduced risk, whereas the changes in the amounts of total cholesterol and triglycerides in the serum were not," stated the researchers. "The risk of coronary heart disease increased with decreasing concentration of HDL."

The study showed that raising your HDL level can have a significant impact on lowering your chances of developing heart disease: for each single percentage point increase in the level of HDL there was a corresponding 3% to 4% decrease in the incidence of heart disease. These same results can be provided by a dietary source like grapeseed oil, which, by increasing your level of HDL by 10% to 13%, as demonstrated in Dr. Nash's studies, can reduce your risk for cardiovascular problems by 30% to 52%.

Low HDL level is also a risk factor for impotence. A 1994 study published in the *Journal of Urology* assessed the risk factors for developing impotence. Based on questionnaires from 1,290 men, 40 to 70 years old, living in Massachusetts, the study found several factors that contributed to a higher probability for impotence. Age was the predominant factor, as the prevalence of complete impotence tripled from 5% to 15% between ages 40 and 70 years. After adjusting for age, the other main factors were heart disease, hypertension, diabetes, and personality type.

Research found that one ounce daily of grapeseed oil raises HDL and lowers LDL and each percentage increase in HDL is correlated with a significant decrease in the incidence of cardiac events.

The researchers also found that the HDL level in the blood was inversely related to the probability of impotence. For the younger men in the study (40 to 55 years old), the likelihood of developing moderate impotence quadrupled from 6.7% to 25% as their HDL level decreased from 90 mg to 30 mg (per deciliter of blood). For the older men in the study (56 to 70 years old), the probability of complete impotence increased from near zero to 16% as their HDL level correspondingly decreased. "The probability of impotence varied inversely with high density lipoprotein cholesterol," stated the researchers.[11]

On the scale of oils which contribute to heart health, grapeseed oil is number one, followed by olive oil, then canola oil.[12] In addition to raising HDL and lowering LDL, which helps maintain the health of the arteries, grapeseed oil reduces platelet aggregation (keeps cells in the blood from sticking together; clustering contributes to heart disease) and helps to prevent high blood pressure caused by sodium excess.

The study results showed that LDL/HDL levels in the blood are an important indicator of health. Over the five-year period of the study, there were 34% fewer incidents of heart disease in the treated group compared to the placebo group and also fewer deaths (14 vs. 19).

The Heart Benefits of Olive Oil

The ancient Greeks knew premium cooking oil when they tasted it, and today Italian, Greek, and Spanish olive oil processors who have been producing oil for generations take great pride in the quality of their oil. The olive tree (*Olea europaea*) was first domesticated around 6,000 B.C. in southern Europe, and olive oil has been a main ingredient in the Mediterranean diet ever since. In recent years, scientific studies have confirmed that olive oil is of considerable health benefit, especially for the heart. That's because it's very low in saturated fats (a major factor in heart disease) and high in omega-3 fatty acids and antioxidants, which are both essential for heart health.

Among the sources of **organic olive oil**, contact: Critelli Olive Oil Co. (CCOF certified), 1009 Factory Street, Unit A, Richmond, CA 94801; tel: 510-412-8990; fax: 510-412-8999. Spectrum Naturals, Inc. (QAI certified), 133 Copeland St., Petaluma, CA 94952; tel: 707-778-8900; fax: 707-765-1026. Sadeg Organic (OCIA certified), 909 Marina Village Parkway, Suite 236, Alameda, CA 94501; tel: 800-400-8851 or 510-521-6548; fax: 510-521-5106.

The chief benefit of using high-quality olive oil is cardiovascular—it's good for your heart because, among commonly available vegetable oils (canola, peanut, corn, soybean, sunflower, safflower) and margarine and butter, it is the highest in *monounsaturated* fats. Studies have demonstrated that this type of fat is excellent for lowering blood cholesterol levels, especially of the harmful LDL variety. Olive oil is also an excellent source of antioxidants, heart-protective substances which must be replenished through the diet.

Saturated and Unsaturated Fat—In 1958, the "Seven Countries" study compared the heart disease rates with dietary content in 13,000 men in seven countries. Researchers found the lowest rate of heart disease on Crete, an island in Greece. Even though the *percentage* of fat in the diet (40%) was the same on Crete as in the country with the highest rate (Finland), the Cretan diet was naturally lower in *saturated* fats. It has since been dubbed the "Mediterranean" diet, and consists primarily of grains, vegetables, bread, and olive oil, with minimal animal protein.

In other words, the *type* of fat can make all the difference, because the Finns ate meat and dairy products, both high in saturated fats, while the Cretans derived much of their fat from olive oil, which is 77% monounsaturated. Saturated fats come mainly from animal sources (meat and butter), but palm and coconut oils are also high in saturated fats. "Saturated fats are the worst threats to the cardiovascular system," says Stephen T. Sinatra, M.D., author of *Optimum Health* and editor of *HeartSense* newsletter. "They are converted to cholesterol in the body and will raise cholesterol levels significantly if consumed in excess."

Conversely, unsaturated fatty acids have been found to lower total cholesterol by reducing LDL (the so-called bad cholesterol) without affecting the level of high-density lipoproteins (HDL, "good" cholesterol). The advantage of monounsaturated fats (olive, canola, and peanut oils) over polyunsaturated fats (corn, sesame, and safflower oils) is that they are less likely to oxidize (become rancid) during cooking. Olive oil also appears to preserve beneficial HDL levels and to exert a mild blood-thinning effect (which prevents clotting within arteries).

The chief benefit of using high-quality olive oil is cardiovascular—it's good for your heart because, among commonly available vegetable oils (canola, peanut, corn, soybean, sunflower, safflower) and margarine and butter, it is the highest in *monounsaturated* fats.

"Given the documented evidence on the positive effects of monounsaturated fats on LDL and HDL levels, it seems likely that the Mediterranean diet, rich in olive oil, plays a significant role" in maintaining a higher level of cardiovascular health, says Dr. Sinatra. "Although it is best to use as little oil as possible, I wholeheartedly endorse the use of olive oil for salads and cooking."

Heart-Protective Antioxidants—Olive oil contains antioxidants, which protect against the development of atherosclerosis (a thickening or hardening of the arteries due to fatty deposits on arterial walls). In a recent study published in *Atherosclerosis*, researchers tested polyphenols (compounds with potential antioxidant properties) extracted from extra virgin olive oil, specifically hydroxytyrosol, oleuropein, and elenolic acid. These substances, it was hypothesized, blocked LDL oxidation.

Atherosclerosis can be caused by many factors, but a prime factor is the oxidation of LDL, according to Dr. Sinatra and a growing body of research. Oxidized LDL leads to the formation of cholesterol blockages. Oxidation, a chemical reaction in the body, can produce free radicals; these are molecules that damage arterial walls and red blood cells.

In the study, three olive oil compounds were incubated with samples of LDL along with copper sulphate, a substance which induces oxidation. To test the results, levels of vitamin E (an antioxidant) were measured periodically (at 30 minutes, one hour, three hours, and six hours) during incubation, as the loss of vitamin E correlates with the degree of oxidation.

Any substance that inhibits this process of oxidation will help prevent the development of atherosclerosis. These substances are called antioxidants and include nutrients such as vitamins E and C, selenium, and beta carotene, among others. Antioxidants are like "friendly guardians or bodyguards," explains Dr. Sinatra. "Sacrificing themselves in chemical reactions, they engulf free radicals before they can do their damage to the body."

The study results demonstrated that all three compounds inhibited free radical formation. They "markedly slowed the loss of vitamin E and retarded the onset of oxidative processes," the researchers concluded. In the control group (without the added compounds), vitamin E disappeared after 30 minutes. The samples incubated with the polyphenols showed 80% protection after 30 minutes and 60% after three hours; and there was still 40% of the original level of vitamin E after six hours incubation time. This antioxidative effect was present even with low concentrations of polyphenols.

The researchers estimated that among olive oil–consuming populations, the daily intake of polyphenols from olive oil alone was about 10 to 20 mg. They concluded that "these amounts of dietary antioxidants, consumed by population groups for several years, are able to reduce the mortality due to CHD [coronary heart disease]."[13]

A Vegetarian Diet Can Prolong Life by 44%

In case you've wondered if following a mostly vegetarian diet that emphasizes the consumption of fresh fruits and vegetables really has long-term health benefits, a new British study provides unarguable evidence that it does.[14] Researchers at the Cancer Epidemiology Unit at Radcliffe Infirmary in Oxford, England, tracked 4,336 men and 6,435 women over a 17-year period to see what effect healthy eating habits produced.

When initially surveyed, the 10,771 subjects described their daily lifestyle and dietary habits: 19% smoked, 43% were vegetarian, 62% ate whole-grain bread, 38% ate nuts or dried fruit, 38% ate raw salads, and 77% ate fresh fruits. The researchers concluded that following healthy eating practices, especially the daily consumption of fresh fruits, was responsible for a much lower death rate from heart and cerebrovascular disease in particular and all causes in general, compared to the general population.

Specifically, only 1,343 individuals died before reaching the age of 80, compared to the expected death rate of about 2,400 from the general population. In other words, a health-conscious diet accounted for a 44% reduction in early deaths. The differences in death rate were especially marked in the areas of cancer, diabetes, heart disease, and gastrointestinal diseases. The death rate from cancer for health-conscious people was only 63% that of the general population; for heart disease, it was 50%; stomach cancer, 48%; lung cancer, 30%; and diabetes, 27%. For those individuals who ate fresh fruit daily, there was a 24% lower premature death rate from heart disease, 32% less cerebrovascular disease, and 21% reduced mortality from all causes.

Lifestyle and Your Heart

There are numerous lifestyle factors aside from diet which have an impact on heart health. High stress levels, smoking, and lack of exercise are probably the greatest contributors to cardiovascular disease.

The Psychology of a Heart Attack

Anxiety increases the risk of sudden cardiac death by 4½ times, even among men free of chronic health problems, according to a 32-year study of 2,280 men, 21-80 years old, as reported in *Circulation* (November 1994). High anxiety is considered a twofold stronger risk factor than cigarette smoking.

Anxiety is a risk factor because it can contribute to the process of plaque buildup in the arteries. "When people are under stress, they form more free radicals, which cause a greater conversion of normal cholesterol into oxidized cholesterol (oxysterols)," says cardiologist W. Lee Cowden, M.D. "These oxysterols then build up in white blood cells and are carried to the site of damage in the arteries." He adds that stress also stimulates the release of adrenalin, which in turn has been shown to cause platelet aggregation (clustering) and

Eliminating the Need for a Heart Transplant

While conventional medicine often relies on the high-risk procedure of heart transplant in treating heart disease, this radical method can often be avoided. William Lee Cowden, M.D., reports the case of a 45-year-old physician who was suffering from pneumonia and an enlarged heart. When given an ejection fraction test (measuring the percentage of the blood contained in the ventricle that is ejected on each heartbeat), his heart was only ejecting 16% of its contents (60% is normal), and his doctor told him his only hope was to receive a heart transplant. When he came into Dr. Cowden's office, he could not walk across the room without becoming short of breath.

Dr. Cowden immediately put him on a detoxification program that included a vegetarian diet and a three-day vegetable juice fast with garlic. Dr. Cowden also had him follow a nutritional supplementation regimen including coenzyme Q10, vitamin C, magnesium, vitamin B complex, trace minerals, omega-3 fatty acids, lauric acid (an essential fatty acid), and the amino acid L-carnitine, as well as the antiviral herbs St. John's Wort, *Pfaffia paniculata*, and *Lomatium dissectum*.

Within three months, Dr. Cowden reports, the patient could jog ten miles a day and, upon repeating the ejection fraction test, his score was up to 30%. Now he works 60 hours a week and continues to jog ten miles daily.

increased blood viscosity (thickness).[15] Increases in blood viscosity can result in spontaneous clot formation. These can either adhere to arterial walls, initiating further plaque formation, or become lodged in narrowed arteries or capillaries, initiating a heart attack or stroke.

Researchers at Duke University Medical Center studied 126 people for five years and found that 27% of those who responded adversely to mental stress in a test situation, such as in public speaking or tight deadlines, later suffered serious heart problems. This means that if a person shows abnormal heart function in response to mental stress, it increases the risk of a future heart problem by two to three times, the researchers reported in the *Journal of the American Medical Association* (June 1996).

In a Danish study (*Circulation*, 1996), 730 men and women followed over a 27-year period showed that, regardless of gender, those with numerous symptoms of depression (such as hypochondria or low self-esteem) had a 70% increased risk of a major heart attack (myocardial infarction). Those who showed strong signs of depression at the beginning of the study were 60% more likely to die early from any cause.

Patients with ischemic heart disease (blood flow shortage to the heart) who had strongly negative thoughts had 1.6 times as many episodes of the disease and were 1.5 times more likely to die from it, a scientist from the U.S. Centers for Disease Control reported in November 1995. About 5% of the 26,000 deaths from this heart problem are due to a patient's negative expectations.

A study of 1,236 men and 538 women found that within the first 24 hours following the death of a loved one, close friends and family members have a 14-fold increased risk of heart attack. The risk of heart attack from grief remains eight times above normal on the second day, six times on the third day, and between two and four times above normal for the next month, according to *Family Practice News* (April 15, 1996).

Stress Reduction

Stress-reduction techniques and exercise have been shown to be highly effective in reversing heart disease. In a study conducted by Dean Ornish, M.D., an experimental group following a routine that combined a low-fat vegetarian diet, stress-management training, the elimination of smoking, and moderate exercise, had a 91% decrease in the frequency

Anxiety increases the risk of sudden cardiac death by 4½ times, even among men free of chronic health problems. High anxiety is considered a twofold stronger risk factor than cigarette smoking.

of angina, as opposed to a control group which experienced a 165% increase in the frequency of angina.[16]

Dr. Cowden also includes stress-reduction exercises as part of his treatment of cardiovascular patients. He believes that deep breathing and imaging techniques aimed at reducing stress should be conducted frequently throughout the day to reduce the output of adrenal hormones and lower the level of platelet aggregation. He encourages patients to do these techniques before meals and at bedtime, as they can not only reduce stress but can improve digestion. "Some of the nutrients we are giving as treatment have to be absorbed out of the gastrointestinal tract. If the gut is in a stressed state, it will not absorb those nutrients nearly as well as if it is in a relaxed state."

Smoking Your Way to Heart Disease

Heart disease specifically related to smoking takes the life of an estimated 191,000 Americans every year. This is 44% more people than are killed by smoking-related lung cancer.[17] In other words, smoking can be worse for your heart than for your lungs. It also endangers the heart health of those around you. An estimated 37,000 to 40,000 people are killed annually by cardiovascular disease caused by secondary smoke, according to the American Heart Association.

Recent research shows that habitual exposure to secondary smoke almost doubles the risk of heart attack and death in nonsmokers. The level of risk (91% higher), determined in a ten-year study of 32,000 women, is far greater than scientists previously thought. The study also found that even occasional exposure produced a 58% higher risk. "The 4,000 chemicals in tobacco smoke just about do everything that we know that is harmful to the heart," Dr. Ichiro Kawachi, of the Harvard School of Public Health, said. "They will damage the lining of the arteries, increase the stickiness of your blood, and therefore increase the chances that you will develop clotting and develop a heart attack."[18]

Until recently, nicotine was thought to be the main culprit in blood vessel constriction, plaque buildup, and reduced blood flow to the heart, and, thus, the link between smoking and heart disease. Now, researchers have identified a substance that is elevated in the blood of smokers and which they believe is behind smoking's damaging effects on the cardiovascular system. Called advanced glycation endproducts (AGEs), these substances are created during the tobacco drying process. AGEs produce sugars which are absorbed from the lungs into the smoker's bloodstream. There, the sugars act like "molecular glue," attaching to arterial walls and eventually creating a blockage.[19]

Exercise is Essential for Heart Health

Research has clearly established exercise as a vital component in maintaining the health of your heart and preventing cardiovascular disease. "Even ten minutes of extra exercise per day can significantly reduce the risk of heart disease," says Dr. Cowden. However, many people have difficulty building a regular program of exercise into their lives. In the following section, **David Essel, M.S.**, provides some helpful tips to accomplish this.

Four Steps to Better Heart Fitness
Through Exercise
As mentioned earlier, cardiovascular disease is the leading cause of death in the United States. The reasons for this are varied, but most

experts believe the main cause has to do with daily lifestyle choices. The way we deal with stress, the foods we eat, and how we take care of our bodies through exercise—all have a health impact on our cardiovascular system.

It has been well documented for more than 30 years that exercise can have a dramatic effect on enhancing heart health. Yet, according to the U.S. Centers for Disease Control and Prevention, only 12%-18% of the U.S. population exercises frequently enough to receive these benefits. One of the reasons the other 82%-88% don't exercise enough is a belief that they do not have enough time to gain any substantial health benefits from exercise.

The fact is, you don't need that much time to benefit. **Here are four hints for how to approach an exercise program and build cardiovascular fitness into your life.**

1. Move at least a little. Set a goal to walk, swim, skate, jump rope, aerobic dance, run or ride a bike three times a week for 20 minutes if possible, but even a ten-minute walk is better than nothing.

2. Exercise can help you control or lose weight. This will likely have a positive effect on your cardiovascular health. Again, the amount of time you exercise is not the most important factor; that you exercise at all is what counts. In a study in the *American Journal of Cardiology*, physicians showed that there was no significant difference in weight loss between a group that walked nonstop for 30 minutes, three times per week, and those who broke a daily walk into three sessions of ten minutes each.

Here's to Your Health: Drinking and the Heart

A number of studies have concluded that moderate alcohol consumption—of red wine in particular—can be beneficial to the heart by raising HDL cholesterol levels and reducing the likelihood of blood clots, which can result in a heart attack. A new study challenges red wine's position as the drink of choice. Coronary heart disease patients who drank liquor, wine, or beer all experienced a lowered risk, although wine and beer lowered it more than liquor.[20]

Before you start imbibing, you might want to consider the results of another recent study. University of Wisconsin-Madison researchers compared purple grape juice, white grape juice, and red wine in terms of their heart-protective effects. Purple grape juice was found to be as beneficial as red wine, and possibly more so.[21] Since alcohol consumption brings health risks along with its heart benefits, purple grape juice can provide a safe alternative.

Therefore, if you are seriously short of time, set a minimum goal of three daily walking sessions of 10 minutes each.

"The 4,000 chemicals in tobacco smoke just about do everything that we know that is harmful to the heart," Dr. Ichiro Kawachi, of the Harvard School of Public Health, said. **"They damage the lining of the arteries, increase the stickiness of your blood, and therefore increase the chances that you will develop clotting and develop a heart attack."**

3. Increasing lean muscle tissue can im-prove your heart's health. A twice-weekly strength-training program using calisthenics, free weights, or exercise machines in which the major muscle groups of the body (chest, back, legs, etc.) are exercised for 1 to 3 sets of 8 to 12 repetitions, can increase lean muscle tissue. This allows the body to burn more calories during the day, thereby assisting in weight loss.

4. Keep to the program because exercise regularity is important. To stick with any program that enhances cardiovascular fitness, consider the following: Invite a friend to exercise with you one or several days each week. Schedule your exercise session in your daily planner so it has the same or higher priority as any other meeting for that day. Or use a walkman with your favorite music, book on tape, or motivational audio to inspire (or entertain) you during your workout.

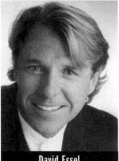

David Essel

David Essel, M.S., is a professional speaker and the host (through Westwood One Entertainment, Ft. Myers Beach, Florida) of the syndicated "positive talk" and lifestyle radio show, "David Essel—Alive!," heard in over 270 U.S. cities each weekend. To contact David: tel: 941-463-7702; fax: 941-463-4019; Internet: http://www.davidessel.com.

By following a regular exercise program, you may achieve a reduction in your blood pressure (if it was high), a reduction in the fatty substance triglyceride and LDL cholesterol levels (which can harm the heart), and an increase in HDL cholesterol (the kind that is beneficial to your system).

A regular exercise program could be one of the most important changes you make to improve your cardiovascular health. However, some people may find the prospect of moving from a sedentary to an active lifestyle daunting, even threatening. It need not be if you tailor your program to your likes and needs, move at your own speed, and respect your limits.

As people become more active, they also start to make healthier choices in the foods they eat and the way they handle stress. The beneficial combination created by this "trickle-down" effect may go far in reducing the number of cardiovascular-related deaths.

The Benefits of Exercise

Many studies provide evidence of the positive effects on the heart of regular exercise, including strengthening the heart muscle, improving blood flow, reducing high blood pressure, and raising HDL cholesterol levels while lowering LDL levels. The British Heart Foundation (BHF) reports that people who do not exercise are twice as likely to develop coronary heart disease as those who exercise on a regular basis. In addition, exercising moderately five times a week reduces your chances of dying from coronary heart disease. If people who exercise suffer a heart attack, their risk of dying from it is half that of those who do not exercise. The BHF recommends 30-minute exercise sessions that are aerobic in nature.[22]

Researchers at the University of Colorado in Boulder demonstrated that exercise is more important than advancing age as a factor in decreased heart function. Comparing older active women (average age of 61), older sedentary women (average age of 62), and young active women (average age of 29), the study showed that the heart health of the younger and older active women was almost the same, as measured by heartbeats per minute, amount of blood pumped with each beat, and the total blood volume pumped by the heart. The heart function of the older sedentary women, on the other hand, was significantly worse, with a six-beat-per-minute faster heartbeat, 24% less blood pumped with each beat, and a 23% lower total blood volume. In addition, the sedentary women were an average of 22 pounds heavier than the older, active women.

Researcher Bryan Hunt observed that this outcome lends weight to the view that "many changes in cardiovascular function typically attributed to aging are likely due to other factors such as age-related reduction in physical activity and increases in body fatness."[23]

As part of a cardiac rehabilitation program, resistive exercises can increase muscle strength and cardiovascular endurance, improve bone density and mineral content, facilitate a return to regular activities, and raise self-confidence.[24]

It is never too late to start exercising. In one study, a regular walking program produced a decrease in the heart rates of previously sedentary people in just 18 weeks.[25] The exercise need not be intensive aerobics. Tai chi, a slow, low-impact activity which never-

The British Heart Foundation (BHF) reports that people who do not exercise are twice as likely to develop coronary heart disease as those who exercise on a regular basis. If people who exercise suffer a heart attack, their risk of dying from it is half that of those who do not exercise.

theless increases the heart rate during practice, has been found to improve overall cardiovascular health.

Get Fit While Running in Place

It is common knowledge that exercising regularly can benefit your health in numerous ways, including losing weight and reducing your risk for cardiovascular disease, prostate cancer, and osteoporosis. But getting that regular exercise can be a problem. Your new year's resolution to join a gym fades quickly or inclement weather has a way of preventing that daily walk you promised yourself. Home exercise on a treadmill—used for walking or running in place—may be the answer.

A study by the Medical College of Wisconsin at Milwaukee[26] compared the effectiveness of the most common exercise machines: a treadmill, exercise cycle, rowing machine, cross-country skier, stair stepper, and combination cycle/upper body machine. The researchers found that "the treadmill machine induced higher rates of energy expenditure [measured by number of calories burned] and aerobic demands than the other exercise machines." Specifically, the treadmill produced the "greatest cardiorespiratory training stimulus during a given duration of exercise" and burned 700 calories/hour compared to 625 calories/hour for the stair stepper, and 500 calories/hour for the exercise bicycle.

In addition, the study measured the "rate of perceived exertion" (RPE) on the treadmill compared to the other exercise machines. RPE means how strenuous the subject felt the exercise was compared to how much energy was used in terms of calories burned.

The 13 subjects (eight men, five women) of the study were given a beginning fitness test and were then acclimated to the machines over a four-week period to establish their individual RPE values. The RPE value of an exercise

The following are a few treadmill manufacturers: Life Fitness, 10601 West Belmont Avenue, Franklin Park, IL 60131; tel: 800-877-3867 or 847-288-3300; fax: 847-288-3741. Precor Inc., 20001 North Creek Parkway, Bothell, WA 98041; tel: 800-4-PRECOR or 206-486-9292; fax: 206-486-3856. True Fitness Technology, Inc., 865 Hoff Road, O'Fallon, MO 63366; tel: 800-426-6570 or 314-272-7100; fax: 314-272-7148. Star Trac by Unisen, Inc., 14352 Chambers Road, Tustin, CA 92780; tel: 800-228-6635 or 714-669-1660; fax: 714-838-6286. Trotter Inc., 10 Trotter Drive, Medway, MA 02053; tel: 800-677-6544 or 508-533-4300; fax: 508-533-5500.

turned out to be a major factor in how strenuously a person exercised. In other words, how hard you think you're exercising determines how many calories you actually burn during the exercise. Treadmills came out on top, with a 40% greater energy expenditure, burning more calories at all levels of perceived exertion than the other exercise equipment.

Whatever your initial fitness level, treadmills can provide the kind of workout you need, from gentle to strenuous. Even a moderate program on the treadmill can help you control your weight, guard against heart disease, and reduce your cholesterol levels by providing a regular cardiovascular workout. It can also improve your muscle tone, reduce your stress level for greater emotional stability, and improve your mood and self-esteem.

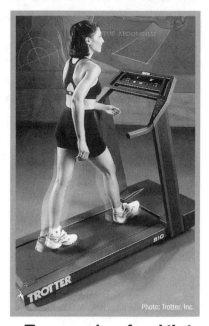

Photo: Trotter, Inc.

Pedal Your Way to a Healthier Heart

A popular choice among types of home exercise equipment is the stationary bicycle because it is easy to use, can accommodate all fitness levels, takes up a small amount of space, and provides the exercise you need for good heart fitness.

That stationary bicycles can be beneficial for any fitness level is demonstrated by the fact that they are used in many physical rehabilitation programs. Stationary bicycles are gentle on the back and joints (hips, knees, and ankles, especially)

The researchers found that "the treadmill machine induced higher rates of energy expenditure [measured by number of calories burned] and aerobic demands than the other exercise machines." Specifically, the treadmill produced the "greatest cardiorespiratory training stimulus during a given duration of exercise."

It is never too late to start exercising. A regular walking program produced a decrease in the heart rates of previously sedentary people in just 18 weeks.

and, unlike running or walking, they provide a nonimpact workout that is nonetheless effective in strengthening the heart and lungs.

A recent French study (*Archives des Maladies du Coeur et des Vaisseaux*, 1996) compared fitness tests of elderly patients (over 65 years old) with a second group 65 years old and younger.[27] Exercise tests were conducted on stationary bicycles during each patient's period of hospital admission for heart surgery.

The results showed a 21% increase in power output and a 28% increase in duration of the elderly patients' exercise periods compared to 25% and 28%, respectively, in the younger group. In other words, the bikes helped both groups of heart patients exercise harder and longer. All patients showed significant improvement in fitness levels without any serious complications.

How Exercise Helps the Heart—One way exercise improves cardiovascular fitness is by increasing the maximum cardiac output. This is the amount of blood pumped by the heart during a heartbeat. Since the maximum heart rate while exercising doesn't change (or may actually lower with continued training), the increase in the amount of blood pumped is due to physiological changes, enabling the heart to work more efficiently by pumping more blood with each beat. This means that your heart rate while at rest will also be lower (a good indicator of your fitness level).

Oxygen consumption—how efficiently your muscles use oxygen—is another measure of cardiovascular fitness. As muscles develop and strengthen through exercise, more capillaries form to supply blood to the muscles; the muscle fibers become more active and can extract more oxygen from the blood with each heartbeat. The increased cardiac output and greater lung capacity that result from regular exercise also support greater oxygen use. When the muscles are not extracting enough oxygen, they deplete their own stores of carbohydrates and lactic acid builds up in the fibers, leading to fatigue and diminished performance.

One of the easiest ways to measure your cardiovascular

fitness—whether or not your heart and muscles are operating at capacity—is by your heart rate. If, after exercising strenuously for ten to 12 minutes, your heart rate is within ten bpm (beats per minute) of the ideal maximum heart rate for your age, then you are probably processing oxygen optimally.

This is why many stationary bikes use heart rate monitors to tailor workout programs to heart rate training "zones." These zones are based on percentages of your maximum heart rate and help you measure your fitness level and set training goals. Using a stationary bike is one of the best ways to get an intense cardiovascular workout because you can focus on heart-rate training without the distractions of road biking.

For those looking for an effective way of recovering from severe congestive heart failure, a regular workout on an exercise bicycle (or treadmill) can be of considerable benefit. German researchers found that 18 patients hospitalized with this condition experienced improvements in

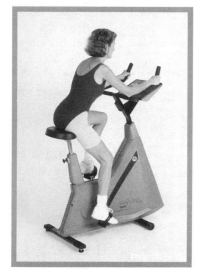

For those looking for an effective way of recovering from severe congestive heart failure, a regular workout on an exercise bicycle (or treadmill) can be of considerable benefit.

their breathing capacity and a reduction in the symptoms of congestive heart failure after only three weeks of specialized exercising.[28] Specifically, they used an exercise bicycle for 15 minutes five times weekly, did treadmill walking for ten minutes, and practiced other exercises for 20 minutes three times weekly.

Lose Weight While Pedaling in Place—Using a stationary bike can also assist weight loss by burning calories. As with other forms of aerobic exercise, there is an additional weight-control benefit from exercising regularly. It increases your basal metabolism rate (BMR). This is the number of calories used by the body at complete rest to maintain basic life processes such as respiration and circulation. It's a bit like gasoline consumption while your car is idling.

Even a moderate exercise schedule—30-40 minutes, three to four times per week—can raise your BMR. Even better, the physiology is such that you burn additional calories for approximately 12 hours immediately after exercise because of having elevated your BMR. This can amount to as much as 15% of the calories burned during your workout, a significant number when you're trying to lose weight.[29]

Stopping a Heart Attack with Your Hands

There are particular locations on your body called "Energy Sphere Points"—when you press on them with your fingers, you can stop a heart attack, seizure, or asthma fit, or give yourself a whole body energy massage, says Glenn King, director of the Glenn King Institute for Better Health in Dallas, Texas.

King is the foremost U.S. practitioner of a little-known Asian art called *Ki-Iki-Jutsu*, which means, literally, "breath of life art." More practically, it's a finger-delivered form of therapy that "allows the body by its own tremendous power to heal itself by unconstricting any stagnation or blockage of the natural energy circulatory patterns," King explains.

Subtle bodily energy (known in Chinese medicine as *Qi*, and presented by King as *Ki*) flows along regular pathways throughout the body. Press on the right points and you can treat seizures (as King experienced personally), chronic pain, insomnia, depression, migraines, memory loss, lymph disorders, and other more serious health conditions.

■ Stopping a Heart Attack—If you are witnessing someone having a heart attack, place your hand on the person's fifth thoracic vertebra (the twelfth vertebra down from the top of the neck, see illustration, p. 68) and with your other hand hold the little finger of the person's left hand. "This prompt action has consistently stopped heart attacks in progress," states King. This process can shift a person from being on the verge of entering cardiac arrest into a state of no sign of heart arrhythmia, pain, or discoloration within two minutes, on average, King says, adding that these results have been confirmed by cardiologists.

■ Whole-Body Energy Tonic—Use this simple exercise to revitalize the circulation of energy throughout your body, relax tension,

To contact some specific manufacturers of **stationary bicycles**: Fitness Master, 504 Industrial Boulevard, Waconia, MN 55387; tel: 800-328-8995 or 612-442-4454; fax: 612-442-5655. Tectrix, 68 Fairbanks, Irvine, CA 92718; tel: 800-767-8082 or 714-380-8082; fax: 714-380-8710; www.tectrix.com. Cateye Ergocisers (Fuji America), 118 Bauer Drive, Oakland, NJ 07436; tel: 800-631-8474 or 201-337-1700; fax: 201-337-1762. Life Fitness, 10601 W. Belmont Avenue, Franklin Park, IL 60131; tel: 800-877-3867 or 847-288-3300; fax: 847-288-3707.

CAUTION

These are emergency, first-aid techniques; they are not curative. If you have any of these conditions, consult a qualified health practitioner for professional long-term treatment.

Original material supplied by **Glenn King**, Glenn King Institute for Better Health, 3530 Forest Lane, Suite 60, Dallas, TX 75234; tel: 214-902-9266; fax: 214-902-0091.

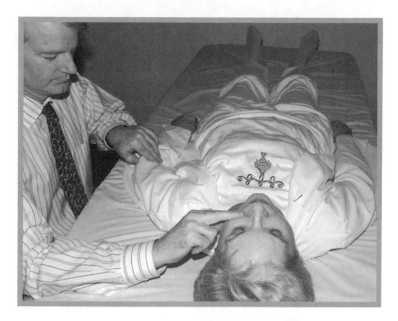

Glenn King demonstrates
Ki-Iki-Jutsu techniques for
stopping a heart attack and
addressing related heart
conditions such as arrhythmia,
fibrillation, and angina.

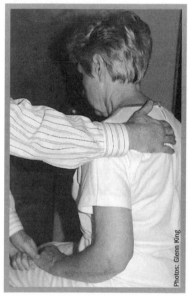

Photos: Glenn King

promote mental alertness, and improve sleep, King advises. Only light finger contact, not pressure, is required. Use the finger pads of your index, middle, and ring fingers. Lie down on a comfortable surface. The sequence of eight steps should take about 24 minutes.

Step 1: Place your right hand on the top center of your head; place your left hand between the eyebrows. Hold for 3 minutes. *Keep your right hand in this location until you reach step 8.*

Step 2: Place your left hand at the tip of your nose; hold for 3 minutes.

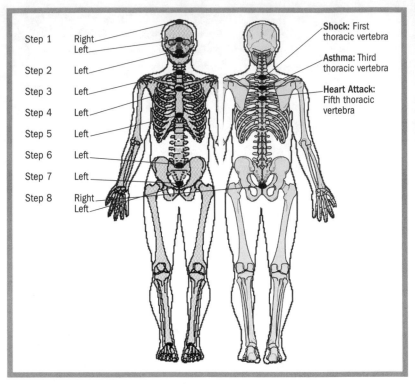

Step 1   Right
          Left

Step 2   Left

Step 3   Left

Step 4   Left

Step 5   Left

Step 6   Left

Step 7   Left

Step 8   Right
          Left

Shock: First thoracic vertebra

Asthma: Third thoracic vertebra

Heart Attack: Fifth thoracic vertebra

Location of *Ki-Iki-Jutsu* treatment points

Step 3: Place your left hand at the center of your collarbone; hold for 3 minutes.

Step 4: Place your left hand at the center of your chest; hold for 3 minutes.

Step 5: Place your left hand at the bottom of your sternum; hold for 3 minutes.

Step 6: Place your left hand at your navel; hold for 3 minutes.

Step 7: Place your left hand at the top center of your pubic bone; hold for 3 minutes.

Step 8: Place your right hand at the tip of your tail bone or coccyx; hold for 3 minutes.

Eating onions and apples and drinking black tea can also contribute to heart health. These items contain high concentrations of quercetin, a bioflavonoid, and are inversely associated with coronary heart disease mortality rates. In other words, the more onions, apples, and black tea you consume, the lower your risk of dying from heart disease. A recent study found that men in the highest third dietary level of the bioflavonoid quercetin had a 53% lower risk of coronary heart disease than those in the lowest third.

Scrubbing the Arteries Naturally

HOW CHELATION THERAPY CAN HELP PREVENT AND TREAT HEART DISEASE

THERE IS MOUNTING EVIDENCE that chelation therapy offers an alternative to the hundreds of thousands of bypass surgeries and angioplasties performed each year. In this therapy, the nontoxic synthesized chemical EDTA (ethylene-diamine-tetra-acetic acid) is given intravenously to remove plaque and calcium deposits from the arterial walls and then the unwanted material is excreted through the urine.

Beginning in the 1940s, the U.S. Navy used EDTA to safely and successfully treat lead poisoning. EDTA was also traditionally used to remove calcium from pipes and boilers. Norman Clarke, Sr., M.D., Director of Research at Providence Hospital in Detroit, Michigan, hypothesized that because calcium plaque is a prominent component in atherosclerosis, EDTA would be an effective treatment for heart conditions. His experiments confirmed his theory, and angina patients treated by Dr. Clarke reported dramatic relief from chest pain. For many patients, memory, sight, hearing, and sense of smell improved, and most reported increased vigor.[1]

In a study completed in 1989, every patient suffering from a vascular disease who was treated with chelation therapy showed a measurable improvement midway through the course of treatment.[2] A second study showed that 88% of the patients receiving chelation therapy exhibited improved blood flow to the brain.[3]

Charles Farr, M.D., Ph.D., of Oklahoma City, Oklahoma, co-founder of the American Board of Chelation Therapy, reports that during the past 20-plus years, he has given more than 500,000 chelation treatments to over 20,000 patients, 60% to 70% of which were for some form of cardiovascular disease or circulatory problems. He reports very positive results in 70% to 80% of the cases. "Many of our patients who were originally scheduled to have bypass surgery or angioplasty continue to be healthy today, some 10 to 15 years past the time they were supposed to die if they did not have the surgery." According to Dr. Farr, chelation is remarkably effective in removing arterial plaque and dissolving clots, as well as in softening up and dilating the blood vessels and allowing nutrients to get to damaged tissues.

> **"Many of our patients who were originally scheduled to have bypass surgery or angioplasty continue to be healthy today, some ten to 15 years past the time they were supposed to die if they did not have the surgery," reports Charles Farr, M.D., Ph.D.**

Dr. Farr reports the case of a man who had several episodes of cardiovascular disease and who had been told by his doctor that he would die if he did not have immediate bypass surgery. Deciding against surgery, the man, who was unable to walk, went to Dr. Farr and, despite the protests of his family, began chelation therapy. Within 45 days, he had gone back to his job of running a construction company and continued to work for many years.

Researchers L. Terry Chappell, M.D., and John P. Stahl, Ph.D., recently reviewed the results of 19 studies evaluating the effectiveness of EDTA chelation therapy on 22,765 patients. They found that 87% registered clinical improvement according to objective tests. In one study, 58 out of 65 bypass candidates and 24 of 27 people scheduled for limb amputation were able to cancel their surgery after chelation therapy. The analysis provides "very strong evidence that EDTA is effective in the treatment of cardiovascular disease," state Chappell and Stahl.[4]

Efrain Olszewer, M.D., and James P. Carter, M.D., reviewed the cases of 2,870 patients with hardening of the arteries and other age-associated diseases who were treated with EDTA chelation therapy and vitamin/mineral supplementation between 1983 and 1985 at the

In one study, 58 out of 65 bypass candidates and 24 of 27 people scheduled for limb amputation were able to cancel their surgery after chelation therapy.

Clinica Tuffik Mattar in Sao Paulo, Brazil. According to their results, marked improvement occurred in 76.9% of patients with ischemic heart disease (coronary artery blockage) and 91% of patients with peripheral vascular disease. In addition, 75% of all patients had reductions in vascular symptoms and, overall, 89% had benefits rated as "good."[5]

Chelation therapy can also relieve chest pain, according to a study involving 18 patients, 45-73 years old, with heart disease, conducted by H. Richard Casdorph, M.D. (*Journal of Advancement in Medicine*, 1989). After 20 chelation infusions, "all patients improved clinically and in all but two there was a complete subsidence of angina during the course of chelation therapy," said Dr. Casdorph.

Chelation Therapy Success Stories

Before we explain in more detail how chelation works, let's look at some actual case studies of successfully treating heart disease with chelation therapy. Michael B. Schachter, M.D., director of the Schachter Center for Complementary Medicine in Suffern, New York, sees many patients who have heart disease and has found chelation extremely useful. Here are two of his cases:

David, 50, had three angioplasties during a six-month period. This kept the veins open twelve, eight, and ten weeks, respectively. When his cardiologist recommended a fourth angioplasty, he chose chelation therapy instead. On his first visit to Dr. Schachter, four months after his last angioplasty, David could walk only two city blocks without severe chest pains. After 24 EDTA infusions, he could walk for 60 to 90 minutes three times weekly with little or no discomfort, and his cardiac-medication use had been reduced by 50%.

Ending 11 Years of Angina

William began suffering from angina pectoris at the age of 25. By 29, bearing a clinical diagnosis of coronary artery disease, William had undergone three balloon angioplasties (which produced short-term improvement, for, respectively, one, three, and 18 months) and a quintuple heart bypass, then, four years later, a heart attack. Following these poor results with conventional medicine, William, then 33, was referred to the Schachter Center for an alternative approach. Dr. Schachter started William on a comprehensive program including EDTA chelation therapy, nutritional supplements, an exercise regimen, and dietary changes. William's intravenous chelation, administered over a 3½ hour period, consisted of the basic EDTA solution and support nutrients such as ascorbic acid, magnesium sulfate, pantothenic acid, potassium chloride, and heparin (a blood thinner), among others. He would receive chelation once weekly for 30 months, then twice monthly for ten months, then once a month indefinitely.

William also began an intensive daily nutritional supplementation program including:

- potassium (99 mg, 4X)
- vitamin C (1,000 mg, 2X)
- vitamin E (400 IU, 4X)
- coenzyme Q10 (60 mg, 2X)
- Ultra Preventive (a multivitamin/mineral, 2 tablets, 3X)
- L-carnitine (250 mg, 2X)
- L-taurine (500 mg, 2X)
- beta carotene (25,000 IU, 1X)
- amino acid capsules (3X)
- vitamin B6 (250 mg, 1X)

To replace the good minerals which are removed along with the toxins in EDTA chelation, William took extra minerals in the form of:

- Tri-Boron Plus (3X) which includes calcium (1,000 mg)
- magnesium (500 mg)
- zinc (25 mg)
- copper (2 mg)
- manganese (10 mg)
- boron (3 mg).

His program also included:

- selenium (250 mcg, 2X)
- zinc picolinate (1X)
- copper (4 mg, 1X)

Finally, Dr. Schachter gave William

Is EDTA Chelation Therapy Cost-Effective?

A recent Danish study says yes. Of 470 cardiovascular patients treated with EDTA chelation therapy, 85% improved. Of 72 patients on a waiting list for coronary bypass surgery, 65 did not require bypass following chelation. Of 30 patients referred for leg amputation, only three required amputation. Aside from the reduced human suffering, the estimated cost savings to the Danish government was $3 million. If EDTA chelation therapy were widely used in the U.S., the estimated cost savings for coronary artery bypass surgery alone would be $8 billion a year.

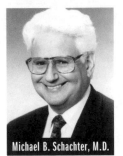

Michael B. Schachter, M.D.

"It was the *combination* of chelation, supplementation, exercise, and diet that gave him such beautiful results," Dr. Schachter says. "I don't think he would have done as well if any one of these four components had been left out."

Ultra GLA (high-potency borage oil rich in gamma linolenic acid, which is important for balancing the essential fatty acids in patients with cardiovascular disease), lecithin capsules (1,350 mg, 4X), lysine (500 mg, 6X), grapeseed extract (50 mg, 1X), and pine bark pycnogenol (50 mg, 1X).

Regarding exercise, the third component of Dr. Schachter's approach, William underwent a cardiac rehabilitation program. His heart rate was monitored as he exercised on a treadmill. As the chelation therapy and nutrient program began to have an effect, William was able to exercise longer and harder without any evidence of heart strain. In medical jargon, his cardiogram showed he had a "negative heart stress test." In fact, William was able to exercise for between 90 and 120 minutes four days a week using aerobic, circuit, and weight-training equipment.

Lastly, Dr. Schachter recommended that William make major dietary changes. These included a low- to moderate-fat, high-fiber diet of whole grains, fruits, and vegetables, with modest amounts of nuts, seeds, fish, and organic chicken, and restricted intake of eggs and dairy products. He was also advised to avoid tobacco smoke, alcohol, sugar, white flour, "junk food," caffeine, artificial sweeteners, preservatives, food additives, pesticides, chlorinated water, fluoride in all forms (including toothpaste), margarine, and aluminum cookware, says Dr. Schachter. This same dietary regimen, he adds, is often given to Schachter Center patients with cancer.

William fared excellently under this fourfold plan, reports Dr. Schachter. It's interesting to note that six years before starting the Schachter program, William had started taking vitamins, watching his weight, and controlling his cholesterol, but this had failed to improve his condition. "It was the *combination* of chelation, supplementation, exercise, and diet that gave him such beautiful results," Dr. Schachter says. "I don't think he would have done as well if any one of these four components had been left out."

"I feel healthier and have a sense of well-being and security that was not there after the bypass," says William. In Dr. Schachter's words, William's treatment resulted in "subjective and objective improvement and full recovery so that he now works full-time and frequently outperforms his law enforcement colleagues in physical endurance activities. He has had no heart attacks in four years and his stress tests keep improving rather than getting worse, as is usual with this disease."

Ironically, William's insurance company refused to reimburse him for the chelation therapy despite the clinical proof of its efficacy. "Yet they loved paying for his dramatic heart surgeries that didn't help him," notes Dr. Schachter. During the course of William's treatments at the Schachter Center, his cardiologist, whom he was still seeing every six months, took him off all his conventional heart drugs except for lovastatin for cholesterol management.

To a large extent, Dr. Schachter's views on complementarity highlight his attitude about how to approach most health problems: "I believe that in many cases, patients who select *only* the alternative program and leave out the more

To contact **Michael Schachter, M.D.:** Schachter Center for Complementary Medicine, 2 Executive Boulevard, Suite 202, Suffern, NY 10901; tel: 914-368-4700; fax: 914-368-4727. Dr. Schachter is coauthor of the forthcoming book, *An Alternative Medicine Definitive Guide to the Prostate* (Future Medicine Publishing).

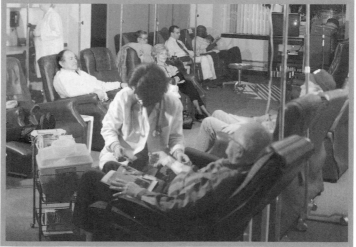

Photo: Schachter Center

Chelation therapy, given intravenously over a 1½- to 3-hour period, is a bit like *gently* scrubbing the inside of approximately 60,000 miles of arteries, veins, and capillaries to remove the deposits that have thickened and hardened the blood vessel walls, blocking blood flow.

The main way chelation reverses atherosclerosis is by removal of calcium plaque. Unabsorbed calcium floating in the bloodstream can build up in the tissues and joints and lead to the formation of plaque lesions on the inner walls of the arteries, making them thick and hardened, producing atherosclerosis.

destructive conventional treatment will do better."

Severe Angina Reversed in Three Months

Guillermo Asis, M.D., of the Marino Center for Progressive Health in Cambridge, Massachusetts, reports similar success treating angina with chelation, as illustrated by the following case study.

Albert, 70, had suffered with severe angina for almost ten years. He had an average of ten searing chest pains daily. In an attempt to correct this, his conventional physicians had performed 14 balloon angioplasties and one heart bypass surgery. By the time Albert came to Dr. Asis, Albert's doctors had essentially written him off as untreatable. They had advised him to take as much nitroglycerin as he needed to get pain relief.

"It was a serious case," says Dr. Asis. "His doctors literally did not know what else to do for Albert." However, in the view of Dr. Asis, Albert was medically treatable.

He put Albert on a once-weekly program of chelation therapy to improve his circulation and heart function. For approximately 3 hours per session, Albert sat comfortably in Dr. Asis' office receiving an intravenous infusion of EDTA, the prime substance used in chelation therapy.

In addition, Dr. Asis gave Albert "a very aggressive" multivitamin supplement called Vitality Plus (with high levels of the B vitamins, zinc, and copper) which he took six times daily. Albert also began taking magnesium aspartate (400 mg, four times daily) and zinc picolinate (50 mg daily). The reason for these two supplements is that the chelation process unavoidably flushes these minerals out of the body, so adequate levels of both must be restored, says Dr. Asis. Albert started taking grapeseed extract (50 mg, twice daily, as an antioxidant to help remove free-radical poisons) and selenium (200 mcg, twice daily, an antioxidant known to benefit the heart).

Within eight weeks, Dr. Asis was able to take Albert off all con-

To contact **Guillermo Asis, M.D.:** The Marino Center for Progressive Health, 2500 Massachusetts Avenue, Cambridge, MA 02140; tel: 617-661-6225; fax: 617-492-2002; Internet: www.allhealth.com. **Vitality Plus** is available from the Marino Health Store; tel: 800-456-LIFE or 617-661-6124.

ventional heart medications. Even better, his angina symptoms were dramatically improved—Albert experienced only one incident of chest pain per month. Albert received a total of 12 chelation treatments. By the end of the three-month treatment, "virtually all of Albert's symptoms and discomfort were gone and he continues to do very well," says Dr. Asis.

Understanding Chelation Therapy

Chelation (key-LAY-shun) comes from the Greek word *chele* meaning "to claw" or "to bind." EDTA circulates through the blood vessels and binds to ("chelates") excess amounts of calcium, iron, copper, lead, or

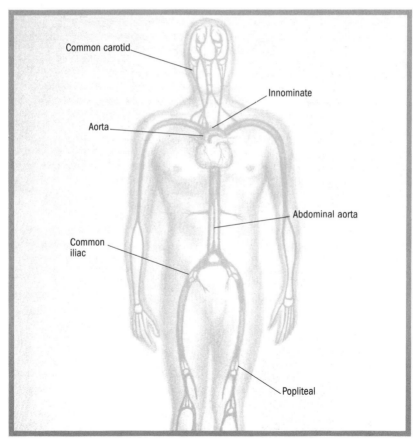

Sites of atherosclerotic lesions in the body

EDTA is nearly three-and-a-half times less toxic than common aspirin and 300 times safer than bypass surgery. Chelation therapy has been used safely on more than 500,000 patients in the United States for the past 40 years, without a single death attributable to EDTA when the American College for Advancement in Medicine (ACAM) protocol is followed.

other heavy metals; the EDTA along with the bound substance is then eliminated in urine.

The main way in which chelation reverses atherosclerosis is by removal of calcium plaque. Unabsorbed calcium floating in the bloodstream can build up in the tissues and joints and lead to the formation of plaque lesions on the inner walls of the arteries, making them thick and hardened, producing atherosclerosis. Calcium acts as a kind of glue that holds the plaque lesions together. These limit the amount of blood flow, reduce the supply of oxygen to body organs, and increase the risk of inappropriate blood clotting. The plaque lesions and the subsequent reduced oxygen supply can lead to heart attacks, coronary heart disease, and chest pain.

If you take an average 80-year-old man and examine his aorta, says Garry F. Gordon, M.D., D.O., a chelation pioneer and co-founder in 1973 of the American College for Advancement in Medicine, now in Laguna Hills, California, you will probably see evidence of 140 times more calcium than he had at age ten. "The abdominal artery shows a 50-fold increase, and the coronary

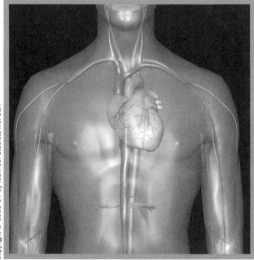

The aorta (the heart's major artery). The aorta of a typical 80-year-old man will probably show signs of 140 times more calcium than that of a 10-year-old; consequently, there will be greatly reduced blood flow.

artery shows a 30-fold increase. This means you're gradually turning to stone in all your arteries. However, we can document that calcium accumulation in the arteries is totally reversible by enough chelation." EDTA is closely related to vinegar, or

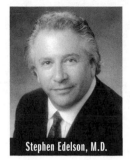

Stephen Edelson, M.D.

"Free radical pathology, it is now believed, is the underlying process triggering the development of most age-related ailments," says Dr. Edelson.

ordinary acetic acid, says Dr. Gordon. "It's actually a weak acid; if you put an eggshell in vinegar, it will dissolve. In the same way, EDTA will take calcium off your arteries. Because EDTA ties up calcium so avidly, it was used by blood banks for 15 years to prevent blood from clotting. Once you tie up calcium, blood cannot clot." At the same time, EDTA does not deplete the body of calcium. By a surprising biochemical mechanism, chelation therapy actually stimulates bone growth and can help prevent osteoporosis. People do not die from atherosclerosis, says Dr. Gordon, but from *preventable* complications of blood vessel spasm (preventable by adequate magnesium intake), irregular heart rhythms (preventable by sufficient mineral intake), or blood clots.

Much of the long-term benefit of chelation therapy derives from its ability to slow down free-radical activity and undo the underlying cause of arterial blockage, says Dr. Gordon. "Damaging free radicals are increased by the presence of heavy metals and act as a chronic irritant to blood vessel walls and cell membranes." This free-radical activity is stimulated by excess heavy metals and minerals in the blood and plays a major role in the development of heart disease. "EDTA removes those metallic irritants, allowing leaky and damaged cell walls to heal."

According to Stephen F. Edelson, M.D., a progressive alternative physician who uses chelation therapy in his practice in Atlanta, Georgia, EDTA's ability to bind with and remove metals, such as iron, copper, lead, mercury, and cadmium, may be a more important factor in reducing heart disease than its effect on calcium plaque. These metals are powerful triggers of excessive free-radical reactions, Dr. Edelson explains. "Free radical pathology, it is now believed, is the underlying process triggering the development of most age-related ailments."

EDTA is nearly three-and-a-half times less toxic than common aspirin[6] and 300 times safer than bypass surgery. Chelation therapy has been used safely on more than 500,000 patients in the United States for the past 40 years, without a single death attributable to EDTA when the American College for Advancement in Medicine (ACAM) protocol is followed.[7] This makes it one of the safest therapies in modern medicine.

However, EDTA, the drug used during the infusions, has yet to receive FDA (Food and Drug Administration) approval for anything other than lead and heavy-metal toxicity. Still, there are over 1,000 physicians who recommend and use chelation therapy for cardiovascular disease and related health problems. Following the treatment protocol set by the American College of Advancement in Medicine and the American Board of Chelation Therapy, FDA-approved studies are currently underway to establish the safety of EDTA.

How Chelation Therapy is Administered

Chelation therapy is performed on an outpatient basis, is painless, and takes approximately $1\frac{1}{2}$ to $3\frac{1}{2}$ hours. For optimal results, physicians who use chelation therapy recommend 20 to 30 treatments given at an average rate of one to three per week, with patient evaluations being made at regular intervals.[8] There is no need to worry about a buildup of EDTA in the body. Chelation therapists state that within 24 hours 99% of the infused EDTA has been excreted.

The patient reclines comfortably while receiving an intravenous solution of EDTA with vitamins and minerals. To monitor the patient's progress, James Julian, M.D., of Los Angeles, California, recommends that the following tests be taken before, during, and after chelation:

- blood pressure and circulation
- cholesterol and other blood components
- pre- and post-vascular
- blood sugar and nutritional
- kidney and organ function
- tissue minerals, if indicated

A whole foods, low-fat diet and appropriate exercise are normally recommended as part of a full treatment program. According to Dr. Gordon, a carefully tailored program of vitamin and nutritional supplements should also be part of the treatment, and can include ascorbic acid (vitamin C), heparin, selenium, chromium, copper, zinc, and manganese. Smoking is strongly discouraged and alcohol should be consumed only in moderation. The cost per treatment can vary, depending in part on the nutritional ingredients the doctor chooses to use.

Conditions Benefited by Chelation Therapy

EDTA chelation therapy has proven safe and effective in the treatment and prevention of ailments linked to atherosclerosis, such as coronary artery disease (which can cause a heart attack), cerebrovascular disease (which can produce a stroke), peripheral vascular disease (leading to pain in the legs and, ultimately, gangrene), and arterial blockages from atherosclerosis elsewhere in the body.

Warren Levin, M.D., of New York City, once administered chelation therapy to a psychoanalyst on the staff of a major New York medical center. "He was in his fifties and looked remarkably healthy, except that he was in a wheelchair," says Dr. Levin. "He had awakened that morning to discover his lower leg was cold, numb, mottled, and blue, with two black-looking toes. He rushed to his hospital and consulted the chief of vascular surgery, who recommended an immediate amputation above the knee. He asked this world-renowned surgeon about the possibility of using chelation in this situation, and was told, 'Don't bother me with that voodoo.'

"The ailing man decided to get a second opinion. This physician also urged him to have an immediate amputation. When asked about chelation therapy, the second doctor's response was, 'You can try it if you want, but it's a waste of time.'

"Through his own tenacity, the psychoanalyst showed up in my office. We started emergency chelation and after approximately nine treatments—one taken every other day—he was pain-free and picking up. After approximately 17 chelation treatments, he was walking on the leg again. He never had an amputation, and he lived the rest of his life without any further complications."

Anecdotal stories of patient success tend to mean little to medical researcher Morton Walker, D.P.M. "But," he writes, "what must an investigative medical journalist do when exposed to story after story of potentially imminent death, blindness, amputation, paralysis, and other problems among people, and upon visiting those people to check their stories, finds them presently free of all signs of their former health problems? About 200 individuals who were victims of hardening of the arteries are ... [now] vibrant, productive, youthful looking, vigorous, full of zest, and enthusiastically endorse chelation therapy as the cause of their prolonged good health. I have turned up not a single untruth."[9]

Medical journalists Harold and Arline Brecher, who have written extensively about chelation therapy, note that physicians who use it not only advise it for their patients, but use it for themselves, unlike many of their orthodox colleagues. "We have yet to find a physician who offers chelation to his patients who does not chelate himself, his family, and friends," they report.

One study documented significant improvement in 99% of patients suffering from peripheral vascular disease and blocked arteries of the legs. Twenty-four percent of those patients with cerebrovascular and other degenerative cerebral diseases also showed marked improvement, with an additional 30% having good improvement. Overall, nearly 90% of all treated patients had marked or good improvement as a result of chelation therapy.[10]

A double-blind study in 1989 revealed that every patient suffering from peripheral vascular disease who was treated with chelation therapy showed a statistically significant improvement after only ten treatments.[11] In another study published in 1989, 88% of the patients receiving chelation therapy showed improvement in cerebrovascular blood flow.[12]

Other documented benefits of chelation therapy include:
- normalization of 50% of cardiac arrhythmias[13]
- improved cerebrovascular arterial occlusion[14]
- improved memory and concentration when diminished circulation is a cause[15]
- improved vision (with vascular-related vision difficulties)[16]
- significantly reduced cancer mortality rates (as a preventive)[17]
- protection against iron poisoning and iron storage disease[18]
- detoxification of snake and spider venoms[19]

According to Elmer Cranton, M.D., of Troutdale, Virginia, chelation therapy has a profound effect on overall health. "In my clinical experience there is no doubt that intravenous EDTA chelation therapy to some extent slows the aging process," says Dr. Cranton. "Allergies and chemical sensitivities also seem to improve somewhat due to a better functioning of the immune system. All types of arthritis and muscle and joint aches and pains seem to be more eas-

CAUTION

EDTA should not be used during pregnancy, severe kidney failure, and hypoparathyroidism (low blood circulation).

Angioplasty and Bypass
Surgery Do Not Extend Life

In 1992, Nortin Hadler, M.D., Professor of Medicine at the University of North Carolina School of Medicine, wrote that none of the 250,000 balloon angioplasties performed the previous year could be justified, and that only 3%-5% of the 300,000 coronary artery bypass surgeries done the same year were actually required. Yet a cost comparison study prepared for the Great Lakes Association of Clinical Medicine in 1993 estimated that $10 billion was spent in the United States in 1991 on bypass surgery alone.[20] At a symposium of the American Heart Association, Henry McIntosh, M.D., stated that bypass surgery should be limited to patients with crippling angina who do not respond to more conservative treatment.[21]

Elmer Cranton, M.D., of Troutdale, Virginia, estimates chelation therapy can help avoid bypass surgery in 85% of cases. He points out that during all the time that chelation therapy has been administered according to established protocol, not one serious side effect has been reported.

A study reported in the *New England Journal of Medicine* demonstrated the ineffectiveness of most angioplasty and bypass surgery procedures to extend life following a heart attack. Scientists at the University of Toronto in Ontario, Canada, studied the death rates for 224,258 U.S. and 9,444 Canadian heart patients. They found that at the end of one year following the heart attack, the death rate was 34% in both countries. The crucial difference, however, is that whereas 12% of U.S. heart attack patients received angioplasty, only 1.5% of Canadian heart patients did; further, while 11% of American heart patients have bypass surgery, only 1.4% of Canadians do.

U.S. patients are also far more likely to have coronary angiography (catherization of heart arteries) than Canadians, 34.9% to 6.7%. The only benefit to the various invasive heart procedures was a slight improvement in 30-day survival rates for Americans, 22.3%, compared to 21.4% for Canadians, a difference that disappeared after 12 months when the mortality rates evened out. The wastefulness and ineffectiveness of these invasive procedures are clearly appreciated in light of the following statistics. Between 1980 and 1992, the rate of coronary angiography in the U.S. grew by 163%, percutaneous coronary revascularization increased by 5946%, and coronary artery bypass surgery increased by 102%.

Comparatively, American patients receive these procedures, within 30 days of a heart attack, at a far higher rate than Canadians: angiography 5.2 times as often; angioplasty, 7.7 times; bypass surgery, 7.8 times. "The strikingly higher rates of use of cardiac procedures in the United States, as compared with Canada, do not appear to result in better long-term survival rates for elderly U.S. patients with acute myocardial infarction [heart attack]," the study directors concluded.[22]

Catheterization After Heart Attacks *Reduces* Lifespan

New data released by William E. Boden, M.D., of the Veterans Affairs Upstate Health Care System in Syracuse, New York, shows that heart surgery (specifically, catheterization, or angiography) given immediately following mild heart attacks does not extend the life of the heart patient. Dr. Boden tracked the health status of 920 heart attack patients for 30 months. Out of this group, 458 received a post–heart attack "conservative strategy," consisting of medications and treadmill and thallium tests as a way of monitoring their condition; the other 462 patients, who received "invasive therapy," underwent catheterization, which was followed by bypass or angioplasty for 45% of these patients.

Dr. Boden found that, within nine days, 21 of the invasive therapy group died, compared to six in the conservative strategy group. After 30 months, 80 patients from the invasive therapy group had died compared to only 59 in the conservative strategy group. This means catheterization, followed in almost half the cases by bypass or angioplasty, *increased* the death rate of heart attack survivors by 36%.[23]

According to Julian Whitaker, M.D., catheterization "leads to a dramatic increase in the use of bypass surgery and angioplasty because physicians then try to open up observed blockages to prevent future heart attacks or death." In catheterization, a catheter is threaded through arteries of the heart; a dye is injected, enabling the arteries to be tracked by X ray to pinpoint blockages in those arteries.[24]

---

ily controlled after chelation, although it is not a cure. In most cases, the progression of Alzheimer's disease will be slowed, and in some cases the improvement is quite remarkable and the disease does not seem to progress. Macular degeneration, a major cause of visual loss in the elderly, is often improved and almost always arrested or slowed in its progression by chelation therapy."

Chelation therapy could save billions of dollars each year by preventing unnecessary coronary bypass surgeries, angioplasties, and other expensive procedures related to vascular disorders.

Chelation Therapy vs. Bypass Surgery and Angioplasty

Each year nearly 300,000 bypass surgeries and 250,000 angioplasties are performed in the United States. Furthermore, nearly 20,000 deaths occur annually as a result of these procedures.[25] The risks of bypass surgery are obvious and, since the benefits are not long-lasting, many people have multiple bypass operations.

Angioplasty is a fairly brutal way of mechanically scrubbing the inside of arteries with an inflated balloon catheter to flatten deposits that have thickened to the point of being dangerous to health. The balloon expands the artery, allowing more blood to pass. The goal is to prevent heart disease and reduce the risk of

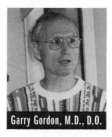

Garry Gordon, M.D., D.O.

"I firmly believe that an oral chelation program can do more for your overall longevity than you can do even with the most prudent lifestyle possible, because of the continuous nutritional protection chelation offers against a stressful and polluted world, " says Dr. Gordon.

heart attack. According to cardiologist W. Lee Cowden, M.D., there is an 80% chance of a person's arteries blocking again within one year of undergoing angioplasty.

Oral Chelation

There are a variety of substances that act as oral chelating agents, according to Dr. Gordon. "Oral chelation is a well-documented, firmly established medical practice," he says. He points out that penicillamine, a drug used to treat heavy-metal poisoning, rheumatoid arthritis, and Wilson's disease (a rare metabolic disorder resulting in an excess accumulation of copper in the liver, red blood cells, and the brain), works in a fashion similar to EDTA. "Some of the benefits derived from penicillamine in the treatment of rheumatoid arthritis are undoubtedly related to the control and removal of excess free radicals.

"Oral chelation is an insurance policy to guarantee that you stay alive long enough to take intravenous chelation when and if you choose to," observes Dr. Gordon. "The oral approach has several major advantages, including convenience, potential long-term continuous health maintenance, and low cost. Its primary shortcoming is that it will take longer and require much more in quantity to get the same benefits as intravenous chelation."

Dr. Gordon notes that for years he has given his cardiac patients 800 mg daily of oral EDTA, of which he estimates only 3%-8% is absorbed compared to 100% of intravenous EDTA. This means it will take about 5 to 8 weeks of daily oral EDTA chelation to get the same effects of a single four-hour intravenous chelation, says Dr. Gordon.

Dr. Gordon also uses many nutritionally-based substances as oral chelators, such as garlic, vitamin C, carrageenan, zinc, and certain amino acids like cysteine and methionine. "Cysteine, for instance, is very effective in the treatment of nickel toxicity," he says, "and it seems to also increase glutathione in the body, which in turn helps to control free radicals." Dr. Gordon recently introduced his own oral chelation product called Garlic-EDTA Chelator™ (each capsule contains 400 mg garlic and 100 mg EDTA).

In his patients who use oral chelation formulas, Dr. Gordon has consistently observed a reduction of serum cholesterol by an average of 20% or more, which he feels significantly decreases the likelihood of atherosclerosis. "The thousands of patients who visit my clinic each year and follow our recommended oral chelation program have all successfully avoided strokes, and heart attack rates were also greatly diminished," he says. "We've never had more than two heart attacks per year among all of our patients, even among those with a history of severe heart disease. I firmly believe that an oral chelation program can do more for your overall longevity than you can do even with the most prudent lifestyle possible, because of the continuous nutritional protection chelation offers against a stressful and polluted world."

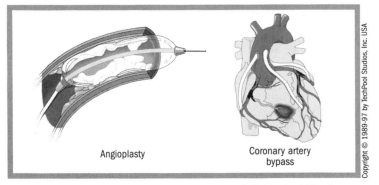

Angioplasty

Coronary artery bypass

Angioplasty is a surgical procedure to open partially-blocked blood vessels. Also known as balloon angioplasty, this procedure inserts a balloon-tipped catheter into the clogged blood vessel, where the balloon is inflated, flattening the plaque causing the blockage against the vessel wall and increasing blood flow.

Coronary artery bypass is a surgical procedure which creates a pathway around a blocked blood vessel. One to five vein grafts (usually from the patient's leg) are attached from the aorta to a point on a coronary artery past the obstruction.

Cardiologist W. Lee Cowden, M.D., argues that a precise combination of nutritional substances and dietary factors can "cause the body to spontaneously, naturally break down the plaque, pull it off the arterial walls, and produce an effect that is equivalent to the chelation process."

Dr. Gordon does not recommend oral chelation as a substitute for intravenous chelation therapy, however. "There is a significant difference in both the rapidity and degree of benefits achieved with intravenous chelation over any currently available oral chelation agents," he says. "And the intravenous approach is clearly the proper choice for patients who have only a few months to get well before facing surgery or worse." But for patients whose conditions are not as drastic, as well as for those who want to optimally safeguard themselves against free radicals and plaque buildup, Dr. Gordon views oral chelation as an effective, noninvasive, inexpensive choice.

However, in Dr. Gordon's view, EDTA-based oral chelation can provide "automatic protection against the clotting process, as well as lowering a patient's lead level, so that they will have a higher functioning immune system, higher IQ, and better coordination."

When platelets, the factors in blood that produce clotting, become "sticky," they tend to clump together or aggregate, and this sets up conditions for excessive and unwanted blood clotting, explains Dr. Gordon. This in turn promotes the formation of vessel-thickening plaque and an increased risk of heart attack and stroke. While conventional drugs such as aspirin and coumadin are given to circumvent this problem, Dr. Gordon notes, these approaches are "dangerous and far less effective" than a comprehensive oral chelation approach.

Dr. Gordon also notes that intravenous chelation cannot provide 24-hour-a-day protection against the main causes of sudden death from heart problems and that this is where oral chelation finds its niche. "Continuous protection is afforded by an oral chelation program," Dr. Gordon says. He claims that "in the last 14 years, new heart attacks and/or strokes have been virtually nonexistent in my patients on this oral chelation program."

Garlic, taken alone, is an excellent chelator of metals such as lead and mercury, says Dr. Gordon. "Now, if you add EDTA to it, you get more removal of lead, but you also enhance the garlic's anti-platelet [anti-blood-clotting] activity. Through this combined action, since

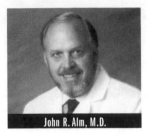

John R. Alm, M.D.

Six weeks after starting the TriCardia+ program, Colin's heart "spontaneously converted to a normal rhythm and has stayed that way for three months," Dr. Alm reports.

EDTA binds with the calcium that is required for blood to clot, you can protect yourself far more effectively against a blood clot, even more so than any aspirin dose you might take."

As a supplement to oral chelation with EDTA, Dr. Gordon recommends OC Packs, a heart nutrient program he originally customized for his patients in the early 1980s. These nutrients represent an "important part of the insurance policy" to prevent death from heart disease, says Dr. Gordon.

A Pill Instead of Angioplasty

John R. Alm, M.D., a physician practicing in Vista, California, views oral chelation as a viable way of "roto-rootering" the cardiovascular system and of detoxifying the liver and kidneys, the system's main filters. Dr. Alm works with the new Cardio-Care line of oral chelation products including Buffer-pH+, TriCardia+, and Systemex. This is a three-step, three-month program designed by Växa International, a maker of homeopathic formulas based in San Diego, California. The concept here is to detoxify, balance, and nourish the cardiovascular system, says Dr. Alm, who is a member of Växa's medical advisory board.

First, Buffer-pH+ helps to restore a more alkaline pH in the body. An acid pH is regarded as the "seed-bed of degenerative disease," including most forms of heart disease. Most people are in a constant state of acidosis, in which their system is overly acidified, primarily from a faulty diet, explains Dr. Alm. This in turn leads to a kind of "corrosion" of the blood vessel linings; in a curious way, hardening of the arteries may emerge as the "body's protective reaction" to this acidic state, Dr. Alm speculates.

"In an acid environment, heavy metals tend to bind with cholesterol which then adheres to vessel linings and attracts fibrin [blood-clotting protein] and other debris, building layer upon layer, eventually becoming a cement of plaque blocking arteries." This decreases blood flow which further acidifies the body's tissues.

However, when the pH is balanced again, heavy metals remain free and unbonded, while those that were previously bonded are easier to remove with EDTA in the program's second element, TriCardia+, says Dr. Alm.

TriCardia+ contains 32 amino acids including EDTA, plus homeopathic ingredients, lipids, enzymes, and herbal ingredients. The product is intended to remove plaque and debris from the circulatory system using EDTA with other orally-delivered chelating agents, says Dr. Alm. Systemex, the third element in Växa's Cardio-Care program, is a liquid meal-replacement formula designed to nutritionally support the cardiovascular system. The formula is fat-free and lactose-free and contains proteins, complex carbohydrates, essential fatty acids, amino acids, and 36 vitamins and minerals.

A reasonable question often raised is whether oral EDTA is absorbed as well as that taken intravenously. According to Gregory C. D. Young, Ph.D., Växa president, "Assimilation of EDTA is effective when it is taken either intravenously or orally." Dr. Young states that, even though EDTA is a synthetic amino acid, "in free form it biochemically behaves and is absorbed in exactly the same way as other free-form (or unbound) amino acids." It bypasses the digestive system entirely and, owing to its small molecular size, enters the bloodstream through the first segment of the small intestine, says Dr. Young. He estimates that, just as with other free-form amino acids, about 80% of oral EDTA is assimilated by the body in the first 20 minutes, the rest following within 90 minutes.

"The notion that EDTA is not absorbed, is in some way destroyed, or suffers from diminished potency when given orally, is unfounded and contradicts the experience of the U.S. Navy in the late 1940s," says Dr. Young. "At that time thousands of sailors benefited from simple oral administration of EDTA for lead toxicity."

Until further definitive research is performed or made public, absorption rates for oral EDTA will have to be placed *somewhere* between Dr. Gordon's 3%-8% and Dr. Young's 80%-100%. Växa's Cardio-Care program has not been on the market long enough—it was introduced in late 1996—for there to be much clinical evidence supporting its claims. However, Dr. Alm offers the following case report showing good results using this approach.

Colin, 74, had chronic high blood pressure and a 20-year history of arrhythmia, and had suffered a series of

QUICK DEFINITION

The term **pH**, which means "potential hydrogen," represents a scale for the relative acidity or alkalinity of a solution. Acidity is measured as a pH of 0.1 to 6.9, alkalinity is 7.1 to 14, and neutral pH is 7.0. The numbers refer to how many hydrogen atoms are present compared to an ideal or standard solution. Normally, blood is slightly alkaline, at 7.35 to 7.45; urine pH can range from 4.8 to 7.5, although normal is closer to 7.0.

Dr. Cowden's Daily Oral Nutritional Chelation Program for Brandon

- Vitamin E: 2,000 IU
- Vitamin C: to bowel tolerance (slightly less than the amount that produces diarrhea)
- Bioflavonoids (vitamin C helpers): 2,000 mg
- Grapeseed extract: 200 mg
- EPA (eicosapentaenoic acid): 1,200 mg
- DHA (docosahaenoic acid): 400 mg
- Fish oils: 400 mg
- Lysine (amino acid): 4,000 mg
- Proline (amino acid): 4,000 mg
- L-taurine (amino acid): 2,000 mg
- Hawthorn berry: 1 capsule, 3X
- *Ginkgo biloba*: 40 mg, 3X
- Cool Cayenne: to bowel tolerance (the amount that causes slight rectal burning on defecation)
- Super Garlic: 3X
- Chorella: 6 capsules, 2X
- Magnesium: 300 mg, 3X
- Vitamin B6: 100 mg
- Vitamin B complex: B1 (thiamine), 100 mg; B2 (riboflavin), 100 mg; B3 (niacin), 100 mg; B5 (pantothenic acid), 100 mg; B6 (pyridoxine), 100 mg; choline, 100 mg; inositol, 100 mg; PABA (para-aminobenzoic acid), 100 mg; B12, 100-400 mcg; folic acid, 400 mcg

strokes after being put on a blood-thinning drug. The strokes produced a partial paralysis and considerable weakness of his right arm and leg, says Dr. Alm. Six weeks after starting the TriCardia+ program, Colin's heart "spontaneously converted to a normal rhythm and has stayed that way for three months," Dr. Alm reports.

Obviously more clinical evidence will be required before it is known for certain if the persuasive theory behind Växa's oral chelation program is borne out.

Chelating Brandon with Diet and Nutritional Substances

Cardiologist W. Lee Cowden, M.D., of the Conservative Medicine Institute in Richardson, Texas, believes that oral EDTA is not "particularly effective" for arterial plaque. But he argues that a precise combination of nutritional substances and dietary factors can "cause the body to spontaneously, naturally break down the plaque, pull it off the arterial walls, and produce an effect that is equivalent to the chelation process."

As evidence, Dr. Cowden cites the case of Brandon, 57, who had severe disease in three coronary arteries. His physicians were strongly urging him to undergo angioplasty and even Dr. Cowden, a long-time advocate of progressive alternatives in medicine,

Patients interested in chelation therapy should choose a doctor who follows the protocol of the American Board of Chelation Therapy or the American College for Advancement in Medicine.

regarded Brandon's condition as dangerous. "I've never had anyone in my office so close to having a heart attack without yet having one," he comments. An echocardiogram revealed that 60% of one heart quadrant was immobilized and the rest was working poorly. Despite the risk, Brandon refused to be hospitalized and asked Dr. Cowden for homecare strategies.

Dr. Cowden put Brandon on a strict vegetarian diet, emphasizing mostly raw fresh foods, whole grains, and beans. Brandon avoided dairy products, red meats, chicken, and turkey, and only occasionally ate fish. The living enzymes in the raw foods probably helped to remove arterial plaque, says Dr. Cowden. Brandon's dietary changes were complemented with several key supplements (see "Dr. Cowden's Daily Oral Nutritional Chelation Program for Brandon," p. 90).

In addition, Dr. Cowden had Brandon wear the negative pole of a small 1,000-gauss magnet against his left chest during all his waking hours. "The magnet dilates blood vessels and increases the blood flow to the coronary arteries," Dr. Cowden says. He emphasizes the importance of using only the negative pole; the positive pole, when placed against the chest, could restrict blood supply and produce a heart attack.

Brandon followed the program faithfully for nine days, then came to Dr. Cowden for another evaluation. "He climbed up the stairs to my office without any chest discomfort," reports Dr. Cowden. "On the heart stress test, performed on a treadmill, Brandon went over 11 minutes, which is probably as far as I could have gone that day. He showed no abnormalities on his electrocardiogram. This means that after nine days we reversed about 90% of his advanced triple-vessel coronary disease. He returned to work the next day and was very healthy." A dental factor (mercury amalgams or infection), which Brandon could not afford to address at the time, probably accounted for the remaining 10% improvement that he failed to achieve, Dr. Cowden adds.

Dr. Cowden cites another case from his practice illustrating how nutritional substances can reverse the symptoms of heart disease. Louisa, 45, had a 75% blockage in the carotid artery in her neck and

A **free radical** is an unstable molecule with an unpaired electron that steals an electron from another molecule and produces harmful effects. Free radicals are formed when molecules within cells react with oxygen (oxidize) as part of normal metabolic processes. Free radicals then begin to break down cells, especially if there are not enough free-radical quenching nutrients, such as vitamins C and E, in the cell. While free radicals are normal products of metabolism, uncontrolled free-radical production plays a major role in the development of degenerative disease, including cancer and heart disease. Free radicals harmfully alter important molecules, such as proteins, enzymes, fats, even DNA. Other sources of free radicals include pesticides, industrial pollutants, smoking, alcohol, viruses, most infections, allergies, stress, even certain foods and excessive exercise.

For more on the health effects of **mercury amalgams,** see Chapter 4: The Dental Connection, pp. 94-105.

For more information about **chelation therapy**, contact: American College for Advancement in Medicine, 23121 Verdugo Drive, Suite 204, Laguna Hills, CA 92653; tel: 714-583-7666 or 800-532-3688. For **TriCardia+, Systemex**, and **Buffer-pH+**, contact: Växa International, Inc., 10307 Pacific Center Court, San Diego, CA 92121; tel: 800-248-8292 (reference RS# 30181-3) or 619-625-8292; fax: 619-625-8272; website: www.vaxa.com/vaxa/vaxa.html. For **John R. Alm, M.D.**, contact: Pacific Immediate Care, 1900 Hacienda Drive, Vista, CA 92083; tel: 760-940-2011; fax: 760-940-0359. For **Garry F. Gordon, M.D., D.O.**: Get Healthy, 901 Anasazi Road, Payson, AR 85541; tel: 520-472-9086; fax: 520-474-1297; e-mail: drgary@netzone.com. For **Garlic-EDTA Chelator™**, contact: Life Enhancement Products, Inc., P.O. Box 751390, Petaluma, CA 94975; tel: 800-543-3873 or 707-762-6144; fax: 707-769-8016. For **Stephen F. Edelson, M.D.**: Environmental and Preventive Health Center of Atlanta, 3833 Roswell Road, Suite 110, Atlanta, GA 30342; tel: 404-841-0088; fax: 404-841-6416. For Dr. Cowden's oral nutritional chelation program [from sidebar] available as **Master-Chel**, contact: Health Restoration Systems, Inc., P.O. Box 832267, Richardson, TX 75083; tel: 972-480-8909; fax: 972-480-8807. For **William Lee Cowden, M.D.**: Conservative Medicine Institute, P.O. Box 832087, Richardson, TX 75083; fax: 214-238-0327. For **Super Garlic**, contact: Metagenics West, Inc., 12445 East 39th Avenue, Suite 402, Denver, CO 80239; tel: 303-371-6848 or 800-321-6382; fax: 303-371-9303.

was told that, unless she had surgery to correct it, she was likely to have a stroke. Dr. Cowden put her on Brandon's nutritional program and after three months a new ultrasound scan of her carotid artery revealed it was only 22% blocked with plaque.

How to Find the Right Doctor

Patients interested in chelation therapy should choose a doctor who follows the protocol of the American Board of Chelation Therapy or the American College for Advancement in Medicine (ACAM).

■ Prior to chelation, a complete physical examination that includes a heart function test, hair mineral analysis, electrocardiogram, stress test, and doppler flow analysis should be conducted. Kidney function must also be checked.

■ EDTA dosage should be individualized for each patient according to age, sex, weight, and kidney function, and should be administered slowly over a period of three or more hours.

■ Treatments should be administered by well-trained staff members who are readily available to deal with any symptoms that might occur during the process, such as weakness or dizziness from low blood sugar levels.

If a patient decides to have chelation therapy, it should be performed by a doctor with several years of experience, who has completed the training conducted by ACAM. If the therapy is administered by a nurse or nonphysician, a qualified physician must be on the premises at all times during the procedure.

Scientists at the
University of Toronto in Ontario, Canada,
studied the death rates for 224,258 U.S.
and 9,444 Canadian heart patients.
They found that at the end of one year
following the heart attack, the death
rate was 34% in both countries.
The crucial difference, however, is that
whereas 12% of U.S. heart attack
patients received angioplasty, only 1.5%
of Canadian heart patients did;
further, while 11% of American heart
patients have bypass surgery,
only 1.4% of Canadians do.

The Dental Connection

PROBLEMS WITH YOUR TEETH CAN AFFECT YOUR HEART—AND HOW TO REVERSE THEM

THERE IS A GROWING RECOGNITION among alternative dentists and physicians that dental health has a strong impact on the health of the body. European researchers estimate that perhaps as much as half of all chronic degenerative illness (including heart disease) can be linked either directly or indirectly to dental problems and the traditional techniques of modern dentistry used to treat them. The well-publicized dangers associated with the use of silver/mercury fillings (amalgams) are only the tip of the iceberg as far as the negative impact that dentistry can have on a person's health.

"One of the big problems in the United States," says Gary Verigan, D.D.S., of Escalon, California, "is that dentists are trained to practice with only the most meager of diagnostic equipment. These instruments, consisting primarily of X rays, are incapable of detecting enough about the tooth and its surrounding environment, giving the dentist only a superficial understanding of the problem and the impact it may be having on the patient's health. People often go through many doctors and therapies in search of answers for their problems, never realizing that their chronic conditions may be traceable to dental complications."

In contrast, biological dentistry treats the teeth, jaw, and related structures with specific regard to how treatment will affect the entire body. According to Hal Huggins, D.D.S., of Colorado Springs, Colorado, a pioneer in this field, "Dental problems such as cavities, infections, toxic or allergy-producing filling materials, root canals,

Dr. Huggins reports the improvement or disappearance of many cardiovascular problems including angina, unidentified chest pains, and tachycardia (rapid heartbeat for no apparent reason) after removing toxic dental amalgams.

and misalignment of the teeth or jaw can have far-reaching effects throughout the body."

How Dental Problems Contribute to Illness

"Dental infections and dental disturbances can cause pain and dysfunction throughout the body," states Edward Arana, D.D.S., former president of the American Academy of Biological Dentistry, "including limited motion and loose tendons, ligaments, and muscles. Structural and physiological dysfunction can also occur, impairing organs and glands."

Dr. Arana cites several major types of dental problems that can cause illness and dysfunction in the body:
- infections under and around teeth
- problems with specific teeth related to the acupuncture meridians and the autonomic nervous system
- root canals
- toxicity from dental restoration materials
- incompatability to dental restoration materials (evidenced by the body's negative reaction)
- temporomandibular joint syndrome (TMJ), a painful condition of the jaw, usually caused by stress or injury

Some of the more common causes of these dental problems are unerupted teeth (teeth that have not broken through the gum), wisdom teeth (both impacted and unimpacted), amalgam-filled cavities and root canals, cysts, bone cavities, and areas of bone condensation due to inflammation in the bone. These conditions can be diagnosed using testing methods such as blood tests, applied kinesiology, electroacupuncture biofeedback, and, in some cases, X rays. A thorough review of the patient's medical and dental histories is also essential.

Infections Under the Teeth
Pockets of infection can exist under the teeth and be undetectable on

Electroacupuncture Biofeedback

Developed in the 1940s by Reinhold Voll, M.D., of Germany, electroacupuncture biofeedback makes use of the acupuncture meridian system to screen for infections and dysfunctions in the body. Today it is employed as a screening tool by alternative health practitioners worldwide, including biological dentists. As employed in biological dentistry, it involves placing an electrode on an individual tooth, then applying a small electrical current and recording the

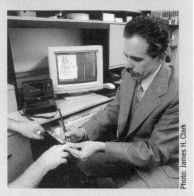

response. Any deviation from the normal reading indicates that there is an infection or disturbance in the vicinity of that particular tooth.[1]

This deviation can also indicate a similar unhealthy state in the organ that shares the same meridian as the tooth. Any determinations using electroacupuncture biofeedback should always be confirmed by a physician.

Photo: James H. Clark

X rays. This is particularly true for teeth that have had root canals, as it is very difficult to eliminate all the bacteria and toxins from the roots during this procedure. These infections may persist for years without the patient's knowledge.

When infections are present, toxins can leak out and depress the function of the immune system, leading to chronic degenerative diseases throughout the body. Once the infection is cleared up, many of the symptoms of disease will disappear. Some dentists use applied kinesiology testing to identify these hidden infections. Applied kinesiology employs a simple strength resistance test on a specific indicator muscle that is related to the organ or part of the body that is being tested. If the muscle tests strong, maintaining its resistance, it indicates health. If it tests weak, it can mean infection or dysfunction.

Relationship Between Specific Teeth and Illness

In the 1950s, Reinhold Voll, M.D., of Germany, discovered that each tooth in the mouth relates to a specific acupuncture meridian. Using his electroacupuncture biofeedback technique (see sidebar), he found that if a tooth became infected or diseased, the organ on the same meridian could also become unhealthy. He found that the opposite held true as well, that dysfunction in a specific organ could lead to a

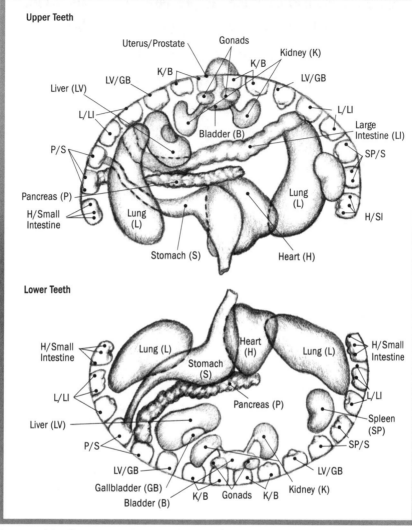

Upper Teeth

Uterus/Prostate
Gonads
Kidney (K)
K/B
K/B
LV/GB
LV/GB
Liver (LV)
L/LI
L/LI
Large Intestine (LI)
P/S
Bladder (B)
SP/S
Pancreas (P)
Lung (L)
H/Small Intestine
Lung (L)
H/SI
Stomach (S)
Heart (H)

Lower Teeth

H/Small Intestine
Lung (L)
Heart (H)
Lung (L)
H/Small Intestine
Stomach (S)
L/LI
Pancreas (P)
L/LI
Liver (LV)
Spleen (SP)
P/S
SP/S
LV/GB
LV/GB
Gallbladder (GB)
K/B
Gonads
K/B
Kidney (K)
Bladder (B)

Organ and tooth correspondences on acupuncture meridians in the mouth

problem in the corresponding tooth. For example, Harold Ravins, D.D.S., of Los Angeles, California, has observed that people who hit their front teeth too hard often have kidney disturbances, as there is a specific relationship between the kidneys and the front teeth.

Ernesto Adler, M.D., D.D.S., of Spain, reports that many diseases can be caused by the wisdom teeth, which have a relationship to

The late Weston Price, D.D.S., former director of research for the American Dental Association, made the astonishing claim that if teeth that have had root canals are removed from patients suffering from heart disease, the disease will resolve in most cases.

almost all organs of the body. When wisdom teeth are impacted, Dr. Adler points out, they press upon the nerves of the mandible (the large bone that makes up the lower jaw), which can result in disturbances in other areas of the body, including heart problems, stammering, epilepsy, pain in the joints, depression, and headaches. He adds that the upper wisdom teeth can cause calcium deficiency, resulting in muscle cramps.

Root Canals as a Cause of Illness

The late Weston Price, D.D.S., M.S., F.A.C.D., former director of research for the American Dental Association, made the astonishing claim that if teeth that have had root canals are removed from patients suffering from kidney and heart disease, these diseases will resolve in most cases. Moreover, implanting these teeth in animals results in the animals developing the same kind of disease found in the person from whom the tooth was taken. Dr. Price found that toxins seeping out of root canals can cause systemic diseases of the heart, kidney, uterus, and nervous and endocrine systems.[2]

Michael Ziff, D.D.S, of Orlando, Florida, points out that research has demonstrated that 100% of root canals result in residual infection. This may be due to the imperfect seal that allows bacteria to penetrate. The oxygen-lacking environment of a root canal can cause the bacteria to undergo changes, adds Dr. Huggins, producing potent toxins that can then leak out into the body. Nutrient materials are also able to seep into the root canal through the porous channels in the tooth, allowing this bacterial growth to flourish.

According to Dr. Ziff, however, there are cases where root canal teeth should not be pulled. It can be difficult to chew without certain teeth intact, and problems can arise if the teeth surrounding the extracted one become misaligned. "The best approach is a conservative one," says Dr. Ziff. "Try other measures first and only remove the tooth as a last resort."

Toxicity from Dental Restoration Materials

"Dental amalgam fillings can release mercury, tin, copper, silver, and sometimes zinc into the body," says Dr. Arana. All of these metals have various degrees of toxicity and when placed as fillings in the teeth can corrode or disassociate into metallic ions (charged atoms). These metallic ions can then migrate from the tooth into the root of the tooth, the mouth, the bone, the connective tissues of the jaw, and finally into the nerves. From there they can travel into the central nervous system, where the ions will reside, permanently disrupting the body's normal functioning if nothing is done to remove them.

Other types of metal-based dental restorations can similarly release toxic metals into the body. According to David E. Eggleston, D.D.S., of the Department of Restorative Dentistry at the University of Southern California in Los Angeles, a patient undergoing dental work developed kidney disease due to nickel toxicity from the dental crowns that were being placed in the patient's mouth. As each successive crown was placed, the disease intensified, verified by blood and urine tests, and physical examinations. Once the nickel crowns were removed, the patient gradually became symptom-free.[3]

Mercury Dental Amalgams

While all metals used for dental restoration can be toxic, the most harmful are the mercury dental amalgams (silver/mercury) used for fillings. According to Joyal Taylor, D.D.S., formerly of Rancho Santa Fe, California, "These so-called 'silver fillings' actually contain 50% mercury and only 25% silver."

Mercury has been recognized as a poison since the

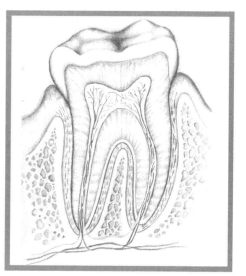

Cross section of a tooth. **The trouble with root canals is that bacteria become trapped within the literally three miles of microscopic dentin tubules inside a single-root tooth and from here can infect the rest of the body.**

Mercury has been recognized as a poison since the 1500s, and yet mercury amalgams have been used in dentistry since the 1820s. They are still being used today even though the Environmental Protection Agency (EPA) declared scrap dental amalgam a hazardous waste in 1988.

To contact **Joyal Taylor's practice,** now under the direction of former colleague Grant Lawton, D.D.S.: P.O. Box 2184, 16095 Avenita de Acacias, San Diego, CA; tel: 619-596-7626; fax: 619-756-7843.

For more on the **hazards of mercury fillings,** see Chapter 1: What Causes Heart Disease?, pp. 40-42.

1500s, and yet mercury amalgams have been used in dentistry since the 1820s. They are still being used today even though the Environmental Protection Agency (EPA) declared scrap dental amalgam a hazardous waste in 1988. Even the American Dental Association, which has so far refused to ban amalgams, now instructs dentists to "know the potential hazards and symptoms of mercury exposure such as the development of sensitivity and neuropathy," to use a no-touch technique for handling the amalgam, and to store it under liquid, preferably glycerin or radiographic fixer solution, in unbreakable, tightly sealed containers.[4]

For some dentists, such as Richard D. Fischer, D.D.S., of Annandale, Virginia, these measures are not enough. Since becoming aware of the health risk amalgams pose, he has refused to work with them and has had his own silver fillings removed. "I don't feel comfortable using a substance designated by the EPA to be a waste disposal hazard," he says. "I can't throw it in the trash, bury it in the ground, or put it in a landfill, but they say it's okay to put it in people's mouths. That doesn't make sense."

According to the German Ministry of Health, "Amalgam is considered a health risk from a medical viewpoint due to the release of mercury vapor."[5] Everyday activities such as chewing and brushing the teeth have been shown to release mercury vapors from amalgams.[6] Amalgams can also erode and corrode with time (ideally they should be replaced after seven to ten years), adding to their toxic output. Studies by the World Health Organization show that a single amalgam can release 3 to 17 mcg of mercury per day,[7] making dental amalgam a major source of mercury exposure.[8]

Since mercury is a cumulative poison, building up in the body with repeated exposure,[9] its effects can be devastating. It can prevent nutrients from entering the cells and wastes from leaving. Mercury can bind to the DNA (deoxyribonucleic acid) of cells as well as to the cell membranes, distorting them and interfering with normal cell

"I don't feel comfortable using a substance designated by the Environmental Protection Agency to be a waste disposal hazard. I can't throw it in the trash, bury it in the ground, or put it in a landfill, but they say it's okay to put it in people's mouths. That doesn't make sense"—Richard D. Fischer, D.D.S.

functions.[10] Mercury poisoning can also lead to symptoms such as anxiety, depression, confusion, irritability, insecurity, and the inability to concentrate. It can cause kidney disease and cardiac and respiratory disorders. Mercury poisoning often goes undetected for years because the symptoms presented do not necessarily suggest the mercury as the initiating cause.

A recent study, directed by Dr. Huggins and sponsored by the Adolph Coors Foundation, showed that mercury filling emissions affected blood hemoglobin levels (the oxygen and iron-carrying molecule), cellular energy production, and white-blood and natural-killer cell activity (our immune system's key agents against infection and disease, including cancer).[11]

CAUTION

If you decide to replace your mercury amalgam fillings, it is essential that you have the procedure performed only by a dentist expert at mercury amalgam removal. Mercury vapor is released in the process and the proper steps must be taken to prevent poisoning from this vapor or from filling fragments.

Dr. Huggins reports the improvement or disappearance of many cardiovascular problems, including angina, unidentified chest pains, and tachycardia (rapid heartbeat for no apparent reason), after removing toxic dental amalgams. Though the ideal replacement for mercury amalgams has not yet been found, there are some less toxic alternatives that biological dentists are working with. The best one so far is the so-called composite amalgam, which is a combination of metals that are less toxic than mercury and slower to break down.

Biological Treatment of Dental Problems

Biological dentists treat dental problems in a variety of ways. They emphasize the conservation of all healthy tooth material and employ the latest techniques of bioenergetic medicine, including neural therapy, oral acupuncture, cold laser therapy, complex homeopathy, mouth balancing, and nutrition.

Neural Therapy

According to neural therapy, the body is charged with electricity or

Dr. Huggins reports the improvement or disappearance of many cardiovascular problems, including angina, unidentified chest pains, and tachycardia (rapid heartbeat for no apparent reason), after removing toxic dental amalgams.

biological energy. This energy flows throughout the body, with every cell possessing its own specified frequency range. As long as this energy flow is unimpeded and stays within its normal range, the body will remain healthy. However, if this balance breaks down, disruptions in the normal function of cells can occur, eventually leading to chronic disorders.

When injury, inflammation, or infection is present in the mouth, there is usually a corresponding blockage in the body's normal energy flow. Injection of a local anesthetic, such as procaine around the tooth to remove the energy blockage, will often resolve the problem. Dr. Adler cites the example of a sports instructor suffering from "tennis elbow." When Dr. Adler injected the man's two upper right premolars with procaine, the instructor received immediate relief from his pain.

Oral Acupuncture

Oral acupuncture, according to Jochen Gleditsch, M.D., D.D.S., of Munich, Germany, has been taught to dentists since 1976, and its use is expanding rapidly. It involves the injection of either saline water, weak local anesthetics, or sterile complex homeopathics into specific acupuncture points of the oral mucous membrane. It can also be combined with neural therapy.

Both Dr. Arana and Dr. Ravins use oral acupuncture to relieve pain during dental procedures with great success. Some dentists also use it to relax patients before any dental procedure. Toothache, tooth sensitivities, jaw pain, gingivitis, and other local problems often respond to oral acupuncture.

Cold Laser Therapy

Cold laser therapy is an alternative form of acupuncture that is especially useful for treating patients who object to the use of needles. The "cold laser" gets its name from the fact that its power output and the light spectrum it uses are incapable of causing any thermal damage to the body's tissues. This therapy kills bacteria, aids in wound healing, reduces inflammation, and helps to rebalance the flow of energy in the body's meridian system.

Selected Health Symptom Analysis of 1,569 Patients Who Eliminated Mercury-Containing Dental Fillings[12]

The following represents a summary of 1,569 patients in six different studies evaluating the health effects of replacing mercury-containing dental fillings with non-mercury fillings. The data was derived from the following sources: 762 Patient Adverse Reaction Reports submitted to the FDA by patients; and 807 patients reports from Sweden, Denmark, Canada, and the United States.

% of Total Reporting	Symptom	Number Reporting	Number Improved or Cured	% of Cure or Improvement
14	Allergy	221	196	89
5	Anxiety	86	80	93
5	Bad temper	81	68	84
6	Bloating	88	70	80
6	Blood pressure problems	99	53	54
5	Chest pains	79	69	87
22	Depression	347	315	91
22	Dizziness	343	301	88
45	Fatigue	705	603	86
15	Intestinal problems	231	192	83
8	Gum problems	129	121	94
34	Headaches	531	460	87
12	Insomnia	187	146	78
10	Irregular heartbeat	159	139	87
8	Irritability	132	119	90
17	Lack of concentration	270	216	80
6	Lack of energy	91	88	97
17	Memory loss	265	193	73
17	Metallic taste	260	247	95
7	Multiple sclerosis	113	86	76
8	Muscle tremor	126	104	82

Homeopathy in Biological Dentistry

According to Dr. Fischer, "Homeopathic first-aid remedies can help alleviate the pain or discomfort of dental emergencies, at least temporarily, until proper dental care can be received. They are not intended to replace regular dental care, but rather to serve as a safe and effective complement."

Mouth Balancing

Dr. Ravins specializes in "balancing" the mouth to improve a wide range of health problems. He believes that structural deformities of the skull influence the entire body. "With the new computerized technology, I can diagnose muscle dysfunction and pick up vibrations from the jaw and movement of the mandible," he says. Often the misalignment has been caused by a prior accident. By analyzing this data and making special orthopedic braces to be worn in the mouth, Dr. Ravins can realign the jaw and remove pain and other symptoms such as headaches, shoulder pain, back problems, and even some eye problems.

Nutrition

Dr. Huggins, like many other biological dentists, makes nutritional supplementation part of his overall protocol for dealing with dental conditions, especially for the patient recovering from mercury amalgam toxicity. According to Dr. Huggins, the basic supplementation program aids in the excretion of mercury from the cells, prevents the exacerbation of further symptoms, and provides the patient with a nutrient base for rebuilding damaged tissues.

Among the nutrients Dr. Huggins uses are magnesium, selenium, vitamin C, vitamin E, and folic acid, along with digestive enzymes. He cautions, however, that the nutrients need to be used in specific ratios, and that supplementation done without proper consultation can actually create further imbalances in the patient's system.

A proper diet is also important for patients suffering from mercury toxicity. Dr. Huggins recommends the avoidance of cigarettes, sugar, alcohol, caffeine, chocolate, soft drinks, refined carbohydrates, milk, cheese, margarine, fish, and excess liquids with meals.

The Politics of Dentistry

Although many new techniques of biological dentistry are available, only 2,000 to 3,000 dentists across the United States are using them in practice. This is due to a deliberate effort by the American Dental Association (ADA) to suppress such practices, even to the point of rescinding the licenses of practitioners using them. Electroacupuncture biofeedback testing by dentists is not allowed in some states and dentists may lose their license for using it, despite its proven effectiveness for screening hidden infections under teeth. For this reason, most dentists are forced to use other methods for detecting hidden infections and other dental problems. Dental acupuncture is also banned in some states.

In 1987, the ADA wrote a provision into their code to declare the removal of clinically serviceable mercury amalgams from patients' teeth to be unethical, according to Dr. Ziff. Any dentist doing so is in violation of the code, and the ADA is assisting state boards in prosecuting these dentists, despite all the evidence of the toxicity of mercury. The financial and legal implications of an admission by the ADA that mercury is toxic and harmful to health may be a possible motive behind this move. If the ADA was to admit that mercury amalgams are toxic health hazards, insurance companies or the government would possibly have to foot the bill for the removal of mercury amalgams from practically the entire population of the United States.

However, the growing number of research studies on biological dental techniques, the information coming out of Europe and Canada on mercury toxicity,[13] and increasing public awareness of some of the dangers of traditional dental practice are combining to build support for the small band of dentists risking their livelihood to practice safe dentistry in the United States. "Biological dentistry will, out of necessity, become the dental medicine of the 21st century," says Dr. Arana.

5 Nutritional Supplements

HOW THEY CAN BENEFIT YOUR HEART

SINCE ATHEROSCLEROSIS and heart disease take many years to develop, a daily regimen of supplements may be helpful in preventing both. The amount of supplements needed varies from one individual to another depending on body weight and absorption levels, and it is best to consult with a nutritionally-skilled physician or naturopathic physician before embarking on a routine of supplements.

Matthias Rath, M.D., author of *Eradicating Heart Disease*, uses a program of supplements to reverse heart disease. "I firmly believe that America's number one killer can be prevented by an optimum intake of essential nutrients," he says. The supplements include vitamin C and other antioxidants, coenzyme Q10, amino acids, B vitamins, and minerals. Vitamin C is an important component because it helps prevent the formation of free radicals, which initiate artery obstruction by damaging arterial walls. It also helps to heal the damaged areas before they fill with cholesterol.

Reversing Heart Failure With Supplements

For example, George, a man in his fifties, came to Dr. Rath after experiencing sudden cardiac failure. This was a severe heart muscle weakness which resulted in decreased pumping function and enlargement of the heart chambers. George was no longer able to work full-time and had to give up

Dr. Rath's book, *Eradicating Heart Disease*, is available from Health Now, 387 Ivy Street, San Francisco, CA 94102; tel: 800-624-2442; fax: 800-582-8000. The nutrients are available as **Cardi-rite** from Carlson Laboratories, 15 College, Arlington Heights, IL 60004; tel: 847-255-1600 or 800-323-4141; fax: 847-255-1605.

most physical activities. Sometimes he felt so weak he had to hold an object with both hands to keep from dropping it and he was unable to climb stairs. His cardiologist recommended a heart transplant.

Dr. Rath put George on his supplement program for heart health. "Soon George could again fulfill his professional obligations on a regular basis and was able to undertake daily bicycle rides," says Dr. Rath. After two months on the program, his cardiologist reported that his heart enlargement had decreased. A month after that, George went on an overseas business trip and reported that physical limitations were no longer interfering with his work.

Vitamins

The following vitamins can help promote heart health:

Beta Carotene (vitamin A precursor)—

Research done at Johns Hopkins University found that there were approximately 50% fewer heart disease cases among those study participants with the highest levels of beta carotene, compared to the group with the lowest levels.[1] A similar study at Harvard University found that of two groups with prior evidence of heart disease, the group given a beta carotene supplement had 40% fewer heart attacks than the group given a placebo.[2]

Vitamin B3 (niacin)—Niacin helps to lower cholesterol levels and lessen the risk of heart disease.[3] It has also

Dr. Rath's Nutrient Recommendations

The following are general supplement guidelines to promote heart health. Keep in mind that each person is unique and has different nutritional requirements. It is always best to consult a qualified health practitioner for assistance in designing a supplement program that meets your individual needs.

Vitamin C: 1,000 mg

Vitamin E: 600 IU

Beta carotene: 8,000 IU

L-proline: 500 mg

L-lysine: 500 mg

L-carnitine: 150 mg

Coenzyme Q10: 25 mg

Vitamin B1: 40 mg

Vitamin B2: 40 mg

Vitamin B3: (niacin) 50 mg

Vitamin B3: (niacinamide): 150 mg

Vitamin B5: (pantothenate): 200 mg

Vitamin B6: 50 mg

Vitamin B12: 0.1 mg

Folic acid: 0.4 mg

Vitamin D: 600 IU

Biotin: 0.3 mg

Calcium: 150 mg

Magnesium: 200 mg

Zinc: 30 mg

Manganese: 6 mg

Copper: 2 mg

Selenium: 0.1 mg

Chromium: 0.05 mg

Molybdenum: 0.02 mg

One of Dr. Abram Hoffer's patients came to him 20 years ago with angina pectoris. He was treated with niacin and has had no signs of angina since.

For more about **homocysteine,** see Chapter 1: What Causes Heart Disease?, pp. 33-37.

been shown to increase the longevity of patients who have suffered one heart attack. Over 8,000 middle-aged men who had suffered a heart attack were given supplements of either niacin, estrogen, thyroid hormone, or a placebo. The study results showed that only niacin was beneficial in lowering the death rate and increasing longevity.[4]

Abram Hoffer, M.D., Ph.D., of Victoria, British Columbia, treated a pilot who had not been able to fly for seven years because of heart problems. Dr. Hoffer put him on 3 g daily of niacin; after one-and-a-half years, he received a clean bill of health and was able to fly again. Another of Dr. Hoffer's patients came to him 20 years ago with angina pectoris. This patient was also treated with niacin and, according to Dr. Hoffer, has had no signs of angina since.

Vitamin B6—Researchers have found vitamin B6 to be a safe and inexpensive supplement which may be helpful in preventing heart attacks, strokes,[5] and atherosclerosis.[6] Recent studies have shown that vitamins B6, B12, and folic acid can dramatically lower homocysteine, a free-radical generator capable of oxidizing cholesterol, one of the major contributing factors in heart disease.[7]

Vitamin B6 is needed for the conversion of homocysteine to the harmless chemical cystathionine, thus preventing the homocysteine-induced oxidation of cholesterol.[8] It has also been suggested that vitamin B6 inhibits the platelet aggregation which occurs in atherosclerosis.[9] The typical American diet, however, leaves many people significantly deficient in this vital nutrient.

In 1949, Moses M. Suzman, M.D., a South African neurologist and internist, gathered a group of pre-cardiac patients who showed signs of arterial damage and had them take 100 mg of vitamin B6 per day, while patients who had already had heart attacks or angina were given 200 mg per day (half in a B complex including choline). In addition, the patients with the most serious conditions were given 5 mg of folic acid, 100-600 IU of vitamin E, magnesium, and zinc.[10]

Over the next 23 years, Dr. Suzman's patients recovered rapidly, as their angina and electrocardiographic irregularities diminished or disappeared. Those who dropped out of the vitamin and diet regimen, however, soon found their cardiac problems returning.[11]

Interest in vitamin B6 deficiency and its relationship to heart disease revived in 1969, when Kilmer S. McCully, M.D., a professor of pathology at Harvard Medical School, found that heart patients had nearly 80% less of the vitamin than healthy individuals did.[12] From this, Dr. McCully postulated that B6 may help the body resist the arterial damage that precipitates heart disease. He also found that patients who had already suffered a heart attack or angina, and were then given 200 mg of B6 daily (half in a B complex including choline) combined with a low-fat, mostly vegetarian diet, recovered rapidly.[13]

Vitamin B12—A deficiency in vitamin B12 is associated with elevated homocysteine levels.[14] When vitamin B12 is supplemented, homocysteine levels decrease.[15] This effect can be increased by also supplementing choline, folic acid, riboflavin, and B6.[16]

Folic Acid—Folic acid is essential for the proper metabolism of homocysteine.[17] Thus, folic acid supplementation can help prevent the arterial plaque buildup caused by an excess of homocysteine in the blood.

Antioxidants—Antioxidants such as vitamin E, vitamin C, selenium, and coenzyme Q10 have also proven in numerous studies to be effective in both the prevention and treatment of heart disease.[18]

Vitamin C—Vitamin C (ascorbic acid) is integral to heart health. It is believed to help prevent the formation of oxysterols.[19] By combining the amino acid lysine with vitamin C, it may be possible to dissolve clots in the bloodstream.[20]

Studies also reveal that vitamin C is required for collagen synthesis and is therefore necessary to maintain the integrity of the walls of arteries.[21] Nobel laureate Linus Pauling, Ph.D., believed that a deficiency of vitamin C may precipitate arteriosclerosis because it causes defects in the arterial walls due to reduced collagen synthesis.[22] Drs. Pauling and Rath have shown in preliminary studies that vitamin C supplementation can reverse arteriosclerosis in humans.[23]

In a study conducted on guinea pigs, it was found that the equivalent of the U.S. Recommended Daily Allowance (RDA) of vitamin C offered virtually no protection against arterial damage. When the amount of vitamin C was increased to a dose equivalent to 2,800 mg for a 154-pound human, the researchers were able to reverse the damage.[24]

"Vitamin C reverses oxidation and prevents free radical forma-

High doses of vitamin C can dramatically reduce your risk of heart attack or death from other degenerative diseases, according to research results from Tufts University. Those individuals who consumed more than 700 mg daily of vitamin C had a 62% reduced risk of dying from heart disease and a 50% reduced mortality rate overall.

CAUTION

High amounts of vitamin C taken over a prolonged period of time can leach calcium and other minerals out of the teeth, bones, and other tissues, according to Dr. Cowden. He recommends that high amounts of vitamin C (ascorbic acid) be balanced by mineral ascorbates containing magnesium, potassium, zinc, and manganese.

tion," states William Lee Cowden, M.D., of Richardson, Texas. "In a diet that involves reducing fats, vitamin C is an integral part of helping the body to repair itself." In patients with existing cardiovascular disease, Dr. Cowden recommends that vitamin C be taken to bowel tolerance (the maximum amount a person can take before causing loose stools or diarrhea). He suggests a minimum of three to four doses daily, increasing the amount until reaching bowel tolerance.

"For example," explains Dr. Cowden, "the first dose could be 1,000 mg, the second dose 2,000 mg, the third dose 3,000 mg, and the fourth dose 4,000 mg. Stay on bowel tolerance until cardiovascular disease is resolved, and then go on a 3,000-mg maintenance dose. For those who are well but want to prevent cardiovascular disease, 3,000 to 10,000 mg daily is sufficient." Higher doses of vitamin C should be taken with adequate amounts of water, magnesium, and vitamin B6, adds Dr. Cowden.

A study conducted by James E. Enstrom, M.D., an epidemiologist at the University of California at Los Angeles, suggests that men who consume vitamin C every day, at levels 500% to 666% of the U.S. RDA, live about six years longer than men who don't.[25]

High doses of vitamin C can dramatically reduce your risk of heart attack or death from other degenerative diseases, according to research results from Tufts University in Boston, Massachusetts. Scientists tracked the health outcomes of 725 volunteers, 60-101 years old (average age of 73), over a 12-year span. Those individuals who consumed more than 700 mg daily of vitamin C had a 62% reduced risk of dying from heart disease and a 50% reduced mortality rate overall, suggesting that adequate vitamin C intake actually increases lifespan. Concurrent blood analyses of the subjects confirmed that those with high levels of vitamin C in their plasma enjoyed these benefits. The scientists also demonstrated that the highest degree of protection was provided by combining vitamin C intake at this level and dietary foods, such as vegetables, high in natural vitamin C.[26]

Vitamin E–Vitamin E is a fat-soluble antioxidant which can help prevent abnormal blood clot formation. Richard Passwater, Ph.D., of Berlin, Maryland, believes that any nutrient that prevents the oxidation of cholesterol, such as vitamin E, beta carotene, and coenzyme Q10, offers a protective factor. Supplementation of vitamin E may also inhibit platelet aggregation[27] and help repair the lining of blood vessels.[28]

Studies published in the *New England Journal of Medicine* suggest that vitamin E can contribute greatly to the prevention of heart disease in both men and women.[29] In a study conducted by Harvard Medical School of 87,245 female nurses, it was found that those who took 100 IU of vitamin E daily for more than two years had a 46% lower risk of heart disease.[30] In another Harvard study, 39,910 male health professionals who took 100 IU of vitamin E daily for an unspecified time period had a 37% lower risk of heart disease.[31] In groups who took higher doses of vitamin E for a longer time, the results were even greater.

In a study of 34,486 postmenopausal women with no tangible signs of heart trouble, those who consumed at least 100 IU of vitamin E daily from their foods were 62% less likely to die of coronary heart disease than those women consuming less vitamin E, according to the *New England Journal of Medicine* in May 1996.[32] An earlier study the same year showed that those with heart problems who took vitamin E experienced a 75% reduction in the rate of heart attacks.

A study funded by the World Health Organization found that among 16 European study populations, those with low serum levels of vitamin E were at greater risk for heart disease than those with high blood pressure and high cholesterol levels.[33] When 1,851 men and women with coronary heart disease, such as angina or atherosclerosis, took natural-source vitamin E at rates between 400 and 800 IU daily, researchers observed that this supplementation reduced the number of clinically significant coronary events. Specifically, the risk of non-

Remember, *oxidized* LDL cholesterol is the kind that leads to plaque formation on the artery walls. Research at the University of Minnesota discovered that subjects taking 800 IU of vitamin E daily for just two weeks had up to three times the resistance to oxidation of LDL cholesterol. Investigators at the University of Texas report that 800 IU of vitamin E is as good as a combination of vitamins E and C and beta carotene for the same purpose—that is, for reducing arterial damage.[36]

fatal heart attack was reduced by 77%. The effects were apparent after about 200 days of vitamin E supplementation.[34]

While it is generally recognized that vitamin E supplementation can reduce the risk of cardiovascular disease, there is some disagreement over what is the most effective dose. A recent study at the University of Texas has concluded that 400 IU daily provides the maximum protection and anything lower may not prevent LDL oxidation.[35]

High dosages of vitamin E are not recommended for people with hypertension, rheumatic heart disease, or ischemic heart disease, except under close medical supervision. However, in hypertensive or ischemic heart disease patients, if the dose of vitamin E is raised gradually, the blood pressure will usually not rise significantly and there will not be a greater workload placed on the heart, according to Dr. Cowden.

Lipoproteins are in two principal forms. *Low-density lipoproteins (LDLs)* are combination molecules of proteins and fats, particularly cholesterol. LDLs circulate in the blood and act as the primary carriers of cholesterol to the cells of the body. An elevated level of LDLs, the so-called "bad" cholesterol, is a contributing factor in causing atherosclerosis (plaque deposits on the inner walls of the arteries). A diet high in saturated fats can lead to an increase the level of LDLs in the blood. *High-density lipoproteins (HDLs)* are also fat-protein molecules in the blood, but contain a larger amount of protein and less fat than LDLs. HDLs are able to absorb cholesterol and related compounds in the blood and transport them to the liver for elimination. HDL, the so-called "good" cholesterol, may also be able to take cholesterol from plaque deposits on the artery walls, thus helping to reverse the process of atherosclerosis. A higher ratio of HDL to LDL cholesterol in the blood is associated with a reduced risk of cardiovascular disease.

Minerals

The following minerals may be effective in the treatment and prevention of heart disease:

Calcium—Calcium supplementation may also decrease total cholesterol and inhibit platelet aggregation.[37] Researchers at the Malmö University Hospital in Malmö, Sweden, studied 33,346 individuals over a 10.8-year period and found direct correlations between calcium levels and heart disease, malignant disorders, and mortality.[38] Too much calcium, they said, can damage health and shorten lifespan. As blood levels of calcium rise, so does the risk of premature death.

According to the study, men under 50 years old who had blood levels of calcium greater than 2.45 mmol/L (the high end of "normal") showed a 20% increase in mortality compared to men with lower levels. Those with calcium levels greater than 2.60 mmol/L died at twice the rate of those with lower levels. Those with levels between 2.51 and 2.55 mmol/L

While it is generally recognized that vitamin E supplementation can reduce the risk of cardiovascular disease, there is some disagreement over what is the most effective dose. A recent study at the University of Texas has concluded that 400 IU daily provides the maximum protection and anything lower may not prevent LDL oxidation.

had a 50% increased risk of premature death from all causes, compared to men with calcium levels at 2.31-2.45 mmol/L, the researchers said. Men with calcium levels exceeding 2.50 mmol/L had a 58% increased chance of dying from cardiovascular disease and a 28% increased risk of dying from malignant disorders, such as cancer.

Chromium—Several studies have linked chromium deficiency to coronary heart disease.[39] Supplementation with chromium has been shown to lower total cholesterol and triglycerides and raise HDL cholesterol.[40] It is even more effective in lowering cholesterol when combined with niacin (vitamin B3).[41]

Magnesium—It has been found that individuals who die suddenly of heart attacks have far lower levels of magnesium and potassium than do control groups.[42] Magnesium deficiency has been implicated in mitral valve prolapse (MVP, also called floppy valve syndrome, a malfunction in the valve between the left atrium and ventricle of the heart) and supplementation with magnesium may reverse symptoms.[43]

A recent study lends new support to these findings.[44] Of 141 people with "heavily symptomatic" MVP, 60% had low magnesium levels, compared to only 5% in the control group. After five weeks of magnesium supplementation, the percentage of those with chest pain dropped from 96% to 47%; with palpitations, from 93% to 51%; with anxiety, from 84% to 47%; low energy, from 74% to 34%; faintness, from 64% to 6%; and difficulty breathing, from 84% to 39%.

Magnesium helps to dilate arteries and ease the heart's pumping of blood, thus preventing arrhythmia (irregular heartbeat). Magnesium may also prevent calcification of the blood vessels, lower total cholesterol, raise HDL cholesterol, and inhibit platelet aggregation.[45] But simply taking oral magnesium supplements may not be sufficient. "Most doctors don't use the best form for optimum absorption," Dr. Cowden explains. "It's more effective to use magnesium

The amino acid L-arginine, when given intravenously at the rate of 20 grams over one hour, can produce significant increases in stroke volume and cardiac output in patients with congestive heart failure. Arginine therapy can also lower arterial blood pressure. Supplementation with the amino acid L-carnitine immediately after an acute heart attack can help damaged heart muscle expand again.

The Meyer's Cocktail is an intravenous vitamin and mineral protocol developed by John Meyers, M.D., a physician in Baltimore, Maryland, in the 1970s. It contains magnesium chloride hexahydrate (5 cc given), calcium gluconate (2.5 cc), vitamin B2 (1,000 mcg/cc; 1 cc given), vitamin B5 (100 mg/cc; 1 cc given), vitamin B6 (250 mg/cc; 1 cc given) the entire vitamin B-complex (100 mg/cc; 1 cc given), and vitamin C (222 mg/cc; 6 cc given). The solution is slowly injected over a 5-15 minute period. The "Cocktail" is indicated for patients with chronic fatigue, depression, muscle spasm, asthma, hives, allergic rhinitis, congestive heart failure, angina, ischemic vascular disease, acute infections, and senile dementia.

glycinate, taurate, or aspartate, or even herbal magnesium such as red raspberry, but some patients need intravenous or intramuscular magnesium to quickly raise their magnesium to ideal levels."

Alan R. Gaby, M.D., of Kent, Washington, has found that cases of congestive heart failure respond well to an intravenous injection of a nutrient "cocktail" composed of magnesium chloride hexahydrate, hydroxocobalamin, pyridoxine hydrochloride, dexpanthenol, B-complex vitamins, and vitamin C. (This is a modification of the nutrient cocktail popularized by John Meyers, M.D.)

Potassium—High blood pressure is often present in heart disease. It has been found that supplements of potassium can help reduce a patient's reliance on blood pressure medication or diuretic drugs.[46] As calcium channel blockers, the most common form of medication for high blood pressure, can increase your risk of heart attack, heart failure, and stroke, lowering blood pressure through natural means is of obvious benefit to heart health.

Selenium—A positive relationship has been found between low serum selenium levels and cardiovascular disease, possibly related to selenium's antioxidant effects.[47] Selenium supplementation also reduces platelet aggregation,[48] and selenium is a cofactor for glutathione peroxidase, an important antioxidant enzyme.

Other Supplements for Heart Health
The following supplements have also proven useful in treating heart

disease and maintaining heart health:

Amino Acids—The amino acid L-arginine, when given intravenously at the rate of 20 g over one hour, can produce significant increases in stroke volume and cardiac output in patients with congestive heart failure. Arginine therapy can also lower arterial blood pressure.[49]

For more about the **dangers of conventional blood pressure medication,** see Chapter 8: What Causes High Blood Pressure?, pp. 152-160, and Chapter 9: Self-Care Options: How to Use Diet, Exercise, and Lifestyle Changes to Lower Your Blood Pressure, pp. 162-171.

Supplementation with the amino acid L-carnitine immediately after an acute heart attack can help damaged heart muscle expand again. In one study, L-carnitine, when given orally at the rate of 2 g daily for 28 days, improved the condition of 51 patients who had undergone heart attacks.[50] Specifically, the amount of damaged heart muscle after 28 days was significantly less, the incidence of angina pectoris and arrhythmia was reduced by 50%, and the number of cardiac events of any kind for those on L-carnitine was 15.6% compared to 26% for those taking a placebo.

Research is needed into the role of nutritional supplements in preventing and reversing heart disease.

In another study of 472 post–heart attack patients, taking 9 g daily of L-carnitine by intravenous infusion for five days, followed by an oral dosage of 6 g daily (in three divided doses) for the next 12 months, improved the ability of the heart muscle to widen to receive incoming blood.[51] A heart attack (myocardial infarction) otherwise leaves portions of the heart muscle (myocardium) dead (infarcted) and thus unable to expand.

For more on **red wine and heart benefits,** see "Here's to Your Health: Drinking and the Heart," Chapter 2: Caring for Yourself, p. 59.

Bioflavonoids—Lower than average dietary intake of bioflavonoids (antioxidants that enhance vitamin C activity), specifically those found in onions and apples, can increase the risk of coronary heart disease, according to a Finnish study of 5,133 men and women, 30-69 years old.[52] Bioflavonoids found in other fruits, black tea, and red wine were also helpful to the heart.

Coenzyme Q10—Coenzyme Q10 is a natural chemical substance essential to the generation of energy in the cells. It's called a "coenzyme" because it enhances the activity of other enzymes. Over 30 years ago, Karl Folkers, Ph.D., a biomedical scientist at the University of Texas in Austin, discovered that coQ10 helps to strengthen the heart muscle and energize the cardiovascular system in many heart patients. Since then, studies have revealed that coenzyme Q10 may protect

Vitamin and Mineral Supplement Ranges

Vitamin	Adult US RDA	Adult Daily Supplement Range

FAT-SOLUBLE VITAMINS

Beta Carotene	**Not Established**	**10,000-50,000 IU**

(Pro-Vitamin A) Converted by the body to vitamin A as needed. Primary antioxidant which helps protect the lungs and other tissues.
Possible side effects: Prolonged ingestion of relatively high doses may cause a benign yellowing of the skin, especially palms and soles. Avoid beta carotene supplement while taking the prescription drug Accutane, especially during pregnancy.

Vitamin E	**12-15 IU**	**200-800 IU**

(Alpha Tocopherol) Primary antioxidant which protects red blood cells and is essential in cellular respiration.
Possible side effects: Prolonged ingestion of vitamin E may produce adverse skin reactions and upset stomach.

WATER-SOLUBLE VITAMINS

Vitamin C	**60 mg**	**300-3,000 mg**

(Ascorbic Acid) Primary antioxidant, essential for tissue growth, wound healing, absorption of calcium and iron, and utilization of the B vitamin folic acid. Involved in neurotransmitter biosynthesis, cholesterol regulation, and formation of collagen.
Possible side effects: Essentially nontoxic in oral doses. However, excessive ingestion may cause abdominal bloating, gas, flatulence, and diarrhea. Acid-sensitive individuals should take the buffered ascorbate form of vitamin C supplement.

Vitamin B3	**16-20 mg**	**20-100 mg**

(Niacin) Essential for food metabolism and release of energy for cellular function. Vital for oxygen transport in the blood, and fatty acid and nucleic acid formation. A major constituent of several important coenzymes.
Possible side effects: Essentially nontoxic in normal oral doses. High doses (100 mg+) may cause transient flushing and tingling in the upper body area as well as stomach upset. Prolonged ingestion of excess vitamin B3 (1,000-2,000 mg+/day) may elevate liver enzymes and cause liver damage.

Vitamin B6	**2.0-2.5 mg**	**5-200 mg**

(Pyroxidine) Involved in food metabolism and release of energy. Essential for amino acid metabolism and formation of blood proteins and antibodies. Helps regulate electrolytic balance.
Possible side effects: Prolonged high doses (500 mg+/day) may be toxic and cause neurological damage. Note: Prescription oral contraceptives may cause deficiency of vitamin B6.

Vitamin	Adult US RDA	Adult Daily Supplement Range
Vitamin B12	3.0-4.0 mg	10-500 mcg

(Cobalamin) Essential for normal formation of red blood cells. Involved in food metabolism, release of energy, and maintenance of epithelial cells (cells that form the skin's outer layer and the surface layer of mucous membranes) and the nervous system.
Possible side effects: Essentially nontoxic in oral doses.

Folate	400 mcg	200-800 mcg

(Folic Acid, Folacin) Essential for blood formation, especially red blood cells and white blood cells. Involved in the biosynthesis of nucleic acids, including RNA and DNA.
Possible side effects: Essentially nontoxic in oral doses. An excess intake of folate can mask a vitamin B12 deficiency. Note: B vitamins should be taken in a B-complex form because of their close interrelationship in metabolic processes.

MINERALS—The functions of minerals are highly interrelated to each other and to vitamins, hormones, and enzymes. No mineral can function in the body without affecting others.

Calcium	800-1,200 mg	200-1,200 mg

(CA ++) Essential for strong bones and teeth. Serves as a vital cofactor in cellular energy production, and nerve and heart function.
Possible side effects: Prolonged ingestion of excess calcium, along with excess vitamin D, may cause hypercalcemia of bone and soft tissue (such as joints and kidneys) and may also cause a mineral imbalance.

Chromium	50-200 mcg	200-500 mcg

(CR +++) Vital as a cofactor of GTF (glucose tolerance factor), which regulates the function of insulin. Involved in food metabolism, enzyme activation, and regulation of cholesterol.
Possible side effects: Essentially nontoxic in oral doses.

Magnesium	300-350 mg	150-600 mg

(MG ++) Essential catalyst for food metabolism and release of energy. A cofactor in the formation of RNA and DNA, and in enzyme activation and nerve function.
Possible side effects: Extremely high doses (30,000 mg+) may be toxic in certain individuals with kidney problems. Doses of 400 mg+ may produce a laxative effect, causing diarrhea.

continued on next page

Vitamin and Mineral Supplement Ranges (cont.)

Vitamin	Adult US RDA	Adult Daily Supplement Range
Potassium	Not established	1,875-5,625 mg*

(K+) A primary electrolyte, important in regulating pH (acidity/alkalinity) balance and water balance. Plays a role in nerve function and cellular integrity.
Possible side effects: Extremely high doses (25,000 mg+/day) of K chloride may be toxic in instances of kidney failure.
*A typical healthy diet contains adequate potassium. Very active individuals may require additional electrolytes.

Vitamin	Adult US RDA	Adult Daily Supplement Range
Selenium	55-200 mcg	100-200 mcg

(SE) Important constituent of the antioxidant enzyme glutathione peroxidase, which is contained in white blood cells and blood platelets.
Possible side effects: Prolonged ingestion of excess selenium may be toxic.

against atherosclerosis and, through its antioxidant properties, may protect against the formation of oxysterols.[53] It can also protect your heart against the damaging effects of the cancer drug adriamycin.

In one study, 17 patients with mild congestive heart failure took 30 mg daily of coQ10; after four weeks, every patient had improved and 53% had become symptom-free. CoQ10 kept 38% of 641 patients from requiring hospitalization for the same condition; they took coQ10 at the rate of 150 mg daily for one year.

Patients with angina pectoris who took 150 mg per day for four weeks had a 53% reduction in chest pain episodes. After 12 weeks on coQ10, patients with cardiomyopathy (a disease of the heart muscle) enjoyed increased strength in their heartbeat and less shortness of breath. Patients undergoing heart surgery who took coQ10 for 14 days before and 30 days after surgery recovered faster and with fewer complications.

Garry F. Gordon, M.D., D.O., reports success in helping infants avoid risky and unnecessary surgery using supplements of coQ10, amino acids, and herbs. "In one case, I went to see a newborn diagnosed with myocardiopathy. I asked the attending doctor if he had tried coenzyme Q10 or carnitine [an amino acid]. He said that he had read about their effects, but would not use either. With the family's permission, I treated the baby with those supplements, as well as

In one study, 17 patients with mild congestive heart failure took 30 mg daily of coQ10; after four weeks, every patient had improved and 53% had become symptom-free.

with magnesium, vitamin C, a multiple vitamin/mineral product, liquid garlic, and the herbal extract of hawthorn berry. The baby recovered without the heart transplant surgery that was being recommended by the university medical center."

Although coenzyme Q10 is present in many foods (such as rice and wheat bran) and the body can make it from the raw materials in foods, many serious health conditions have now been linked to a shortage of coQ10 in the body's nutritional stocks. Some conventional medications can also deplete the supply. For example, Mevacor, taken to lower cholesterol, also dangerously lowers body levels of coQ10.

While coQ10 is not yet generally prescribed by physicians in the U.S., in Japan it is among the most widely used of drugs. Animal studies prove that even at high doses, coQ10 has no toxic side effects and is safe as a nutritional supplement. Generally it takes four to eight weeks for coQ10 to build up a peak concentration in the body and to produce noticeable effects. CoQ10 is best absorbed as a supplement when it's prepared dissolved in oil rather than as a powdered capsule; in fact, one of the leading authorities on the substance states that the body cannot absorb coQ10 unless it is made fat-soluble. Chewable wafers of coQ10 combined with fatty acids are available and work well.[54]

For more about **coenzyme Q10**, see Chapter 10: Preventing & Reversing High Blood Pressure: One Doctor's Approach, pp. 172-182.

CoQ10 is available as capsules from: Stan Jankowitz, 730 Galloping Hill Road, Franklin Lakes, NJ 07417; tel: 201-891-1104; fax: 201-848-1867.

Essential Fatty Acids (EFAs)—Omega-3 and omega-6 oils are the two principal types of essential fatty acids, which are unsaturated fats required in the diet. The digits "3" and "6" refer to differences in the oil's chemical structure with respect to its chain of carbon atoms and where they are bonded. A balance of these oils in the diet is required for good health. The primary omega-3 oil is called alpha-linolenic acid (ALA) and is found in flaxseed (58%), canola, pumpkin and walnut, and soybeans. Fish oils, such as salmon, cod, and mackerel, contain the other important omega-3 oils, DHA (docosahexaenoic acid) and EPA (eicosapentaenoic acid).

Omega-3 oils help reduce the risk of heart disease. Linoleic acid or cis-linoleic acid is the main omega-6 oil and is found in most plant

Is Fish Oil as Effective as Aspirin in Preventing Heart Attacks?

In the early 1980s, physicians began prescribing aspirin as a preventative to those patients at risk for heart attacks and strokes. Many cited aspirin's anticoagulant effects, noting that aspirin prevents the blood from clotting in plaque-occluded arteries. Dr. Cowden suggests that this approach may be misguided, since aspirin has been known to cause gastrointestinal bleeding and even perforated ulcers in some cases, whereas eicosapentaenoic acid (EPA), an omega-3 essential fatty acid from fish oils, has no such risks and has also been shown to significantly reduce death from coronary heart disease.[55]

In addition, EPA (especially when taken in conjunction with adequate antioxidant nutrients like vitamins E and C and beta carotene) works on reducing stickiness of clotting cells in the blood by affecting prostaglandin ratios (as aspirin does). However, EPA also favorably alters blood lipid ratios and helps to lower blood pressure (which aspirin does not).[56]

and vegetable oils, including safflower (73%), corn, peanut, and sesame. The most therapeutic form of omega-6 oil is gamma-linolenic acid (GLA), found in evening primrose, black currant, and borage oils. Once in the body, omega-6 is converted to prostaglandins, hormone-like substances that regulate many metabolic functions, particularly inflammatory processes.

Supplementing the diet with essential fatty acids may help to lower the level of homocysteine.[57] Omega-3 EFAs are useful in reducing high LDL cholesterol levels and may prevent heart attacks by eliminating clotting and arterial damage.[58] Omega-6 EFAs have been shown to decrease the aggregation or stickiness of platelets, allowing them to pass through the arteries without danger of clotting.[59] Evidence suggests that gamma-linolenic acid may help to regulate the cardiovascular system.[60] Dr. Cowden recommends taking at least equal amounts of omega-3 whenever taking omega-6 fatty acids.

FOS (Fructo-oligosaccharides)—A Japanese study found that when 23 hospital patients, 50-90 years old, took 8 g of fructo-oligosaccharides (FOS) daily for two weeks, the *Bifidobacteria* (beneficial bacteria) levels in their intestines increased by ten times. Benefits from increasing *Bifidobacteria* levels include cholesterol reduction, control of blood sugar levels, immune function enhancement, and a reduction of the detoxification load on the liver, among others. FOS also has been shown to lower blood pressure by 9% when taken at 11.5 g daily by people with high blood pressure.

Under the best of conditions, the estimated 100 trillion bacteria that live in the human intestines do so in a delicate balance. Certain bacteria such as *Lactobacillus* and *Bifidobacteria* are "friendly" bacteria that support numerous vital physiological processes. Other bacteria such as *E. coli*, *Staphylococcus*, and *Clostridrium* may be present in smaller numbers, but they are considered "unfriendly," even dangerous bacteria.

A healthy intestine maintains a balance of the various intestinal flora, but with current lifestyles and the use of antibiotics, drugs, and processed foods, this balance is often upset. For example, people who eat a high-fat, low-fiber diet have reduced *Bifidobacteria* populations in their intestines. Practitioners of alternative medicine often recommend using probiotics, which means deliberately introducing live "friendly" bacteria into the system through food products (yogurt or *Acidophilus* milk) or through special supplements.

A new approach, developed in Japan in the mid-1980s, is called *prebiotics*. Here you introduce nutrients that directly feed the beneficial bacteria already in place in a person's large intestine, most typically, *Bifidobacteria* and *Lactobacilli*. Japanese researchers determined that FOS, a naturally occurring form of carbohydrate found in certain foods in minute amounts, could be a perfect food for *Bifidobacteria*. FOS acts like an intestinal "fertilizer," selectively feeding the friendly microflora in the large intestine so that their numbers can usefully increase. *Bifidobacteria* work to lower the pH (acidity/alkalinity balance) in the large intestine to a slightly more acidic condition; this discourages the growth of unfriendly bacteria.

In recognition of the health benefits of FOS, in Japan today over 500 commercially prepared foods contain FOS (known there as "neo-sugar"), with the endorsement of Japan's Minister of Health. FOS, which is made by fermenting sucrose with a fungus called *Aspergillus niger* (*Aspergillus oryzae*, for example, is used to make miso and soy sauce), is about 30% as sweet as sucrose.[61]

QUICK DEFINITION

Friendly bacteria, or probiotics, refer to beneficial microbes inhabiting the human gastrointestinal tract where they are essential for proper nutrient assimilation. The human body contains an estimated several thousand billion beneficial bacteria comprising over 400 species, all necessary for health. Among the more well-known of these are *Lactobacillus acidophilus* and *Bifidobacterium bifidum*. Overly acidic bodily conditions, chronic constipation or diarrhea, dietary imbalances, overly processed foods, and the excessive use of antibiotics and hormonal drugs can interfere with probiotic function and even reduce their numbers, setting up conditions for illness.

For more information about **FOS,** contact: GTC Nutrition Company, 1400 W. 122nd Avenue, Suite 110, Westminster, CO 80234; tel: 303-254-8012; fax: 303-254-8201.

The standard American diet has been continually cited by numerous studies conducted since the 1960s as a contributing, causative factor in a variety of "killer" diseases, including coronary heart disease, atherosclerosis, strokes, and high blood pressure.

Why Do We Need Nutritional Supplements?

Ever since the term "vitamins" was coined almost 100 years ago to describe the discovery of the essential life substances in foods, scientists have debated the issue of nutritional adequacy. Medical science has long held that healthy adults do not need supplementation if they consume a healthful, varied diet. Until recently, it was widely believed that supplements were only considered necessary if a person had an outright, or "severe," nutrient deficiency, usually manifested by overt illness.

Today, research indicates that people can have "mild" or "moderate" nutrient deficiencies, and that nutritional supplements are necessary to maintain health, according to nutritionist D. Lindsey Berkson, M.A., D.C., of Santa Fe, New Mexico. These mild disorders may not cause tangible health disorders, making them difficult to diagnose, but can result in a variety of symptoms along with a general decrease in wellness. Unaddressed, these deficiencies can often put the body at risk for future health problems. Therefore, it is important for individuals to be sure they are receiving the proper amounts of nutrients for overall emotional and physical well-being.

The standard American diet has been continually cited by numerous studies conducted since the 1960s as a contributing, causative factor in a variety of "killer" diseases, including coronary heart disease, atherosclerosis, strokes, high blood pressure, diabetes, arthritis, and colitis. Additionally, other contributing factors such as environmental pollution and stressful life patterns are creating even greater nutrient requirements. As the typical American diet is resulting in dangerous deficiencies, people are requiring more nutrients to maintain good health, even though they may appear to be adequately fed.

The United States Department of Agriculture (USDA) has found that a significant percentage of the United States population receives well under 70% of the U.S. Recommended Daily Allowance (RDA) for vitamin A, vitamin C, B-complex vitamins, and the essential minerals calcium, magnesium, and iron.[62] A separate study found that most typical diets contained less than 80% of the RDA for calcium, magnesium, iron, zinc, copper, and manganese, and that the people most at risk were young children and women, adolescent to elderly.[63]

A new Healthy Eating Index study of 4,000 Americans, conducted by the USDA, reveals that 88% of the population does not get good grades for proper nutrition. More than 80% eat too much saturated fat and too little fruits, vegetables, and fiber-rich grains. The worst eaters are between 15 and 39 years old. In all, the American diet of the 1990s achieves only 63% of what the USDA considers good nutrition.

Recommended Daily Allowances

The generally accepted reference standard for nutritional adequacy in the United States is the RDA. Developed by a group of government-sponsored scientists, its function is to provide levels of essential nutrients that prevent classic deficiency diseases and to set marginal daily guidelines for average population groups. As it was difficult for the scientists to agree upon the RDAs, they built within the guidelines instructions to keep reviewing and changing the RDAs every four years as new information is discovered. Today, in the wake of overwhelming clinical evidence that shows a wide variance in each person's individual nutritional needs, a growing number of scientists have begun to dispute the validity of RDA standards.

While a diet adequate in RDAs may be appropriate to avoid severe nutritional deficiency diseases such as rickets, scurvy, or beriberi, it may not be appropriate to avoid more mild deficiency reactions such as nervousness, insomnia, mental exhaustion, improper immune function, or proneness to injury. Emmanuel Cheraskin, M.D., D.M.D., suggests that IDAs—Ideal Daily Allowances—should replace RDAs, to make up for the limiting nature inherent in the current method.

Scientists have increasingly begun to examine whether the standardized RDA guidelines are sufficient for individual nutritional needs. One of the first to question the guidelines was Roger Williams, Ph.D., a pioneering biochemist who discovered vitamin B5 (pantothenic acid) in the 1930s. In his book *Nutrition Against Disease*, Dr. Williams express-

Since the current U.S. RDAs are an inadequate guide to the therapeutic benefits of nutritional supplements, research should be conducted to determine accurate supplementation ranges.

The United States Department of Agriculture (USDA) has found that a significant percentage of the United States population receives well under 70% of the U.S. Recommended Daily Allowance (RDA) for vitamin A, vitamin C, B-complex vitamins, and the essential minerals calcium, magnesium, and iron.

es his belief that each person is genetically unique, and therefore requires slight variations in nutrient intake to function optimally. He calls this principle biochemical individuality. Dr. Williams also believes that all living creatures are greatly affected by the overall quality, balance, and quantity of food ingested.

The concept of biochemical individuality has brought about many changes, including the emergence of new preventive diagnostic procedures, such as nutrition assessment and risk factor analysis. These utilize physiological data, personal and family health history, dietary intake analysis, and scientifically advanced biochemical screenings to help nutritional practitioners determine individual biochemistry and nutritional status.

The current challenge for medicine and nutritional science is to look beyond statistical guidelines in order to gain a greater understanding of the role of nutrients and determine the levels appropriate for each individual to achieve and maintain a high level of wellness. Through education and involvement, people can develop an understanding of the proper diet and nutritional needs specifically suited to their individual chemistries, and make this knowledge an integral part of living well.

Essential Nutrients

"Essential nutrients are those nutrients derived from food that the body is unable to manufacture on its own," says Jeffrey Bland, Ph.D., of Gig Harbor, Washington. These are absolutely necessary for human life and include eight amino acids, at least 13 vitamins, and at least 15 minerals, plus essential fatty acids, water, and carbohydrates.

Amino acids are the building blocks of protein. The essential amino acids are L-isoleucine, L-leucine, L-valine, L-methionine, L-threonine, L-phenylalanine, and L-tryptophan.

Essential vitamins are broken up in two groups: fat-soluble and water-soluble. The essential vitamins classified as fat-soluble include A, D, E, and K. The water-soluble essential vitamins are C (ascorbic acid), B1 (thiamine), B2 (riboflavin), B3 (niacin), B5 (pantothenic acid), B6 (pyridoxine), B12, folic acid, and biotin.

The essential minerals include calcium, magnesium, phosphorus, iron, zinc, copper, manganese, iodine, chromium, potassium, sodium, and a number of trace elements. They make up part of the necessary elements of body tissues, fluids, and other nutrients and play an active role in the body's regulatory functions. Low levels of these nutrients have been linked to such conditions as heart disease, high blood pressure, cancer, osteoporosis, depression, schizophrenia, and problems relating to menopause.

Essential fatty acids (EFAs) required for proper metabolism include linoleic and linolenic acid, found in seafood and unrefined veg-

Today, an estimated 46% of adult Americans take nutritional supplements, many on a daily basis.

etable oils, plus oleic and arachidonic acids, found in peanuts and most organic fats and oils. As mentioned earlier, EFAs play an important role in reducing heart disease.

Accessory Nutrients

There are also many nonessential nutrients, called accessory nutrients or cofactors, that work in harmony with the essential nutrients to aid in the breakdown and conversion of food into cellular energy, and that also help support all of the body's physical and mental functions.

According to Dr. Bland, some of the accessory nutrients that help support metabolism include vitamin B-complex cofactors choline and inositol, as well as coenzyme Q10 (a close relative of the B vitamins) and lipoic acid.

Other accessory nutrients which have demonstrated preventative functions include B-complex cofactor PABA (para-aminobenzoic acid) and substance P, bioflavonoids which work with vitamin C. Certain amino acids found in protein are also considered nonessential because they can be synthesized by the body from the essential amino acids.

How Nutrients Work Together

Vitamins and minerals help regulate the conversion of food to energy in the body, according to Dr. Bland, and can be separated into two general categories: energy nutrients, which are principally involved in the conversion of food to energy, and protector nutrients, which help defend against damaging toxins derived from drugs, alcohol, radiation, environmental pollutants, or the body's own enzyme processes.

Nutritional supplements are not a panacea, however, and it is important to be aware of some potential risks. Prolonged intake of excessive doses of vitamins A, D, and B6, for example, may produce toxic effects. Other vitamins, minerals, and accessory nutrients can also sometimes cause side effects when they interact with medications, or due to health condition, or simply a person's biochemical individuality.

"The B-complex vitamins and magnesium are examples of energy nutrients," says Dr. Bland, "for they activate specific metabolic facilitators called enzymes, which control digestion and the absorption and use of proteins, fats, and carbohydrates. These nutrients often work as a team, their mutual presence enhancing each other's function."

In the process of converting food to energy, oxygen–free radicals are produced that can damage the body and set the stage for degenerative diseases, including heart disease, arthritis, certain forms of cancer, and premature aging. Protector nutrients, such as vitamin E, beta carotene, vitamin C, and the minerals zinc, copper, manganese, and selenium, play a critical role in preventing or delaying these degenerative processes. Vitamins E, A, and C work together as a team, protecting against breakdown and helping each other maintain adequate tissue levels.

Dr. Berkson notes that vitamins and minerals are what make the chemical and electrical circuitry of the body work, and that the body's functioning is therefore profoundly affected by how nutrients either work together or against each other. Nutrients can help each other or inhibit each other when taken simultaneously. For example, iron is best absorbed when taken separately from pancreatic enzymes and also should not be taken with vitamin E, says Dr. Berkson. There are also certain nutrients that can help "potentiate" the other nutrients. For example, vitamin C taken with iron provides the maximum absorption of the iron.

Using Nutritional Supplements

Today, an estimated 46% of adult Americans take nutritional supplements, many on a daily basis.[64] It is no longer just a fad, but part of a growing trend as more and more people take a proactive approach to their own health care.

Although researchers are learning more every day about the connection between nutrients and health, there is still no definitive scientific "how-to guide" for the complexity of nutritional supplementation, especially since each individual's needs are different.

While it is always recommended that a person try to obtain as many nutrients as possible through the consumption of a variety of nutrient-dense foods, this can be unrealistic for many, due to: reduced calorie intake; the dislike of certain foods; loss of nutrients in cooking; the variable quality of food supply; lack of knowledge, motivation, or time to plan and prepare balanced meals; and nutrient depletion caused by stress, lifestyle, and certain medications. This is where nutritional supplements can play an important role in filling nutrient gaps.

Alternative practitioners may sometimes recommend dosages higher than those currently considered safe by conventional medicine. The scientific literature and numerous clinical trials support these elevated dosages for short periods of time and only under medical supervision. "For example," says Dr. Berkson, "many alternative practitioners use extremely elevated levels of vitamin A for several days to a week to act as a natural antibiotic for acute infection."

Nutritional supplements should also never take the place of appropriate medical care when warranted. If you are currently under medical care, taking any medications, or have a history of specific problems, it is important to consult with a physician before making any changes in diet or lifestyle, including the use of supplements.

It can take years of personal research and experimentation to put together a good dietary and supplement program. To eliminate a lot of guesswork and frustration, it is advisable to consult a qualified health professional trained in the intricacies of nutritional biochemistry for assistance in determining your individual needs and developing an effective dietary and nutritional supplement program tailored to those needs.

How to Take Nutritional Supplements

Before taking any nutritional supplement, you should ask what scientific data supports its safety and what are the safe intake levels. Drs. Bland and Berkson make the following recommendations:

■ Nutritional supplements should be taken with meals to promote increased absorption. Fat-soluble vitamins (such as vitamin A, beta carotene, and vitamin E) and the essential fatty acids linoleic and alpha linolenic acid should be taken during the day with the meal that contains the most fat.

Since nutritional supplements cannot be patented, there is little financial incentive for pharmaceutical companies to invest the millions of dollars needed to meet the government's stringent research requirements and thus receive FDA approval for their use in the treatment of specific conditions. Alternative sources of funding must be found in order to make nutritional supplements an accepted part of mainstream medicine.

■ Amino acid supplements should be taken on an empty stomach at least an hour before or after a meal, with fruit juice to help promote absorption. When taking an increased dosage of one particular amino acid, be sure to supplement with an amino acid blend.

■ If you become nauseated when you take tablet supplements, consider taking a liquid form, diluted in a beverage.

■ If you become nauseated or ill within an hour after taking nutritional supplements, consider the need for a bowel cleanse or rejuvenation program prior to beginning a course of nutritional supplementation.

■ If you are taking high doses, do not take the supplements all at one time, but divide them into smaller doses taken throughout the day.

■ Take digestive enzymes with meals to assist digestion. If you are taking pancreatic enzymes for other therapeutic reasons, be sure to take them on an empty stomach between meals.

■ Take mineral supplements separately from the highest fiber meals of the day as fiber can decrease mineral absorption.

■ When taking an increased dosage of a particular B vitamin, be sure to supplement with a B complex.

■ When taking nutrients, be sure to take adequate amounts of liquid to mix with digestive juices and to prevent side effects.

The standard American diet has been continually cited by numerous studies conducted since the 1960s as a contributing, causative factor in a variety of "killer" diseases, including coronary heart disease, atherosclerosis, strokes, high blood pressure, diabetes, arthritis, and colitis. As the typical American diet is resulting in dangerous deficiencies, people are requiring more nutrients to maintain good health, even though they may appear to be adequately fed.

CHAPTER 6

How Herbs Can Aid Your Heart

THE WORD "HERB" as used in herbal medicine (also known as botanical medicine or, in Europe, as phytotherapy or phytomedicine) means a plant or plant part that is used to make medicine, food flavors (spices), or aromatic oils for soaps and fragrances. An herb can be a leaf, a flower, a stem, a seed, a root, a fruit, bark, or any other plant part used for its medicinal, food-flavoring, or fragrant property.[1]

Herbs for the Heart

According to David L. Hoffmann, B.Sc., M.N.I.M.H., of Sebastopol, California, past president of the American Herbalist Guild, "Some herbs have a potent and direct impact upon the heart itself, such as *Digitalis purpurea* (foxglove), and form the basis of drug therapy for heart failure."

While it's best to consult a skilled herbalist before taking herbs, the following is an example of a cardiac tonic that Hoffmann recommends: an equal combination of tinctures of hawthorn berries, *Ginkgo biloba*, and linden flowers (one-half teaspoon three times a day). He also suggests the addition of tincture of motherwort, to prevent palpitations, and garlic, to help manage cholesterol.

The following herbs can be beneficial to the heart and circulatory system:

Cayenne (*Capsicum annuum*)

Cayenne or red pepper is the most useful of the systemic stimulants. It stimulates blood flow, strengthening the heartbeat and metabolic rate.[2] A general tonic, it is helpful specifically for the circulatory and digestive systems. If there is insufficient peripheral circulation, leading to cold hands and feet and possibly chilblains (a form of cold injury characterized by redness and blistering), cayenne may be used. It is also useful for debility as well as for warding off colds.[3]

Chlorella

In Japan, *Chlorella pyrenoidosa*, a freshwater single-celled green algae, is more popular as a regular supplement than vitamin C. An estimated five million Japanese use this medicinal algae every day. Chlorella's broad spectrum health benefits, amply researched by Japanese scientists, include the impressive fact that it contains 60% protein, including all the essential amino acids, and high levels of beta carotene and chlorophyll.

It is to chlorella's high chlorophyll content (more chlorophyll per gram than any other plant) that many researchers (and enthusiastic users) attribute its multiple health benefits, but new research from Japan suggests that chlorella's secret might lie elsewhere—in its effect on albumin.

Albumin, continually secreted by the liver, is the most abundant protein found in the blood. It acts as a major natural antioxidant, contributing an estimated 80% of all neutralizing activity against free radicals in the blood that would otherwise damage cells and tissues. Albumin transports key nutritional substances and detoxifies the fluid surrounding cells in the connective tissue. But most important, at least 38 recent scientific studies have demonstrated the strong relationship between high blood levels of albumin and the lifespan of cells.

This research, says Tim Sara, president of Nature's Balance, a major U.S. supplier of chlorella, "has confirmed that serum levels of albumin are extremely accurate indicators of overall health status and that low albumin levels exist at the onset and progression of virtually every nonhereditary, degenerative disease process, including cancers and cardiovascular heart disease." A series of studies with rats demonstrated that chlorella supplementation increases albumin levels by 16% to 21%.

For more information on **chlorella**, contact: Nature's Balance, Inc., 635A Southwest St., High Point, NC 27260; tel: 910-882-4102; fax: 910-882-4119; orders: 800-858-5198. Sun Wellness, Inc., 4025 Spencer Street, Unit 104, Torrance, CA 90503; tel: 800-829-2828 or 310-371-5515; fax: 310-371-0094.

For more about **albumin** and **longevity**, see "A New Marker for Longevity: How's Your Albumin Level?" *Digest* #20, pp. 112-116.

Garlic

Garlic has many properties that make it valuable in treating heart disease. It helps control cholesterol and contains sulfur compounds that work as antioxidants and aid in dissolving blood clots.[4]

For more about garlic's heart benefits, see Chapter 12: Lower Your Blood Pressure with Herbs, pp. 200-202.

Ginger (*Zingiber officinalis*)

In addition to its popular food flavoring qualities, ginger is well known for its cardiotonic properties.[5] It has been shown to lower cholesterol levels and make the blood platelets less sticky.[6]

Ginkgo (*Ginkgo biloba*)

Ginkgo is an excellent example of why protecting plants and animals from extinction can help create new medicine. Ginkgos are the oldest living trees on earth. They first appeared about 200 million years ago and, except for a small population in northern China, were almost completely destroyed in the last Ice Age. Ginkgo leaves contain several compounds called ginkgolides that have unique chemical structures. A standardized extract was developed in the past 20 years in Germany to treat a number of conditions associated with peripheral circulation.[7] It is currently licensed in Germany as a supportive treatment for peripheral arterial circulatory disturbances, such as intermittent claudication (a severe pain in the calf muscles resulting from inadequate blood supply).[8] Ginkgo leaf extracts are also used for heart diseases.[9]

One study found that a garlic-ginkgo combination lowered cholesterol rates in 35% of patients with levels ranging from 230 to 390—even during the Christmas holiday season when people tend to eat more high-fat foods. The supplement contained 150 mg of garlic and 40 mg of ginkgo (from a 50-to-1 extraction). Upon discontinuing the supplement, cholesterol levels rose again.[10]

Green Tea

Green tea (*Camellia sinensis*) is a highly popular beverage in China, Japan, and Korea, and may constitute 20% of the world's consumption of tea. In recent years, food scientists have identified health benefits connected to drinking tea. The primary chemical compounds found in green tea are called polyphenolic catechins and represent 17% to 30% of the dry weight of green tea leaves.

Catechins are many times stronger than vitamin E in defending the body against free radicals, thus supporting the immune system's responsiveness. They can reduce the risk of stroke and cardiovascular disease as well as stomach, pancreatic, and possibly lung cancers. A

No More Arrhythmia

John Sherman, N.D., of the Portland Naturopathic Clinic in Oregon, relates the case of Jolene, who came to his clinic complaining of heart palpitations. She was also concerned about the drugs she'd been prescribed for her heart arrhythmia. Jolene told Dr. Sherman that the drugs had been "sapping" her energy and only partially helping her heart problem. Dr. Sherman prescribed a combination herbal tincture of cactus, hawthorn, valerian, and lily of the valley, which is a standard combination naturopathic physicians use to combat arrhythmia and a "feeble" heart. He also analyzed her diet to determine her intake of specific minerals which affect the heart, including calcium, potassium, and sodium.

Jolene returned to Dr. Sherman's clinic two weeks later, still complaining of heart palpitations and feeling even more frustrated. Dr. Sherman decided to change the herbal formula slightly by adding Scotch broom. Within a few days, she happily reported the absence of any heart symptoms and was subsequently able to wean herself off the prescription drugs.

Japanese study showed that green tea can significantly lower blood pressure, reduce serum levels of LDL cholesterol, and keep blood sugar levels from rising inappropriately (as in diabetes and chronic weight-gain conditions).

To maximize the health benefits of catechins, Chemco Industries of Los Angeles, developed Polyphenon 60™ Green Tea Extract (under the Opti-Pure™ brand), a highly concentrated mixture obtained through organic nontoxic solvents, that contains 65.4% catechins. To put this in perspective, it takes about 909 pounds of green tea to extract 2.2 pounds of catechins. Optio™ Health Products, also in Los Angeles, uses Polyphenon 60 (a minimum of 20 mg in each tea bag) in its line of therapeutic green teas, which also contain *Ginkgo biloba*, bilberry, rose hips, and *Panax ginseng*.

For more information about **Polyphenon 60™ Green Tea Extract**, contact: Opti-Pure Brand, Chemco Industries, Inc., 500 Citadel Drive, No. 120, Los Angeles, CA 90040; tel: 213-721-8300; fax: 213-721-9600. For **Ginkgo Plus, Supreme Green Tea, Antioxidant Plus,** and **Ginseng Plus**, contact: Optio Health Products, Inc., 500 Citadel Drive, No. 120, Los Angeles, CA 90040; tel: 213-721-7400 or 800-678-4692; fax: 213-721-9600.

Hawthorn

One of the most promising herbal remedies for the treatment of heart disease is the extract from the hawthorn berry, a commonly found shrub. Hawthorn berry has been found to help improve the circulation of blood to the heart by dilating the blood vessels and relieving spasms of the arterial walls.[11] According to Garry F. Gordon, M.D., D.O., "Hawthorn berry may render unnecessary medications that decrease the rate and force of heart contraction in

A Japanese study showed that green tea can significantly lower blood pressure, reduce serum levels of LDL cholesterol, and keep blood sugar levels from rising inappropriately as in diabetes and chronic weight-gain conditions.

For more on the **olive's heart benefits**, see Chapter 2: Caring for Yourself, pp. 52-54.

For a source of **olive leaf extract**, contact: Allergy Research Group (Prolive™ or Alive and Well™), 400 Preda Street, San Leandro, CA 94577; tel: 800-782-4274 or 510-639-4572; fax: 510-635-6730; e-mail: info@nutricology.com.

the treatment of heart disease as it performs a similar function to these drugs."

Olive Leaf Extract

Long a staple of Mediterranean cuisine, the olive and its oil have been linked to a lower incidence of heart disease in people of that region. Now evidence is mounting that an extract from olive leaves—oil comes from olive pulp—also has extensive therapeutic benefits, including lowering blood pressure, working against free-radical activity (which causes cell damage and leads to degeneration), repelling bacteria and viruses, and enhancing the immune systems of AIDS patients.

The active component of the olive leaf is oleuropein (the bitter element removed from olives when they are processed). The leaf also contains natural vitamin C helpers called bioflavonoids, such as rutin, luteolin, and hesperidin, which are needed for maintenance of the capillary walls and for protection against infection.[12] Analysis of oleuropein at the University of Messina in Italy demonstrated that olive leaf extract has distinct heart benefits. Researchers concluded that oleuropein increased blood flow to the heart and lowered blood pressure. Oleuropein found in olive leaf extracts had a stronger effect than oleuropein and the flavonoids in their isolated, purified form.[13]

Olive leaf extract may also have a heart-protecting effect due to its antioxidant ability, according to a study at the University of Milan in Italy. A high level of low-density lipoproteins (LDLs, the so-called bad cholesterol) in the blood—a result of a diet high in saturated fat—is considered a major risk factor for coronary heart disease. Oxidation of LDL (an undesirable chemical change produced by exposure to oxygen) is one of the factors that leads to the development of atherosclerotic lesions. Researchers found that oleuropein "interferes with biochemical events that are implicated in atherogenetic [heart] disease," such as blocking LDL oxidation by retarding the loss of vitamin E, a heart-protecting nutrient.[14]

The olive leaf's oleuropein may be effective against viruses. Some years ago, researchers at Upjohn, the pharmaceutical giant based in Kalamazoo, Michigan, reported that the main component in oleuropein, a salt extract called calcium elenolate, was "virucidal (virus-killing) for all viruses against which it has been tested." These include encephalomyocarditis, which attacks the brain and heart muscles. Upjohn researchers believed that calcium elenolate, interacting with the protein coat of the virus, managed to reduce the ability of these organisms to convey infections.

"The leaf and its extract may be of excellent nutritional value and will gain wide acclaim," says Stephen Levine, Ph.D., President and Director of Research at the Allergy Research Group in San Leandro, California. His company now markets an olive leaf extract in two forms: Alive and Well™ (for consumers) and Prolive™ (for medical professionals); both in 500-mg capsules. Dr. Levine suggests taking one capsule per day with meals for health maintenance, noting that it's advisable to consume extra amounts of pure water while taking the extract, to help the body flush out toxins released under the influence of the olive leaf extract.

Olive leaf extract has distinct heart benefits. Researchers concluded that oleuropein increased blood flow to the heart and lowered blood pressure.

Herbs and Modern Medicine

Herbs have always been integral to the practice of medicine. The word drug comes from the old Dutch word *drogge* meaning "to dry," as pharmacists, physicians, and ancient healers often dried plants for use as medicines. Today, approximately 25% of all prescription drugs are still derived from trees, shrubs, or herbs.[15] Some are made from plant extracts; others are synthesized to mimic a natural plant compound. The World Health Organization notes that of 119 plant-derived pharmaceutical medicines, about 74% are used in modern medicine in ways that correlate directly with their traditional uses as plant medicines by native cultures.[16]

Yet, for the most part, modern medicine has veered from the use of pure herbs in its treatment of disease and other health disorders. One of the reasons for this is economic. Since herbs cannot be patented and drug companies cannot hold the exclusive right to sell a particular herb, they are not motivated to invest any money in that herb's

Of 119 plant-derived pharmaceutical medicines, about 74% are used in modern medicine in ways that correlated directly with their traditional uses as plant medicines by native cultures.

testing or promotion. The collection and preparation of herbs for medicine cannot be as easily controlled as the manufacture of synthetic drugs, making the profits less dependable.

In addition, many of these medicinal plants grow only in the Amazonian rain forest or politically and economically unstable places, which also affects the supply of the herb. Most importantly, the demand for herbal medicine has decreased in the United States because Americans have been conditioned to rely on synthetic, commercial drugs to provide quick relief, regardless of side effects.

However, the current viewpoint seems to be changing. "The revival of interest in herbal medicine is a worldwide phenomenon," says Mark Blumenthal, Executive Director of the American Botanical Council in Austin, Texas. This renaissance is due to the growing concern of the general public about the side effects of pharmaceutical drugs, the impersonal and often demeaning experience of modern health-care practices, as well as a renewed recognition of the unique medicinal value of herbal medicine.

Herbs Can Be Used in Many Forms

Herbs and herbal products are now available not only in natural food stores, but also grocery stores, drugstores, and gourmet food stores. Also, a number of multilevel marketing organizations sell a variety of herbal products, as do mail-order purveyors. Herbs come in many forms, including:

Whole Herbs: Whole herbs are plants or plant parts that are dried and then either cut or powdered. They can be used as teas or other products.

Teas: Teas come in either loose or tea-bag form. Because of the obvious convenience, most Americans today prefer to purchase their herbal teas in tea bags, which include one or a variety of finely cut herbs. When steeped in boiled water for a few minutes, the fragrant, aromatic flavor and the herbs' medicinal properties are released.

Capsules and Tablets: One of the fastest growing markets in herbal medicine in the past 15 to 20 years has been capsules and tablets. These offer consumers convenience and, in some cases, the bonus of not having to taste the herbs, many of which have undesirable flavor profiles, from intensely bitter (e.g., goldenseal root) due to the presence of certain alkaloids to highly astringent (e.g, oak bark) due to the presence of tannins.

Extracts and Tinctures: These offer the advantage of a high concentration in low weight and volume. They are also quickly assimilated by the body in comparison to tablets. Extracts and tinctures almost always contain alcohol. The alcohol is used for two reasons: as a solvent to extract the non-water-soluble compounds from an herb and as a preservative to maintain shelf life. Properly made extracts and tinctures have virtually an indefinite shelf life. Tinctures usually contain more alcohol than extracts (sometimes 70% to 80% alcohol, depending on the particular herb and manufacturer).

Essential Oils: Essential oils are usually distilled from various parts of medicinal and aromatic plants. Some oils, however, like those from lemon, orange, and other citrus fruits, are expressed directly from fruit peels. Essential oils are highly concentrated, with one or two drops often constituting adequate dosage. Thus, they are to be used carefully and sparingly when employed internally. Some oils may irritate the skin and should be diluted in fatty oils or water before topical application. Notable exceptions are eucalyptus and tea tree oils, which can be applied directly to the skin without concern of irritation.

Salves, Balms, and Ointments: For thousands of years, humans have used plants to treat skin irritations, wounds, and insect and snake bites. In prehistoric times, herbs were cooked in a vat of goose or bear fat, lard, or vegetable oils and then cooled in order to make salves, balms, and ointments. Today, a number of such products, made with vegetable oil or petroleum jelly, are sold in the United States and Europe to treat a variety of conditions. These products often contain aloe, marigold, chamomile, St. John's Wort, comfrey, or gotu kola.

How to Make an Herb Tea

Loose teas are usually steeped in hot water: three to ten minutes for leaves and flowers (this method is called infusion), or 15 to 20 minutes at a rolling boil for denser materials like root and bark (called a decoction).

Infusions: Infusions are the simplest method of preparing an herb tea and both fresh or dried herbs may be used, such as peppermint, chamomile, and rosehips. Due to the higher water content of the fresh herb, three parts fresh herb replace one part of the dried herb. To make an infusion:

- Put about one teaspoonful of the dried herb or herb mixture for each cup into a teapot.
- Add boiling water and cover. Let steep for five to ten minutes. Infusions may be taken hot, cold, or iced. They may also be sweetened.
- Infusions are most appropriate for plant parts such as leaves, flowers, or green stems where the medicinal properties are easily accessible. To infuse bark, root, seeds, or resin, it is best to powder them first to break down some of their cell walls before adding them to the water. Seeds like fennel and aniseed should be slightly bruised to release the volatile oils from the cells. Any aromatic herb should be infused in a pot that has a well-sealing lid to reduce loss of the volatile oil through evaporation.

Decoctions: For hard and woody herbs, ginger root and cinnamon bark for example, it is best to make a decoction rather than an infusion, to ensure that the soluble contents of the herb actually reach the water. Roots, wood, bark, nuts, and certain seeds are hard and their cell walls are very strong, requiring more heat to release them than in an infusion. These herbs need to be boiled in the water. To make a decoction:

- Put one teaspoonful of dried herb or three teaspoonfuls of fresh material for each cup of water into a pot or saucepan. Dried herbs should be powdered or broken into small pieces, while fresh material should be cut into small pieces.
- Add the appropriate amount of water to the herbs.
- Bring to a boil and simmer for 10 to 15 minutes.

When using a woody herb that contains a lot of volatile oil, it is best to make sure that it is powdered as finely as possible and then used in an infusion, to ensure that the oils do not boil away. Decoctions can be used in the same way as an infusion.

The Politics of Herbal Medicine

Additional research into the medicinal benefits of herbs will speed the integration of herbal medicine into the American health care system.

According to James Duke, Ph.D., a scientist and former USDA (United States Department of Agriculture) specialist in the area of herbal medicine, one of the reasons that research into the field of herbal medicine has been lacking is the enormous financial cost of the testing required to prove a new "drug" safe. Dr. Duke has seen that price tag rise from $91 million over ten years ago to the present figure of $231 million. Dr. Duke asks, "What commercial drug manufacturer is going to want to prove that

A 2,000-Year-Old Multi-Medicine from Deer Antlers

The cartilage of antlers from the velvet deer is poised to be one of the most versatile multipurpose natural remedies to arrive in the West. The Chinese have known about it for at least two millennia, according to an ancient medical scroll that recommends it for 52 health problems. Russians have used velvet deer antler for decades, especially as an endurance-building supplement for athletes, called Pantocrine. And for those living in Asia, Korea, and New Zealand, velvet deer antler is a medicinal food in high demand.

The medicinal claims for velvet deer antler are comprehensive and ambitious, and preliminary research tends to support most of them. Among the numerous claims, velvet deer antler can: improve blood circulation, reverse atherosclerosis, and possibly reduce the incidence of fatal heart attacks; increase the quality and quantity of blood production in treating kidney disorders and anemia; modulate the immune system, bringing it back to an even keel when it is depressed or overactive; increase muscular strength and nerve function; and generally boost energy.

For information about **velvet deer antlers**, contact: Life Extension Foundation, P.O. Box 229120, Hollywood, FL 33022; tel: 1-800-544-4440.

What's in the antlers that can produce these effects? Cartilage, for one, which contains a substance called N-acetyl-glucosamine, which speeds up wound healing. The antlers also contain chondroitin sulfate, an anti-inflammatory substance that in concentrated form has been shown to reduce the incidence of fatal heart attacks reportedly by 400%, according to a six-year study. A natural growth hormone called IGF-1 is found in high levels in velvet deer antlers; this substance helps to keep the body lean and the muscles well-developed.[17]

Velvet deer antler is available as a powdered capsule (250 mg each) from the Prolongevity brand. The recommended dosage is one to four capsules a day for four weeks followed by one week off; users are advised that it may take 6 to 12 weeks to notice effects.

saw palmetto is better than his multimillion dollar drug, when you and I can go to Florida and harvest our own saw palmetto?"

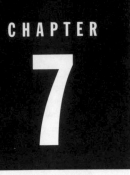

Other Alternatives for Heart Health

I N   C O N T R A S T to conventional medicine, alternative medicine is providing exciting new options in treating heart disease. Instead of complicated, costly, and often dangerous surgery and drugs, many health-care professionals who practice alternative medicine work to correct the nutritional and biochemical imbalances that can affect the function of the heart and cause plaque deposits in the arteries.

In addition to the diet, exercise, and lifestyle recommendations and therapies covered in the preceding chapters, the following alternative medical techniques can be useful in restoring and maintaining heart health.

Ayurvedic Medicine

In treating heart disease, Ayurvedic physicians use several methods that can result in the reduction of the generation of free radicals, which, as we have discussed, can contribute to the disease process in the arteries and heart. "Meat, cigarette smoke, alcohol, and environmental pollutants all generate free radicals," explains Hari Sharma, M.D., president of Maharishi Ayurveda Medical Association. By using specific herbal food supplements and *pancha karma* (detoxification and purification techniques), says Dr. Sharma, "free radicals and lipid peroxides are reduced." As it is especially important for those with heart disease to lower their level of stress, Dr. Sharma also recommends a program of Transcendental Meditation.

Virender Sodhi, M.D. (Ayurveda), N.D., director of the American School of Ayurvedic Sciences in Bellevue, Washington, reports an interesting case of heart disease. Soram, a 55-year-old Asian male, had chest pain so severe that he could not walk more than ten steps before having to sit down. He came to Dr. Sodhi's office after receiving word from the local hospital that he needed immediate bypass surgery. The doctors told him that refusing the surgery would mean certain death.

Before beginning treatment, Soram underwent a battery of tests ordered by Dr. Sodhi. Angiographic studies showed that his coronary arteries were blocked—the left main coronary artery was 90% narrowed, the anterior descending was 80% narrowed, and the right coronary was 30% blocked. Blood tests indicated elevated cholesterol levels at 278 and decreased HDLs (high-density lipoproteins) at 38. Dr. Sodhi determined Soram's metabolic type according to Ayurvedic principles and started him on an appropriate cleansing program that included dietary changes and appropriate herbs.

After three months, Soram's cholesterol levels reportedly dropped more than 30% and his HDL level rose to 48. More importantly, though, his exercise tolerance had dramatically improved. "He was doing the treadmill exercise at the speed of five miles per hour for 45 minutes without any angina," reports Sodhi. More than two years later, Soram is doing fine. He now jogs up and down hills with no symptoms and his EKG has shown improvement. According to Dr. Sodhi, there is a hospital in Bombay, India, which has treated some 3,300 cases of coronary heart disease using this method with about 99% success.

Magnetic Field Therapy

The world is surrounded by magnetic fields: some are generated by the earth's magnetism, while others are generated by solar storms and changes in the weather. Magnetic fields are also created by everyday electrical devices: motors, televisions, office equipment, computers, microwave ovens, the electrical wiring in homes, and the power lines that supply them. Even the human body produces subtle magnetic

QUICK DEFINITION

Ayurveda is the traditional medicine of India, based on many centuries of empirical use. Its name means "end of the Vedas" (which were India's sacred scripts), implying that a holistic medicine may be founded on spiritual principles. Ayurveda describes three metabolic, constitutional, and body types (doshas), in association with the basic elements of Nature in combination. These are *vata* (air and ether, rooted in intestines), *pitta* (fire and water/stomach), and *kapha* (water and earth/lungs). Ayurvedic physicians use these categories (which also have psychological aspects) as the basis for prescribing individualized formulas of herbs, diet, massage, breathing, meditation, exercise and yoga postures, and detoxification techniques.

For information about **Ayurvedic health products**, contact: Maharishi Ayur-Ved Products International Inc., P.O. Box 49667, Colorado Springs, CO 80949; tel: 719-260-5500; fax: 719-260-7400; e-mail: postmaster@mapi.com.

fields that are generated by the chemical reactions within the cells and the ionic currents of the nervous system.[1]

Recently, scientists have discovered that external magnetic fields can affect the body's functioning in both positive and negative ways, and this observation has led to the development of magnetic field therapy.

What is Magnetic Field Therapy?

The use of magnets and electrical devices to generate controlled magnetic fields has many medical applications and has proven to be one of the most effective means for diagnosing human illness and disease. For example, MRI (magnetic resonance imaging) is replacing X-ray diagnosis because it is safer and more accurate, and magnetoencephalography is now replacing electroencephalography as the preferred technique for recording the brain's electrical activity.

In 1974, researcher Albert Roy Davis, Ph.D., noted that positive and negative magnetic polarities have different effects upon the biological systems of animals and humans. He found that magnets could be used to arrest and kill cancer cells in animals, and could also be used in the treatment of arthritis, glaucoma, infertility, and diseases related to aging.[2] He concluded that negative magnetic fields have a

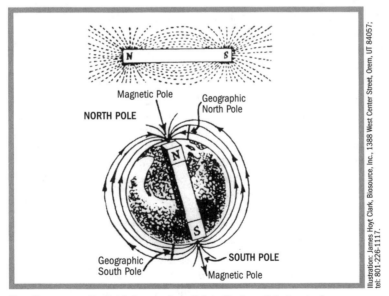

Illustration: James Hoyt Clark, Biosource, Inc., 1388 West Center Street, Orem, UT 84057; tel: 801-226-1117.

Negative *magnetic fields* have a beneficial effect on living organisms, whereas positive magnetic fields have a stressful effect.

"Symptoms of cardiac atherosclerosis and brain atherosclerosis have been observed to disappear after six to eight weeks of nightly exposure to a negative static magnetic field," reports Dr. Philpott.

beneficial effect on living organisms, whereas positive magnetic fields have a stressful effect.

"Scientifically designed, double-blind, placebo-controlled studies, however, have not been done to substantiate the claims of there being different effects between positive and negative magnetic poles," says John Zimmerman, Ph.D., president of the Bio-Electro-Magnetics Institute in Utah. "But numerous anecdotal, clinical observations suggest that such differences are real and do exist. Clearly, scientific research is needed to substantiate these claims."

Robert Becker, M.D., an orthopedic surgeon and author of numerous scientific articles and books, found that weak electric currents promote the healing of broken bones. Dr. Becker also brought national attention to the fact that electromagnetic interference from power lines and home appliances can pose a serious hazard to human health. "The scientific evidence," writes Dr. Becker, "leads only to one conclusion: the exposure of living organisms to abnormal electromagnetic fields results in significant abnormalities in physiology and function."[3]

According to Wolfgang Ludwig, Sc.D., Ph.D., director of the Institute for Biophysics in Horb, Germany, "Magnetic field therapy is a method that penetrates the whole human body and can treat every organ without chemical side effects." Magnetic field therapy has been used effectively in the treatment of atherosclerosis, circulatory problems, environmental stress, cancer, rheumatoid disease, infections and inflammations, headaches, sleep disorders, and fractures and pain. Dr. Ludwig notes that magnetic changes in the environment can affect the electromagnetic balance of the human organism and contribute to disease. Researchers suggest that magnetic therapy can be used to counter the effects caused by the electromagnetic pollution in the environment.

Kyoichi Nakagawa, M.D., director of the Isuzu Hospital in Tokyo, Japan, believes that the time people spend in buildings and cars reduces their exposure to the natural geomagnetic fields of the earth, and may also interfere with health. He calls this condition magnetic field deficiency syndrome, which can cause headaches, dizziness, muscle stiffness, chest pain, insomnia, constipation, and general fatigue.[4]

How Magnetic Field Therapy Works

"The healing potential of magnets is possible because the body's nervous system is governed, in part, by varying patterns of ionic currents and electromagnetic fields," reports Dr. Zimmerman. There are numerous forms of magnetic field therapy, including static magnetic fields produced by natural or artificial magnets, and pulsating magnetic fields generated by electrical devices. The magnetic fields produced by magnets or electromagnetic generating devices are able to penetrate the human body and can affect the functioning of the nervous system, organs, and cells. According to William H. Philpott, M.D., an author and biomagnetic researcher based in Choctaw, Oklahoma, magnetic fields can stimulate metabolism and increase the amount of oxygen available to cells. When used *properly*, magnetic field therapy has no known harmful side effects.

Metabolism is the biological process by which energy is extracted from the foods consumed, producing carbon dioxide and water as by-products for elimination. Biochemically, metabolism involves hundreds of different chemical reactions, necessitating the involvement of hundreds of different enzymes, each of which handles a specific reaction. There are two kinds of metabolism constantly underway in the cells: anabolic and catabolic. In anabolic metabolism, the upbuilding phase, larger molecules are constructed by joining smaller ones together; in catabolic metabolism, the deconstructing phase, larger molecules are broken down into smaller ones. The anabolic function produces substances for cell growth and repair, while the catabolic function controls digestion (called hydrolysis), disassembling food into forms the body can use for energy.

All magnets have two poles: one is called positive, and the other negative. However, as there are conflicting methods of naming the poles of a magnet, a magnetometer should be used as a standard method of determination (if one is using a compass to locate the poles, the arrowhead of the needle marked "N" or "North" will point to the magnet's negative pole). Dr. Philpott and other researchers claim that the negative pole generally has a calming effect and helps to normalize metabolic functioning. In contrast, the positive pole has a stressful effect, and with prolonged exposure interferes with metabolic functioning, produces acidity, reduces cellular oxygen supply, and encourages the replication of latent microorganisms.

The strength of a magnet is measured in units of gauss (a unit of the intensity of magnetic flux) or tesla (1 tesla=10,000 gauss), and every magnetic device has a manufacturer's gauss rating. However, the actual strength of the magnet at the skin surface is often much less than this number. For example, a 4,000-gauss magnet transmits about 1,200 gauss to the patient. Magnets placed in pillows or bed pads will render even lower amounts of field strength at the skin surface because a magnet's strength quickly decreases with the distance from the subject.

"A negative magnetic field can function like an antibiotic in helping to destroy bacterial, fungal, and viral infections," says Dr. Philpott, "by promoting oxygenation and lowering the body's acidity."

How Magnets are Used Therapeutically

Magnetic therapy can be applied in many ways, and devices range from small, simple magnets to large machines capable of generating high magnitudes of field strength (used for treating fractures and pseudoarthrosis, a false joint forming after a fracture). Magnetic blankets and beds have also been manufactured for the purposes of promoting sleep and reducing stress. Specially designed ceramic, plastiform, and neodymium (a rare earth chemical element) magnets can be placed either individually or in clusters over the various organs of the body, on lymph nodes, or on various points of the head.

Research into the therapeutic benefits of magnetic field therapy is needed. This type of therapy could provide a safe and effective way to curb rising health care costs.

In Japan, small *tai-ki* magnets have been designed to stimulate acupuncture points, but no clinical studies have yet explored this procedure. Magnetic devices are popular in Germany, where the use of certain devices is covered by medical insurance. After simple instruction is given to the patient, these devices can be used at home.

Magnetic Field Therapy Treatment

Treatment can last from just a few minutes to overnight and, depending upon the situation and severity, may be applied several times a day or for days or weeks at a time. The following cases illustrate both the potential for success and wide range of application of magnetic field therapy. Sometimes the results can be dramatic, as in this case of heart flutter cited by Dr. Ludwig:

Heart Flutter—A 46-year-old man had suffered for years from severe heart flutter, diarrhea, and nausea. No treatment seemed to help, but when a magnetic applicator with less than one gauss of energy was placed upon his solar plexus for only three minutes, his symptoms immediately ceased. Two years later, he had experienced no relapse.

Atherosclerosis—According to Dr. Philpott, "Symptoms of cardiac atherosclerosis and brain atherosclerosis have been observed to disappear after six to eight weeks of nightly exposure to a negative static magnetic field." A man, 70, with atherosclerotic heart disease, underwent a multiple bypass operation. Two years later his heart pain returned, leaving him unsteady on his feet and subject to disorientation in familiar surroundings; his speech grew thick and he became chronically depressed.

Dr. Philpott had him sleep with the negative pole of several magnets (ferrous ceramic, 2,000-4,000 gauss in strength) placed at the crown of his head. During the day, the man also wore a magnet strapped to the skin over his heart. Within a week, his symptoms improved and after one month of this treatment, he had no heart pain, his balance returned, his speech became distinct, and his depression was gone. Through this method, "the mental confusion, disorientation, and depression of cerebral atherosclerosis is remarkably reduced or even completely relieved," reports Dr. Philpott.[5]

Stress—A negative magnetic field applied to the top of the head has a calming and sleep-inducing effect on brain and body functions, due to the stimulation of the production of the hormone melatonin, according to Dr. Philpott. Melatonin has been shown to be antistressful, anti-

aging, anti-infectious, and anticancerous, and to have control over respiration and the production of free radicals.[6] A free radical is a highly destructive molecule that is missing an electron and readily reacts with other molecules. Free radicals contribute to the aging of cells, hardening of muscle tissue, wrinkling of skin, and, in general, decreased efficiency of protein synthesis.

As there are literally hundreds of diseases that are related to stress, infections, and aging, magnetic field therapy could be considered an important adjunct in their treatment and researchers are currently studying its contributions.

For more information about **magnetic therapy**, contact: William Philpott, M.D., P.O. Box 50655, Midwest City, OK 73140; tel: 405-390-1444.

Bacterial, Fungal, and Viral Infections—"A negative magnetic field can function like an antibiotic in helping to destroy bacterial, fungal, and viral infections," says Dr. Philpott, "by promoting oxygenation and lowering the body's acidity." Both these factors are beneficial to normal bodily functions but harmful to pathogenic (disease-causing) microorganisms, which do not survive in a well-oxygenated, alkaline environment.

Dr. Philpott theorizes that the biological value of oxygen is increased by the influence of a negative electromagnetic field, and that the field causes negatively charged DNA (deoxyribonucleic acid) to "pull" oxygen out of the bloodstream and into the cell. The negative electromagnetic field keeps the cellular buffer system (pH or acid-alkaline balance) intact so that the cells remain alkaline. The low acid balance also helps maintain the presence of oxygen in the body, which is essential to the health of the cells, blood and circulation, and all organs including the heart.

Pain Relief—A negative magnetic field normalizes the disturbed metabolic functions that cause painful conditions such as cellular edema (swelling of the cells), cellular acidosis (excessive acidity of the cells), lack of oxygen to the cells, and infection.

Dr. Philpott cites the case of a woman in her seventies who for 33 years had experienced pain and weakness in her left leg stemming from a blood clot in the groin area. She could not climb stairs without stopping several times due to pain. After a year of sleeping on a negative magneto-electric pad, the woman found that she could walk up a long flight of stairs without any pain or weakness in her leg.

While a negative magnetic field may relieve pain, a positive magnetic field can increase pain due to its interference with normal metabolic function. However, magnetic therapy should not be considered a replacement for local anesthetics or pain relievers.

Oxygen Therapy

Studies at Baylor University in the 1970s found that an intravenous drip of hydrogen peroxide into leg arteries of atherosclerotic patients cleared arterial plaque.[7] In cardiopulmonary resuscitations, hydrogen peroxide infusions often stopped ventricular fibrillation (rapid, ineffective contractions by ventricles of the heart), the heart's response to insufficient oxygen.[8] Charles Farr, M.D., reports success alternating treatments of intravenous diluted hydrogen peroxide and chelation therapy to bring patients out of high-output heart failure (where the heart fails even though it is pumping a high amount of blood).

CAUTION The body's subtle electromagnetic fields can be affected by even the weakest of magnets. Since even minor alterations in the fields can cause mild to serious symptoms, magnetic therapy should be practiced only under the supervision of a qualified professional.

Dr. Philpott adds the following precautions:

■ Industrial magnets often have different positive and negative pole identifications than the magnets used in medicine and therapy. Use a magnetometer or compass to confirm proper identification.

■ Don't use magnets on the abdomen during pregnancy.

■ Don't use a magnetic bed for more than eight to ten hours.

■ Wait 60 to 90 minutes after meals before applying magnetic therapy to the abdomen, to prevent interference with peristalsis (wavelike contractions of the smooth muscles of the digestive tract).

■ Do not apply the positive magnetic pole unless under medical supervision. It can produce seizures, hallucinations, insomnia, and hyperactivity; stimulate the growth of tumors and microorganisms; and promote addictive behavior.

Traditional Chinese Medicine

For more on **oxygen therapy**, see Chapter 16: Oxygen Therapy, pp. 244-256; for **traditional Chinese medicine**, see Chapter 11: Chinese Medicine, pp. 184-199.

Traditional Chinese medicine (TCM) views heart disease as a problem stemming from poor digestion, which causes the buildup of plaque in the arteries. Harvey Kaltsas, Ac. Phys. (FL), D. Ac. (RI), Dipl. Ac. (NCCA), president of the American Association of Acupuncture and Oriental Medicine, recommends herbs to strengthen digestive functioning. "It has been understood in China for thousands of years that the circulation needs to flow unimpeded," states Dr. Kaltsas.

An herbal extract made from a plant known as *mao-tung-ching* (*Ilex puibeceus*) is often used to dilate the blocked vessels. According to Dr. Kaltsas, a study was conducted in China in which *mao-tung-ching* was administered daily (4 ounces orally, 20 mg intravenously) to 103 patients suffering from coronary heart disease. In 101 out of the 103 cases, there was significant improvement.[9]

Maoshing Ni, D.O.M., Ph.D., L.Ac., vice president of the Yo San University of Traditional Chinese Medicine in Santa Monica, California, views heart disease as either a weakness or block in the body's energy system. He generally refers patients with acute heart problems to a Western physician, stating that TCM is more suited to the treatment of chronic heart problems. For these, Dr. Ni uses a combination of acupuncture and herbs to dissolve plaque, lower cholesterol levels, raise blood flow rates, and relieve angina.

One patient came to Dr. Ni after having an angioplasty because of 70% blockage of the coronary arteries. After the angioplasty, he still had 55% blockage. Dr. Ni treated him with herbs and acupuncture and, within four months, the blockage was reduced to 35%.

Additional Alternative Therapies

Self-Care

The following therapies for the treatment and prevention of heart disease can be undertaken at home under appropriate professional supervision:

- Fasting
- Yoga
- Aromatherapy: To strengthen heart muscle—garlic, lavender, peppermint, marjoram, rose, rosemary. For palpitations—lavender, melissa, neroli, ylang-ylang.
- Juice Therapy: Carrot, celery, cucumber, beet (add a little

garlic or hawthorn berries); Blueberries, blackberries, black currant, red grapes.
■ Hydrotherapy: Constitutional hydrotherapy two to five times weekly.

Professional Care

The following therapies can only be provided by a qualified health professional:
■ Alexander Technique
■ Biofeedback Training
■ Cell Therapy
■ Environmental Medicine
■ Guided Imagery
■ Hypnotherapy
■ Meditation
■ Osteopathy
■ Body Therapy: Acupressure, reflexology, *shiatsu*, massage.
■ Chiropractic: To improve mid-back mobility and breathing.
■ Hydrotherapy: Leon Chaitow, N.D., D.O., reports that the neutral bath (patient immersed in water 35°C for two hours) has been effective in treating mild heart failure problems that result in fluid retention.

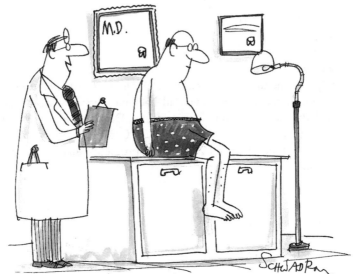

"YOUR HEART'S GREAT. IT'S ALL THOSE ASPIRIN COMMERCIALS THAT ARE MAKING YOU SICK."

PART TWO

High
Blood
Pressure

(Hypertension)

CHAPTER 8

What Causes High Blood Pressure?

HIGH BLOOD PRESSURE (clinically known as hypertension) is the most common cardiovascular disease in industrialized nations and is a major cause of heart attack, stroke, and congestive heart failure. In 1994 alone, high blood pressure killed 38,130 Americans and was a factor in 180,000 additional deaths.[1] Hypertension accounts for an estimated 28.3 million annual office visits to conventional physicians, or about 7.2% of all doctors' appointments in a year. This amount is twice that for acute upper respiratory infection, the next most prevalent health condition on a list of the top ten, according to data compiled by *Scott-Levin's Physician Drug and Diagnosis Audit* in 1996.

Approximately 50 million Americans (nearly one out of five) currently suffer from high blood pressure and two-thirds of them are under 65 years of age, which indicates that hypertension is not an inevitable result of aging but rather a condition affected by a number of risk factors, including smoking, obesity,[2] stress,[3] excessive alcohol consumption, and a diet high in fats and sodium chloride (table salt).[4] According to William Lee Cowden, M.D., of Richardson, Texas, "Individuals with diabetes are especially susceptible, as are those with a family history of hypertension. Stress and a sedentary lifestyle are other factors to consider when diagnosing and treating this condition."

The Heart Under Pressure

To understand high blood pressure, you need to know a few facts about the heart. The human heart beats on average 70 times per minute, 100,000 times a day, and 2.5 billion times in a lifetime. With each heartbeat, about 2.5 ounces of blood are pumped through the heart—that is 1,980 gallons every day.

The term blood pressure refers to the force of the blood against the walls of arteries, veins, and the chambers of the heart as it is pumped through the body. Greater than normal force

Approximately 50 million Americans (nearly one out of five) currently suffer from high blood pressure and two-thirds of them are under 65 years of age.

exerted by the blood against the arteries (when high blood pressure is present) begins to weaken the cellular walls and makes it easier for harmful substances, such as toxins and oxidized cholesterol, to form dangerous deposits on the arterial walls.

Hypertension takes two forms: essential hypertension, when the cause is unknown; and secondary hypertension, when damage to the kidneys or endocrine dysfunction causes blood pressure to rise. Of

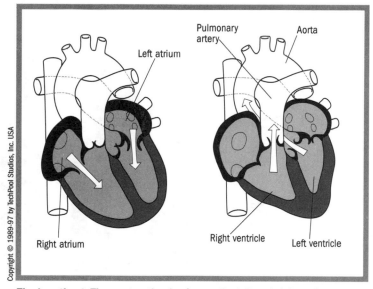

The heartbeat. **The contraction begins as the left and right atria squeeze blood downward into the ventricles and then continues as both ventricles squeeze upward. The right ventricle pumps blood into the pulmonary artery, then to the lungs to be re-oxygenated. The left ventricle pumps oxygenated blood into the aorta, then out to all parts of the body.**

The symptoms of hypertension are far-reaching and include dizziness, headache, fatigue, restlessness, difficulty breathing, insomnia, intestinal complaints, and emotional instability.

the diagnosed cases of hypertension in the United States, over 90% are essential hypertension.[5] The symptoms of hypertension are far-reaching and include dizziness, headache, fatigue, restlessness, difficulty breathing, insomnia, intestinal complaints, and emotional instability. In advanced stages, the hypertensive patient often suffers from other forms of cardiovascular disease as well as damage to the heart, kidneys, and brain.

Diagnosing High Blood Pressure

Blood pressure is measured by placing an inflatable cuff around the

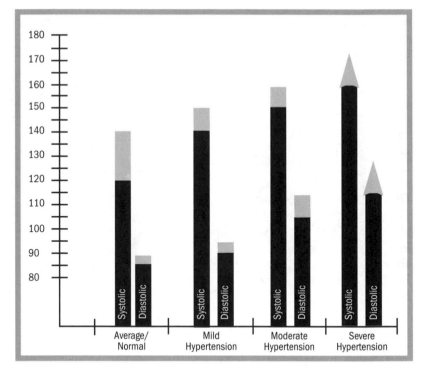

High blood pressure (hypertension) is usually measured as a range of the systolic (when the heart contracts) and diastolic (when the heart rests, filling with more blood) values.

upper arm. As the cuff is inflated, the arm is squeezed tight. At this point the pulse cannot be heard through the stethoscope. As the cuff is slowly deflated, the pulse is heard again. This is the high number and measures the systolic pressure, when the heart is contracting to pump blood into the body. A second reading is taken as the cuff is deflated even further.

The pulse sound disappears again and when it returns, that reading is the low number and measures the diastolic pressure, when the heart is relaxing to refill with blood. The ratio of the two numbers represents blood pressure, as in 120/85, an "average" or healthy reading. A patient has hypertension if the high reading is above 140 and the low reading is above 90, when tested on two separate occasions.

Causes of High Blood Pressure

"High blood pressure often occurs due to a strain on the heart, which can arise from a variety of conditions, including diet, atherosclerosis [narrowing and hardening of the arteries], high cholesterol, diabetes, environmental factors, as well as lifestyle choices," according **Hypertension is closely associated with the Western diet and is found almost exclusively in developed countries.** to Dr. William Lee Cowden. When these factors combine with a genetic predisposition, hypertension can occur in two out of three individuals.[6]

Dietary Factors

Hypertension is closely associated with the Western diet and is found almost exclusively in developed countries.[7] Recent studies of residents in remote areas of China, New Guinea, Panama, Brazil, and Africa show virtually no evidence of hypertension, even with advanced age. But when individuals within these groups moved to more industrialized areas, the incidence of hypertension among them rose. The studies concluded that changes in lifestyle, including dietary changes and increased body mass and fat, significantly contributed to the higher levels of blood pressure.[8]

"Although a combination of genetic and environmental factors such as behavior patterns and stress are believed to contribute to hypertension, the main cause appears to be a diet high in animal fat and sodium chloride, especially if high in relation to potassium and magnesium organic salts," says Dr. Cowden.

Research concurs that a diet high in sodium chloride and deficient in potassium has been associated with hypertension. Lack of potassium and other nutritional deficiencies play a significant role in the development of hypertension. Magnesium levels have also been found to be consistently low in patients with high blood pressure.[9] High blood pressure can also develop as a symptom of adult-onset diabetes (see Chapter 11: Chinese Medicine: How It Can Help Reverse High Blood Pressure).

Lifestyle Factors

Lifestyle choices, including smoking and consumption of coffee and alcohol, have been shown to cause hypertension. A recent study conducted in Paris, France, showed higher systolic and diastolic levels in coffee drinkers compared to nondrinkers, with levels rising in direct correlation to the amount of coffee consumed each day.[10] Even moderate amounts of alcohol can produce hypertension in certain individuals, and chronic alcohol intake is one of the strongest predictors of high blood pressure.[11] In the face of this evidence, restricting alcohol and avoiding caffeine are recommended.

Smoking is a contributing factor to hypertension, due in part to the fact that smokers are more prone to increased sugar, alcohol, and caffeine consumption.[12] However, even smokeless tobacco (chewing tobacco, snuff, etc.) causes hypertension through its nicotine and sodium content.[13]

Atherosclerosis and High Blood Pressure

Atherosclerosis involves the accumulation of plaque in the blood vessels, which restricts blood flow and increases blood pressure. Consequently it is a common cause of hypertension as well as the main cause of coronary heart disease and strokes.

According to Leon Chaitow, N.D., D.O., of London, England, "Blood pres-

Blood Pressure Drug May Cause Cancer

According to a study involving 5,000 patients over 70 years old, conducted by scientists at the University of Tennessee in Memphis, the regular use of calcium channel blockers, the most widely prescribed group of high blood pressure drugs, is associated with a 72% higher rate of cancer. In research published in The Lancet (August 1996), this percentage increase is equal to eight new cancers per 100 people using the drugs for five years.

sure rises when the blood leaving the heart has to be pumped more vigorously due to a thicker consistency of the blood or to a greater resistance from the blood vessels themselves. The vessels may have become narrower, less elastic, or the muscles which surround them may be exerting more tension. The function of the muscles and breathing apparatus may also be inefficient in helping the heart to function properly. The relative health of the kidneys and liver (which filter the blood) also influences blood pressure."

Environmental Factors

Environmental factors such as lead contamination from drinking water, as well as residues of heavy metals such as cadmium, have also been shown to promote hypertension.[14] People whose hypertension has been left untreated have been shown to have blood cadmium levels three to four times higher than those with normal blood pressure.[15] It is important to check for both lead and cadmium toxicity when treating hypertension.

Lead Contamination and High Blood Pressure

A low level of lead exposure and accumulation in tissues in adults is now linked to both hypertension and impaired kidney function, according to the *Journal of the American Medical Association* (April 1996). In two studies involving over 1,000 men, the exposure to lead was at levels previously considered safe. Those with the highest levels of bone lead were 50% more likely to have hypertension than those with the lowest.

Researchers at the Harvard School of Public Health found that high levels of childhood exposure to lead are linked to adult obesity, according to their 1995 study of 79 overweight adults.[16] Adults who had absorbed high lead levels as children gained the most weight between the ages of 7 and 20. Both excess weight and high lead concentrations are associated with high blood pressure in adults.

Reversing High Blood Pressure Caused by Heavy Metal Toxicity

Jonathan Wright, M.D., of Kent, Washington, treated Jonas, who had unexplained high blood pressure (156/100). His blood, urine, and kidney examinations were all normal and his lifestyle habits were exemplary. He avoided sugar, refined flour, caffeine, and excess salt; his diet was high in vegetables and fruits; and he took vitamin C and E supplements. He also exercised regularly and did not smoke.

However, Jonas was an industrial painter and Dr. Wright suspected that heavy metals in the paints were the problem. Pubic hair analysis confirmed his suspicions, showing higher than usual amounts of lead, cobalt, and cadmium. Dr. Wright started Jonas on a zinc supplement, to force the cadmium out of his system, and increased his vitamin C intake to bowel tolerance. He also recommended extra vitamin B6 to prevent the increased vitamin C from causing kidney stones, and added selenium, which is known to protect against cadmium toxicity.

Dr. Wright further suggested linseed oil, which contains essential fatty acids noted for reducing hypertension. After six months, Jonas' blood pressure had dropped to 154/96; after 12 months to 142/90; and after 18 months to 134/80. At that point, Dr. Wright cut the supplement dosages, but zinc and vitamin C were continued to prevent recurrence since Jonas continued in his profession.

For more about the thyroid, see "The Reason Behind Weight Gain, Fatigue, Muscle Pain, Depression, Food Allergies, Infections...." *Digest* #16, pp. 52-56.

The Hypothyroidism Connection

According to Broda O. Barnes, M.D., low thyroid function (hypothyroidism) is correlated with a tendency to develop high blood pressure.[17] "I have seen many patients

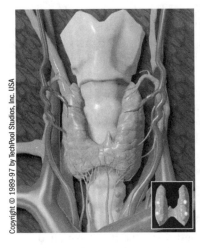

The thyroid gland, one of the body's seven endocrine glands, is located just below the larynx in the throat with interconnecting lobes on either side of the trachea. The thyroid is the body's metabolic thermostat, controlling body temperature, energy use, and, for children, the body's growth rate. The thyroid controls the rate at which organs function and the speed with which the body uses food; it affects the operation of all body processes and organs. Of the hormones synthesized in and released by the thyroid, T3 (triiodothyronine), represents 7%, and T4 (thyroxine), accounts for almost 93% of the thyroid's hormones active in all of the body's processes. Iodine is essential to forming normal amounts of thyroxine. The secretion of both these hormones is regulated by thyroid-stimulating hormone, or TSH, secreted by the pituitary gland in the brain. The thyroid also secretes calcitonin, a hormone required for calcium metabolism.

Drugs Associated with a Higher Incidence of High Blood Pressure (Hypertension)

According to the *Physicians' Desk Reference*, the following drugs are associated with hypertension. (Statistics refer to the percentage of individuals affected.)

- Alfenta Injection (18%)
- Aredia for Injection (up to 6%)
- Clozaril Tablets (4%)
- Dobutrex Solution Vials (most patients)
- Epogen for Injection (0.75% to approximately 25%)
- Habitrol Nicotine Transdermal System (3%-9%)
- Lupron Depot 3.75 mg (among most frequent); Injection (5% or more)
- Methergine Injection, Tablets (most common)
- Orthoclone OKT3 Sterile Solution (8%)
- Polygam, Immune Globulin Intravenous (Human) (3-6%)
- Procrit for Injection (0.75%-24%)
- Sandimmune IV Ampules for Infusion, Oral Solution (13%-53%)
- Sandimmune Soft Gelatin Capsules (13%-53%)
- Sufenta Injection (3%)
- Tolectin (200, 400, and 600 mg) (3%-9%)
- Velban Vials (among most common)
- Ventolin Inhalation Aerosol and Refill (less than 5%)
- Wellbutrin Tablets (4.3%)

with hypertension—mild, moderate, and even severe—respond to thyroid therapy," Dr. Barnes said.

Hypothyroidism is a condition of low or underactive thyroid gland function that can produce numerous symptoms. Among the 47 clinically recognized symptoms: fatigue, depression, lethargy, weakness, weight gain, low body temperature, chills, cold extremities, general inappropriate sensation of cold, infertility, rheumatic pain, menstrual disorders (excessive flow or cramps), repeated infections, colds, upper respiratory infections, skin problems (itching, eczema, psoriasis, acne, skin pallor, dry, coarse, and scaly skin), memory disturbances, concentration difficulties, paranoia, migraines, oversleep, "laziness," muscle aches and weakness, hearing disturbances, burning/prickling sensations, anemia, slow reaction time and mental slug-

See "Hyperthyroidism," p. 934; "Hypothyroidism," pp. 936-937.

Based on a long-term study of 1,500 of his own patients, Dr. Barnes concluded that thyroid treatment (supplementation with an oral thyroid extract) yielded considerably fewer cases of high blood pressure than would be expected in a population of that age and health status.

gishness, swelling of the eyelids, constipation, labored and difficult breathing, hoarseness, brittle nails, and poor vision. A resting body temperature (measured in the armpit), below 97.8°F, indicates hypothyroidism; menstruating women should take the underarm temperature only on the second and third days of menstruation.

Based on a long-term study of 1,500 of his own patients, Dr. Barnes concluded that thyroid treatment (supplementation with an oral thyroid extract) yielded considerably fewer cases of high blood pressure than would be expected in a population of that age and health status. Patients on thyroid therapy had "marked protection against the development of elevated blood pressure" despite their age, and those who were initially hypertensive experienced a reduction in their high blood pressure from thyroid therapy alone (without antihypertensive medications).

"High blood pressure often occurs due to a strain on the heart, which can arise from a variety of conditions, including diet, atherosclerosis [narrowing and hardening of the arteries], high cholesterol, diabetes, environmental factors, as well as lifestyle choices," according to William Lee Cowden, M.D., of Richardson, Texas. When these factors combine with a genetic predisposition, hypertension can occur in two out of three individuals.

Self-Care Options

HOW TO USE DIET, EXERCISE, AND LIFESTYLE CHANGES TO LOWER YOUR BLOOD PRESSURE

ONVENTIONAL HIGH BLOOD pressure medications treat hypertension by reducing the heart output, lowering the blood pressure, or reducing fluid retention through the use of diuretics. These medications may relieve the symptoms of hypertension but do little to address the cause. As many of these drugs have unwanted side effects and can actually increase the risk of life-threatening heart disease, an alternative for reducing blood pressure is warranted.

Alternative medical approaches inevitably begin with a careful evaluation of the factors[1] contributing to the patient's illness. Such an evaluation often reveals a need for dietary changes and lifestyle changes such as increased exercise, weight loss, and stress management.

Diet

A diet low in fat, sugar, and salt, and rich in foods containing potassium, calcium, magnesium, and fiber is highly recommended for hypertensives. Also, garlic and other members of the onion family should be included in any diet that aims to lower high blood pressure, as they significantly reduce both systolic and diastolic pressure.[2]

Making relatively simple changes in diet, such as eating less fat and more fruits and vegetables, can lower blood pressure as effectively as conventional hypertension drugs. This conclusion comes from a

There was a significant reduction in both systolic and diastolic blood pressures in the subjects eating fish and/or taking fish-oil supplements, particularly those on a low-fat diet.

study directed by the Kaiser Permanente Center for Health Research in Portland, Oregon, in cooperation with researchers at Johns Hopkins, Harvard, and Duke Universities.[3]

The study enrolled 459 adults (50% women, 60% African American) with a starting blood pressure of less than 160/80-95 (high blood pressure was considered 140/90 or higher). The participants were divided into three groups, each of which followed a different diet. The first group ate a conventional American diet (typically high in fats, sugar, meat, and processed foods); the second group ate the same diet complemented with a high level of fruits and vegetables. The third group practiced a diet low in fats, fat comprising only 31% of the total calories compared to 37% in a typical American diet. This group kept their consumption of fats and cholesterol low and their consumption of fruits, vegetables, and low-fat dairy products high.

Changes in blood pressure were noticeable within two weeks. For those in the third group, blood pressure values dropped by an average of 5.5/3, while for those in the second group, the readings declined an average of 2.8/1.1. In the view of the researchers, both changes were significant. Even more impressive, those in the third group who started with high blood pressure experienced drops of 11.4/5.5.

Another study compared the effects of omega-3 fatty acids in fish or fish-oil supplements on 125 men with moderately high blood pressure consuming high-fat or low-fat diets. The subjects ate fish, took fish-oil supplements, or had a combination providing an average total of 3.65 g per day of omega-3 fatty acids. There was a significant reduction in both systolic and diastolic blood pressures in the subjects eating fish and/or taking fish-oil supplements, particularly those on a low-fat diet, compared with control subjects.[4]

A third study of 2,300 middle-aged people, all moderately overweight and with blood pressure in the high

QUICK DEFINITION

Omega-3 and omega-6 oils are the two principal types of essential fatty acids, which are unsaturated fats required in the diet. The digits "3" and "6" refer to differences in the oil's chemical structure with respect to its chain of carbon atoms and where they are bonded. A balance of these oils in the diet is required for good health. The primary omega-3 oil is called alpha-linolenic acid (ALA) and is found in flaxseed (58%), canola, pumpkin and walnut, and soybeans. Fish oils, such as salmon, cod, and mackerel, contain the other important omega-3 oils, DHA (docosahexaenoic acid) and EPA (eicosapentaenoic acid). Omega-3 oils help reduce the risk of heart disease. Linoleic acid or cis-linoleic acid is the main omega-6 oil and is found in most plant and vegetable oils, including safflower (73%), corn, peanut, and sesame. The most therapeutic form of omega-6 oil is gamma-linolenic acid (GLA), found in evening primrose, black currant, and borage oils. Once in the body, omega-6 is converted to prostaglandins, hormone-like substances that regulate many metabolic functions, particularly inflammatory processes.

Within two weeks of starting a nutritional supplement program, Dr. Braverman's patient was off medication and his blood pressure had dropped from 150/90 to 128/82.

normal range, found that those who lost around ten pounds within six months and cut the sodium in their diet experienced a 60% lowering of their blood pressure.[5]

Lowering Hypertension with Diet and Supplements

Eric R. Braverman, M.D., director of Place for Achieving Total Health (PATH) in New York City, treats hypertension with a program centered around diet and nutritional supplementation.

To contact **Eric Braverman, M.D.**, or order his book, *How to Lower Your Blood Pressure and Reverse Heart Disease Naturally* (1995), contact: PATH, 274 Madison Ave., 4th Floor, Room 402, New York, NY 10016; tel: 212-213-6155; fax: 212-213-6188.

Dr. Braverman's diet is low in sodium, low in saturated fat, high in vegetables from the starch group, and high in protein (particularly fish). In addition, the diet features large amounts of fresh salad. Simple sugar, alcohol, caffeine, nicotine, and refined carbohydrates are reduced dramatically or eliminated altogether. His nutritional supplement program for a typical hypertensive patient includes fish oil (containing omega-3 fatty acids), garlic, evening primrose oil, magnesium, potassium, selenium, zinc, vitamin B6, niacin, vitamin C, tryptophan, taurine, cysteine, and coenzyme Q10.

One of Dr. Braverman's patients had been treated with medication for hypertension for two years and his blood pressure was still 150/90. Dr. Braverman started him on multivitamins and supplements of B6, folic acid, B12, magnesium, taurine, garlic, and evening primrose oil. Within two weeks, he was off medication and his blood pressure had dropped to 128/82.

When John, 62, first came to Dr. Braverman, he had suffered from high blood pressure for ten years. His levels for total cholesterol, triglycerides, and high-density lipoproteins (HDLs), which are key indicators of heart health, were highly imbalanced. He was taking strong daily doses of three conventional medications. When John began Dr. Braverman's program, his blood pressure was 140/90.

First, Dr. Braverman put John on a low-carbohydrate, high-protein diet to help him lose weight. Next, he started John on daily supplementation with evening primrose and fish oils, a niacin-garlic formula, safflower oil, and a hypertension nutrient formula Dr. Braverman had specially developed for his blood pressure–lowering program. The formula consisted of:

High Blood Pressure Drugs—
Another Heart Disease Risk Factor

For adults with borderline to mild high blood pressure, the use of conventional antihypertensive drugs is not only often unneeded, but also can increase the risk of heart attack by nearly four times, according to physicians at Malmö University Hospital in Malmö, Sweden. Lead researcher Juan Merlo noted that despite mounting doubt about the effectiveness of high blood pressure drugs in preventing heart attacks, the trend of physicians routinely prescribing them continues to grow. In the Malmö University Hospital study, 484 men, born in 1914, were tracked between 1969 and 1992, and their use of antihypertensive drugs recorded.

Out of this group, 13% who had a diastolic blood pressure below 90 mm Hg (mild high blood pressure) and were taking antihypertensive drugs experienced a rate of heart attacks 3.9 times greater than men with similar blood pressures not taking any heart drugs. For men with blood pressures exceeding 90 mm Hg (high blood pressure) and who were taking antihypertensive drugs, the risk of having a serious heart attack was doubled.[6]

Calcium channel blockers also pose threats to heart health. A study of 900 elderly people with high blood pressure found that taking one kind of calcium channel blocker (the short-acting form of nifedipine, marketed as Procardia and Adalat) doubled the likelihood of dying within five years after using the drug, typically from heart attacks, heart failure, and strokes. American doctors wrote two million prescriptions for this drug in 1994, despite the lack of rigorous scientific trials by either the FDA or drug companies to prove its safety.[7]

- garlic powder (200 mg)
- magnesium (oxide, 50 mg)
- zinc (chelate, 4 mg)
- niacinamide (50 mg)
- molybdenum (40 mg)
- beta carotene (1222.33 IU)
- amino acid taurine (200 mg)
- potassium (chloride, 6.7 mg)
- chromium (chloride, 26.7 mcg)
- vitamin C (40 mg)
- vitamin B6 (50 mg)
- selenium (sodium selenite, 20 mcg)

John took six pills daily of this formula along with a magnesium formula, containing vitamin B6 (65 mg), magnesium (oxide, 470 mg), and zinc (chelate, 15 mg).

Two weeks into the program, John's cholesterol had dropped from 264 to 131, his triglycerides had decreased from 161 to 100, his blood pressure was 120/80, and his HDLs increased positively from 59 to 64. John was able to stop taking his conventional medications. After another week on the nutrients, his blood pressure was a healthier 110/80. Over the following months, Dr. Braverman reduced John's nutrient program and adjusted his diet. John continued to be

Researchers at Johns Hopkins University in Baltimore stated that "the higher the oats intake, the lower the blood pressure," regardless of other factors such as age and weight, or alcohol, sodium, or potassium intake, which are known to affect blood pressure.

medication-free, his energy level and sexual drive had increased, and he was "doing fantastically well," reports Dr. Braverman.

What a Bowl of Oatmeal Can Do for Your Heart

While people living in the British Isles may take it for granted, making oatmeal a mainstay of the diet makes smart nutritional sense. In recent years, at least 37 clinical studies have affirmed the ability of oatmeal and oat bran to reduce blood cholesterol levels, lower blood pressure, and generally reduce the long-term risk of heart disease.

In recognition of these now well-established benefits, in 1996, the U.S. FDA granted manufacturers or packagers of oatmeal (as a food category) the right to make specific health claims about this food. It was the first such permissible health claim ever accorded to a food by the FDA, an agency that generally has favored drugs over natural substances. The FDA's proposed health claim (now in the process of public review) states that diets high in oatmeal or oat bran may reduce the risk of heart disease.

Among the numerous studies that have demonstrated the health benefits of oatmeal, at least four put the food's health advantages in clear focus. In 1995, researchers at Johns Hopkins University in Baltimore, Maryland, reported that people who regularly consumed even a modest portion of oatmeal (one ounce, cooked, daily) had lower blood pressure and cholesterol readings than those who never ate oatmeal.[8] The study was based on evaluation of 850 men, 17-77 years old, living in China; their oatmeal consumption ranged from 25-90 g daily.

The researchers stated that "the higher the oats intake, the lower the blood pressure," regardless of other factors such as age and weight, or alcohol, sodium, or potassium intake, which are known to affect blood pressure.

According to chief researcher Michael Klag, M.D., it is oatmeal's high content of water-soluble fiber (called beta glucan) that produces the heart benefits. A six-year study involving 22,000 middle-aged Finnish males showed that consuming as little as three g daily of soluble fiber (from the beta-glucan fiber component of oats, barley, or rye) reduced the risk of death from heart disease by 27%.[9]

Another study of oatmeal's heart benefits was conducted by scientists at the Chicago Center for Clinical Research in Illinois. The researchers enlisted 156 adults, all of whom had a diagnosis of high cholesterol or multiple heart risk factors, and had them consume differing amounts of oatmeal or oat bran. In this case, more was not necessarily better. Those who ate 56 g (two ounces, dry weight) of oat bran daily for six weeks achieved the best results (15.9% reduction of low-density lipoprotein cholesterol), followed by those who consumed 84 g (three ounces) daily of oatmeal (11.5% reduction).[10]

A related study involved 206 adults, 30-65 years old, who consumed 60 g daily of oatmeal or oat bran, in addition to reducing their fat intake, for 12 weeks. The results also showed that eating oats at a "moderate and practical level" produced important decreases (at least 5.2%) in blood cholesterol levels.[11]

Studies have also certified the widely circulated folk saying that a bowl of oatmeal "sticks to your ribs" throughout the morning. William Evans, Ph.D., director of the Noll Physiological Research Center at Pennsylvania State University at State College, tested oatmeal's ability to sustain athletic performance in 18 college students.

Lifestyle plays a major role in the development of hypertension, and any program to reduce blood pressure must take this into consideration.

The study participants were divided into three groups, each consuming equal-calorie portions of oats in three different forms: oatmeal; oat rings, a snack food; and dry oat cereal. Then they exercised on stationary bicycles as long as they could, stopping just short of exhaustion. Students who had oatmeal were able to exercise for five hours compared to four hours for the other two groups, according to Dr. Evans. The results confirm that oatmeal at breakfast can help keep you feeling "energized" throughout the morning.

This same advantage translates into benefits for diabetics, too. A recent study enrolled eight men, with an average age of 45, who had diabetes but did not require insulin injections.[12] Over a 12-week period, those eating oat bread (34 g of oat fiber intake) daily had more stability in their blood sugar (glucose) levels. Large fluctuations in glucose often lead to serious problems in diabetics. The men reported a "longer delay in the return of hunger" after eating oatmeal than

Meditation is so effective in reducing stress that in 1984 the National Institutes of Health recommended meditation over prescription drugs for mild hypertension.

with other foods, particularly white bread, indicating oatmeal helped them achieve more control of their daily blood sugar levels.

Lifestyle and Exercise

Lifestyle plays a major role in the development of hypertension, and any program to reduce blood pressure must take this into consideration. Dr. Cowden notes that any changes that are implemented must be maintained if blood pressure is to be controlled on a long-term basis. Smoking should be moderated or, preferably, totally avoided, and alcohol intake should be kept to a minimum. Weight loss reduces blood pressure in those with and without hypertension, and should be a primary goal for hypertensives who are obese or moderately overweight. Other lifestyle factors important in reducing and controlling hypertension are stress management and increased exercise.

For more about **biofeedback,** see Chapter 13: Alternative Medicine Options for Lowering High Blood Pressure, pp. 217-221.

Biofeedback training is a method of learning how to consciously regulate normally unconscious bodily functions (such as heart rate, blood pressure, and breathing). It uses a monitoring device to measure and report back immediate information about the heart rate, for example, transmitting one blinking light or beep per heartbeat. The person being monitored learns techniques such as meditation, relaxation, and visualization to slow their heart rate and then uses the flashes or beeps to check their progress and make adjustments accordingly.

Stress Management

Stress-reduction techniques from the various disciplines of mind/body medicine such as biofeedback, yoga, meditation, *qigong*, relaxation exercises, and hypnotherapy have all proven successful in lowering blood pressure.[13] In fact, meditation is so effective in reducing stress that in 1984 the National Institutes of Health recommended meditation over prescription drugs for mild hypertension.[14]

To reduce stress and improve digestion and thus improve absorption of nutrients from food and supplements, Dr. Cowden has his patients perform stress-reduction techniques before meals and at bedtime. Says Dr. Cowden, "The nutrients we recommend have to be absorbed out of the gastrointestinal tract. But if the gut is in a stressed state, it will not absorb those nutrients nearly as well as if it is in a relaxed state."

Biofeedback has proven particularly valuable in working to lower hypertension. Patients in one study were able to sustain lower blood pressure readings than those registered prior to treatment after three years of using biofeedback.[15] Combining biofeedback with other stress-reduction techniques can also help patients achieve optimum results. A study of mildly hypertensive males treated with either biofeedback, autogenic training, or breathing relaxation training showed a significant reduction in both systolic and diastolic blood pressure. The higher the pretreatment blood pressure, the greater the effects of relaxation training.[16]

Self-guided relaxation techniques can be a quick and effective way to lower blood pressure, according to researchers at the National Taiwan University in Taiwan.[17] Hypertension is widespread there with 27% of men and 13% of women having readings of at least 140/90.

Based on a study group of 590 individuals with high blood pressure, Taiwanese researchers found that practicing progressive relaxation techniques (from a taped cassette) coupled with home study of healthful practices led to an average drop of blood pressure to 130/85 after two months. No drugs or other treatments were involved other than the power of self-directed relaxation.

Exercise

Regular exercise reduces stress and blood pressure, so it is highly recommended that it be an integral part of your life. Consistent aerobic exercise can both prevent and lower hypertension.[18] In a study of 902 people, 45 to 69 years old, with hypertension, positive long-term effects on blood pressure and all cholesterol levels were achieved with increased exercise along with a lower-fat diet.[19]

Swimming, which is frequently prescribed as a non-impact exercise to lower high blood pressure, can produce a significant decrease in resting heart rate (a sign of cardiovascular health) and resting systolic blood pressure in previously sedentary people with elevated blood pressure.[20]

Exercise Lowers High Blood Pressure in Black Men

Seventy-one percent of black men over age 60 have high blood pressure. In a study conducted by the Veterans Affairs Medical Center in Washington, D.C., 46 black men with hypertension rode an exercise bicycle strenuously for 45 minutes daily for 32 weeks, after which time, their blood pressure had dropped and the men were able to reduce their medications by 30%-40%.

CAUTION

Before undertaking any exercise program, an individual with hypertension should consult a physician.

For more about **herbal medicine**, see Chapter 12: Lower Your Blood Pressure With Herbs, pp. 200-206; for **nutritional supplements**, see Chapter 13: Alternative Medicine Options for Lowering High Blood Pressure, pp. 208-226.

Rebounding and the Benefits of Aerobic Exercise

Aerobic training of any kind, including rebounding, improves your cardiovascular fitness in a variety of ways, according to John A. Friedrich, M.D., of Duke University, who first reported on the effects of aerobic exercise on the body in the *Journal of Physical Education* (May/June 1970).

Aerobics can strengthen heart muscles and produce other cardiovascular changes so that the heart can pump more blood with fewer beats. This means your resting (normal) heart rate will be lower, which is good. By regularly working your heart harder during exercise, you improve its overall function so that it doesn't have to work as hard during your normal activities, Dr. Friedrich wrote.

"A conditioned person may have a resting heart rate 20 beats per minute slower than a deconditioned person," says Dr. Morton Walker. "He saves 10,000 beats in one night's sleep." Reducing the day-to-day workload of your heart can lessen your chances of developing heart disease, Dr. Walker adds.

Aerobic exercises such as rebounding increase red blood cell count, allowing faster oxygen transport through the body, and can help lower elevated blood pressure. According to Dr. Friedrich's research, aerobic exercise helps dissolve blood clots and increases the amount of high-density lipoproteins (HDLs, the so-called good cholesterol and a major factor in the prevention of atherosclerosis) in the blood.

The capacity of the lungs also increases, enabling them to process more air and replenish oxygen in the cells of the body's tissues and organs more quickly. Metabolism (conversion of food into energy) is enhanced and you tend to absorb nutrients from your food more efficiently. Any tendency towards constipation, kidney stones, or diabetes is reduced by this form of exercise.

Lower Your High Blood Pressure Naturally

Here are easy alternatives to blood-pressure-lowering drugs for mild to moderate hypertension, according to naturopath Michael T. Murray, N.D.

If you have mild hypertension (140-160/90-104):
- Reduce your weight.
- Eliminate your salt intake and avoid alcohol, caffeine, and smoking.
- Exercise more and practice stress-reduction techniques (such as biofeedback, self-hypnosis, yoga, meditation, and muscle relaxation).

■ Change your diet to include more potassium-rich foods (such as potatoes, avocado, cooked lima beans, bananas, flounder), fiber, and complex carbohydrates.

■ Eat more celery, garlic, onions, and vegetable oils high in omega-3 fatty acids, but eat less animal fats.

■ Take supplements, including calcium (1,000-1,500 mg/day), magnesium (500 mg/day), vitamin C (1-3 g/day), zinc (in picolinate form, 15-30 mg/day), and flaxseed oil (1 tablespoon/day).

■ Maintain this program for at least three months, and preferably for six months; if your blood pressure isn't normal after this period, see a doctor.

If you have moderate hypertension (140-180/105-114):

■ Do all of the above.

■ Take hawthorn herbal extract (100-250 mg, 3 times daily, provided the extract contains 10% procyanidins).

■ Take coenzyme Q10 (20 mg, 3 times daily).

■ Follow this program for three months; if there is no change in your blood pressure, see a physician.[21]

10

Preventing & Reversing High Blood Pressure

ONE DOCTOR'S APPROACH

WHEN IT COMES to heart disease, prevention is easier than cure, says cardiologist Stephen T. Sinatra, M.D., executive director of the New England Heart Center in Manchester, Connecticut. Based on 20 years of experience as a board-certified cardiologist, Dr. Sinatra strongly believes that "if you do have heart disease, you can slow its progression and even reverse it." One of the best places to start is to reduce high blood pressure, a major risk factor for cardiovascular illness, says Dr. Sinatra. It may be major, but it's also *controllable*, using natural nondrug approaches, he adds.

To accomplish this, Dr. Sinatra offers a comprehensive alternative program of dietary change, nutritional supplements, exercise, and psychological counseling, in addition to some conventional prescription of beta blockers and other "antihypertensive" drugs. Dr. Sinatra's approach addresses the mind and body, the physiology and emotions, of the individual with high blood pressure. "There is definitely a heart/brain 'hotline,'" he notes in his book *Heartbreak & Heart Disease*. "The identification of people at risk for sudden death depends not only on the hidden possibilities of heart disease, but also on the psychological and emotional status of the one afflicted."

Coenzyme Q10:
An Energy Nutrient for the Heart

For more on coenzyme Q10, see Chapter 5: Nutritional Supplements, pp. 115-119.

Pamela, 47, came to Dr. Sinatra with a seriously high blood pressure of 205/105. About two years earlier, physicians had placed her on standard antihypertensive drugs, including beta blockers, calcium channel blockers, and ACE inhibitors. These had left her excessively fatigued, coughing, and dissatisfied with the results.

Dr. Sinatra immediately started Pamela on coenzyme Q10, at a dosage of 30 mg, three times daily; at the same time he reduced her intake of high blood pressure drugs by half. CoQ10, a substance found naturally in sardines, salmon, mackerel, and beef heart (but not made by the human body) is an essential feature of Dr. Sinatra's program because it helps prevent the depletion of substances that recharge the cellular energy system in the body.

"As the heart muscle continually uses oxygen and consumes huge amounts of energy, heart muscle cells can greatly benefit from the energy boost of coenzyme Q10," says Dr. Sinatra. In fact, levels of coQ10 are usually ten times higher in the healthy heart than in any other organ. This is why a coQ10 deficiency is most likely to primarily affect the heart and contribute to heart failure. It is estimated that 39% of patients with high blood pressure have a coQ10 deficiency.

The heart requires a constant supply of coQ10 to meet its energy needs. It is both "extremely vulnerable to nutritional deficiencies" and highly receptive to the

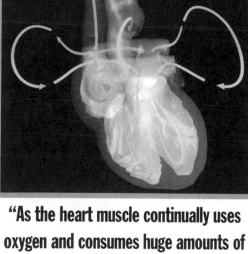

"As the heart muscle continually uses oxygen and consumes huge amounts of energy, heart muscle cells can greatly benefit from the energy boost of coenzyme Q10," says Dr. Sinatra.

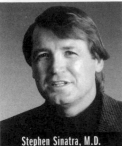

Stephen Sinatra, M.D.

"The identification of people at risk for sudden death depends not only on the hidden possibilities of heart disease, but also on the psychological and emotional status of the one afflicted," says Dr. Sinatra.

benefits of "targeted nutrition," Dr. Sinatra says. Clinical research indicates it usually takes 4 to 12 weeks for coQ10 to have a noticeable effect on blood pressure.

"I regard coQ10 as one of the best medical discoveries of the 20th century," he states. "I've been using it for ten years and have probably thousands of patients on it now. It is absolutely essential for strengthening the biochemistry of the heart cells." CoQ10 functions like a vitamin, "rescuing" body tissues that have been damaged by free radicals. "CoQ10 taken for cardiovascular conditions may enable some patients to reduce the dosage of their medications by up to 50%," notes Dr. Sinatra.

For these reasons, Dr. Sinatra starts almost all his cardiovascular patients on coQ10 at the initial low dose of 90 mg daily, then gradually increases it. "Extremely few people are oversensitive to it and may experience nausea—very rarely do I see side effects," says Dr. Sinatra. After one week, he increased Pamela's coQ10 dosage to 60 mg, three times daily. The standard dose for coQ10, as commonly prescribed by physicians, is "sub-therapeutic" and probably too low to be effective, says Dr. Sinatra. If you take 90-120 mg daily, you're likely to have a blood level of 1.5 ug/ml of usable coQ10, while what the body requires for a strong therapeutic response is 2.5 to 3.5 ug/ml.

As a general heart-protective dose, Dr. Sinatra himself takes 180 mg daily, but for high blood pressure, he usually builds toward a daily dose of 180 to 360 mg, and for serious congestive heart failure, 360-400 mg daily. For preventive maintenance for someone without a specific heart problem, Dr. Sinatra recommends a dosage of 30 to 90 mg daily.

The Value of a Mediterranean Diet

Dr. Sinatra also recommended that Pamela institute major changes in her diet. Specifically, he said her diet should consist of 30% fats, 20%-

A coenzyme Q10 deficiency is most likely to primarily affect the heart and contribute to heart failure. It is estimated that 39% of patients with high blood pressure have a coQ10 deficiency.

25% protein, and 45%-50% carbohydrates. The fats should come from fish such as salmon, mackerel, Greenland halibut, cod, and bluefish, but not tuna because of possible mercury contamination. Large amounts of red meat should be avoided while fresh fruits and vegetables are emphasized. Dr. Sinatra calls this the traditional Mediterranean diet.

For more about **olive oil**, see Chapter 2: Caring for Yourself, pp. 52-54.

A now classic study conducted in the 1980s investigating the rate of heart attacks over a ten-year period for individuals in European nations revealed that the island of Crete reported zero heart attacks as a cause of death, even though many of the residents had dangerously high cholesterol levels, a presumed risk factor for heart disease.

According to Dr. Sinatra, "the Mediterranean diet, rich in monounsaturated fat (olive oil) and antioxidants, has proved to be crucial in cardiovascular protection." Dr. Sinatra says this diet is low in saturated fats (such as dairy products and meats), high in fiber and antioxidants (from fresh fruits and vegetables) such as vitamin C, beta carotene, and vitamin E, and high in essential fatty acids, found in flax and other omega-3 oils. Avocados and asparagus, commonly eaten in this diet, are rich in L-glutathione, an amino acid that can scavenge harmful free radicals, while garlic and onions have ingredients that help protect the heart, and olive oil is "the healthiest of oils, no doubt."

Underlying the success of the Mediterranean diet is a biochemical principle, Dr. Sinatra says. It is called insulin resistance or hyperinsulinism. Insulin is a key digestive hormone, secreted by the pancreas for regulating the absorption of glucose (blood sugar) and the metabolism of carbohydrates and fats. In general, most Americans are eating too many carbohydrates, which in turn leads to excess insulin secretion (hyperinsulinism) and to insulin resistance, says Dr. Sinatra.

"When you've had too much insulin circulating in your bloodstream for too long—as is often the case when people doggedly stick to high-carbohydrate, low-fat diets—specialized receptor cells lose their ability to respond to insulin." The resulting insulin resistance can lead to higher blood pressure, thickened, less elastic arterial walls, increased cravings for carbohydrates, and higher blood sugar levels, says Dr. Sinatra.

This factor contributes to heart disease in two ways. First, as insulin secretion increases, so does the level of arachidonic acid. (This is a fatty-acid precursor to prostaglandins and is found almost entirely in animal foods.) Further biochemical changes resulting from this cause blood vessels to constrict and blood to clot, and this sets up a risk factor for both higher blood pressure and serious heart problems.

The second problem with too much insulin is that it is antagonistic to the cells (called endothelial) that line the blood vessels and keep them free of obstructions, Dr. Sinatra says. As insulin levels rise, the structural integrity of the endothelial cells suffers and the type of muscles in the blood vessels changes. The result can be blood vessels that are prone to developing plaque deposits, which again can lead to high blood pressure, he adds.

"The benefit of the Mediterranean diet is that everything in it helps prevent excess insulin release," says Dr. Sinatra. The diet, through saltwater fish, shellfish, and flaxseed, contains high levels of alpha-linolenic and omega-3 fatty acids, which are "the most important essential fatty acids for the protection of cardiovascular health."

Dr. Sinatra also generally recommends minimizing the consumption of "high glycemic carbohydrates." This means foods such as flour pastas, white potatoes, and white rice, whose carbohydrate portion enters the bloodstream quickly, leading to higher levels of insulin to handle the sudden glucose load. Examples of fruits with a low-glycemic index (slow absorption by the blood) include grapefruit, cherries, peaches, plums, kiwi, and rhubarb. Pamela was also instructed to avoid preservatives, processed foods and meats, canned vegetables, diet soft drinks, and chemical ingredients.

Under Dr. Sinatra's supervision, Pamela added tofu, navy beans, and seaweeds to her diet for their magnesium content. She also started taking an antioxidant vitamin-mineral formula (containing no copper or iron) developed by Dr. Sinatra under the brand name Optimum Health. Pamela started taking a daily formula containing 1,000 mg of calcium and 500 mg of magnesium. These amounts were in addition to the vitamin-mineral supplement which contained lower amounts of both (280 mg of magnesium, 250 mg of calcium). "Magnesium prevents spasming of blood vessels which is why it's one of the most important mineral treatments for high blood pressure," says Dr. Sinatra.

Dr. Sinatra also encouraged Pamela to begin a regular exercise program, preferably vigorous walking. "I don't recommend jogging. If you can do a brisk walk lasting 15 minutes twice a day, that's all the exercise you really need," says Dr. Sinatra. As an alternative, he advises dancing (and practices it himself) as a "heart nurturing" form of daily rhythmic exercise. Regularity, not intensity, of exercise is paramount, he says.

At Pamela's next appointment two weeks later, her blood pressure had dropped to 170/90, "a big improvement," says Dr. Sinatra. He kept her on the diet and supplement program, including coQ10 at 180 mg daily; he took her off calcium channel blocker but kept her on a low dose of beta blocker. She maintained a daily walking program of one to two miles. After about three months on the Sinatra program, Pamela's blood pressure had come down to a safe 140-145/80-85. "I was satisfied with that," Dr. Sinatra says.

Hawthorn Helps Colin's Heart Relax

Dr. Sinatra offers another case involving Colin, 65, who came to him with a history of heart attacks and progressive heart failure. His problem was that his heart's pumping ability was severely reduced. Colin's blood pressure was 180/90, he was unable to tolerate most conventional heart drugs, and his mitral valve (one of the heart's four valves) was leaking blood as a result of his high blood pressure. Colin had chronic shortness of breath and was unable to walk much without getting winded.

Dr. Sinatra started Colin on the Mediterranean diet; coQ10, magnesium, calcium, and potassium supplements; and hawthorn herbal extract (from hawthorn berries) beginning at 500 mg daily, then increasing to 1,000 mg. Clinical studies have shown that hawthorn can help reduce blood pressure by reducing or blocking the constriction of blood vessels directly serving the heart. This is crucial because when blood vessels constrict, blood pressure rises. "I gave Colin hawthorn to reduce his blood pressure, strengthen his heart, and give him a good quality

EDITOR'S NOTE
Dr. Sinatra is board certified in Internal Medicine and Cardiology and is a certified bioenergetic therapist in the tradition of Alexander Lowen, M.D. Dr. Sinatra has served as chief of cardiology at the Manchester Memorial Hospital in Connecticut and as assistant clinical professor at the University of Connecticut. He is the editor of the monthly newsletter, *HeartSense*, and the author of *Heartbreak & Heart Disease* (1996), Keats Publishing, Inc., 27 Pine Street, New Canaan, CT 06840; tel: 203-966-8721; fax: 203-972-3991; and *Optimum Health* (1997), Bantam Doubleday, New York, NY.

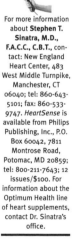

For more information about **Stephen T. Sinatra, M.D., F.A.C.C., C.B.T.,** contact: New England Heart Center, 483 West Middle Turnpike, Manchester, CT 06040; tel: 860-643-5101; fax: 860-533-9747. *HeartSense* is available from Philips Publishing, Inc., P.O. Box 60042, 7811 Montrose Road, Potomac, MD 20859; tel: 800-211-7643; 12 issues/$100. For information about the Optimum Health line of heart supplements, contact Dr. Sinatra's office.

"Magnesium prevents spasming of blood vessels which is why it's one of the most important mineral treatments for high blood pressure," says Dr. Sinatra.

For more on **homocysteine**, see Chapter 1: What Causes Heart Disease?, pp. 34-37.

of life," which means improved health without the unpleasant side effects of drugs.

Colin also began taking B vitamins, specifically 40 mg each of B1, B2, and B6, 40 mcg of B12, and 800 mcg of folic acid. "I recommend B vitamins for anybody with heart disease because they are the antidote to a condition we call hyperhomocysteinemia," says Dr. Sinatra.

Here is how it works: Red meat contains methionine, an essential amino acid and protein building block. But if your system is deficient in B vitamins, methionine does not get broken down into simpler substances and instead forms homocysteine. Too much homocysteine contributes to premature heart disease and aging, explains Dr. Sinatra.

After about six weeks on the program, Colin's blood pressure dropped to 140-145/90-95. There was less leakage at his mitral valve; he was not taking any conventional drugs; he was able to walk, play golf, and exercise more freely; and "he felt he was in terrific control of his life," says Dr. Sinatra.

Often an individual with high blood pressure or heart disease suffers from depression and sexual dysfunction, including impotence, Dr. Sinatra notes. Sometimes these conditions are caused by conventional drugs; other times, they result from diminished nutrition and unresolved emotional issues. To help shift the depression that can accompany heart problems, Dr. Sinatra prescribes the amino acid L-tyrosine. Getting a person off conventional heart drugs and onto a solid nutritional support program often completes the turnaround, he adds.

"When you empower patients with nutritional support, diet, and exercise, they have control over their destiny and develop a much greater optimism. When you have this optimism about participating in your health, you become alive sexually. I've seen this many times. I tell them I am not their doctor but their nurse. In other words, I will nurse them along and nurture their healing, but *they* have the power to get well."

Uncovering the Anger in Ray's Blood Pressure

It's important not to overlook the crucial role that emotions can play in the development of high blood pressure, notes Dr. Sinatra. "The psychological risk factors can be just as lethal as the more accepted

Clinical studies have shown that hawthorn can help reduce blood pressure by reducing or blocking the constriction of blood vessels directly serving the heart.

physical risk factors," he says. Unresolved emotions, such as anger, hostility, and rage, and the way one reacts to stress, are hidden risk factors in heart disease that many cardiologists fail to acknowledge.

To many, both physicians and patients, these emotions represent the "dark side" or shadow portion of the personality that tends to get denied or suppressed. "But I think that getting in touch with these powerful hidden emotions and becoming aware of their contribution to heart disease is critical to healing and protecting the heart," Dr. Sinatra says. Ray's case perfectly demonstrates this point.

Ray, 44, was a corporate executive in a position of high responsibility and stress. His blood pressure was "horrendous" at 220/115 and was not responding at all to conventional antihypertensive drugs when he first came for treatment. Dr. Sinatra performed an emotional stress test on Ray, using a computerized device called a Cardiac Performance Laboratory (CPL) that in effect measures anger by evaluating the degree to which the blood vessels are constricted from hypertension. The CPL measures 17 dynamic circulatory changes inside the heart and blood vessels.

Dr. Sinatra asked Ray to perform mental arithmetic, put his hands in ice-cold water, and answer stressful questions. The test registers the changes in blood pressure, literally with each heartbeat, in accordance with these requests. If you are a reasonably calm person, putting your hands in ice water will elevate your blood pressure five to ten points, says Dr. Sinatra, but if you are what is called a "hot reactor" or physiological overreactor, the jump may be 30-40 points.

"With Ray, I was dealing with a man who was very calm on the outside, but on the inside, he was a hot reactor. When I asked him questions about his mother or his personal life, he virtually went off the walls with his blood pressure." He saw it rise dangerously to 240/125 under stress. "Ray was a young man but in tough shape—a risk for sudden death."

During his interview with Ray, Dr. Sinatra observed how much anger Ray held in his body, as evidenced by his clenched jaw and shallow breathing. Dr. Sinatra then understood why the antihypertensive drugs were having no useful effect on Ray: his anger was the prime cause of his high blood pressure.

"Are you aware of how much anger you have?" Dr. Sinatra asked

How Well is Your Heart Working?
The Cardiac Performance Lab Can Tell You

The Cardiac Performance Lab (CPL) from SoftQue Inc. of Mesa, Arizona, is a noninvasive diagnostic system that measures heart and circulatory performance. CPL, which looks at heart stroke volume, cardiac output, total systemic resistance, and 14 other heart functions, provides more information than the standard electrocardiogram (EKG) yet is not as expensive or invasive as heart catheterization.

Impedance cardiography (as this process is called) originated in the 1930s and was used by NASA during the Apollo space program. It uses elec-

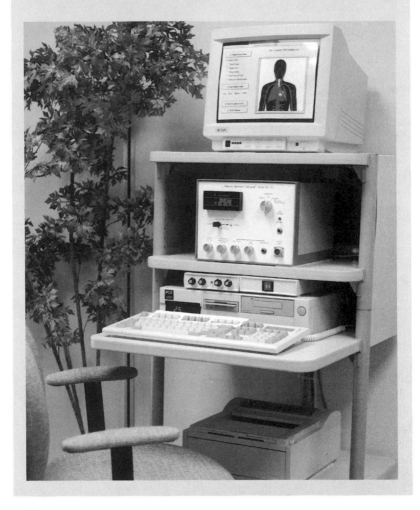

trical resistance (impedance) to measure cardiac performance. All substances, including body tissues, have a higher or lower opposition (resistance) when an electrical current passes through them. Copper, the most common conductor, has a low resistance to electricity; that is to say, it has a low electrical impedance. In body tissues, electrical resistance is lower in wet tissue than in dry, and blood is a particularly good electrical conductor because it has low resistance compared to other tissues.

CPL in effect turns the chest cavity into an electrical conductor and then measures changes in resistance which reflect changes in blood flow. A high-frequency, low-intensity alternating current is conducted through the chest of the subject (with no discomfort) from electrodes attached to the forehead and abdomen. EKG leads attached to the body monitor resistance levels throughout the area and send this information to the CPL computer. As blood is pumped through the heart and into the body, resistance in the chest cavity fluctuates because of the changing concentration of blood. These changes are recorded by the CPL computer, which displays heart and circulatory performance along with blood pressure fluctuations in wave patterns on a continuous graph giving an accurate picture of cardiac activity.

The CPL test is adjusted for each individual to accommodate for demographic information, such as age, sex, height, and weight. These values help establish normal ranges for the individual. Changes in cardiac performance under stress are induced using five standard tests: the subject goes through a series of different postures and movements and performs mental tests to simulate "real world" stress. The results are then compared to normal ranges for the individual to evaluate heart function under these conditions.

Some of the heart and circulatory factors measured by CPL include blood pressure (systolic, diastolic, and mean); cardiac output (stroke volume times heart rate); left ventricular ejection time (time for blood to be pumped from the left ventricle); stroke volume index (stroke volume divided by body surface area); vascular rigidity index (pulse pressure per change in stroke volume per body surface area); and total systemic resistance (mean arterial pressure times 80 then divided by cardiac output).

For more information about **Cardiac Performance Laboratory**, contact: SoftQue Inc., 2427 East Huber, Mesa, AZ 85213; tel: 602-834-1318; fax: 602-835-6559.

him. Ray responded: "Yes, but I can't get it out or show it." He then admitted he had never shared this secret with anybody nor had he ever allowed himself to show his anger. "Then Ray started to cry because he was seeing this side of himself for the first time. Crying is very healthy for the heart. I try to reframe a patient's anger and make it a healing rather than a destructive energy."

After this meeting, Ray started psychotherapy with a practitioner trained in the way emotions can be lodged in the body. Soon after,

Ray's corporation transferred him to another city, but when Dr. Sinatra heard from him about six months later, Ray reported that his blood pressure was completely normal.

Ray's case underscores another important insight gained from the heart study of the Cretans, particularly the men, says Dr. Sinatra. Equally as important as their Mediterranean diet is the fact that men in that region tend to talk more openly with other men about their feelings, families, dreams, and spiritual beliefs.

Men in this Mediterranean culture tend not to wear social masks, but feel comfortable arguing, crying, supporting, even holding one another, says Dr. Sinatra. This quality of comradery and the respect for the "healing powers of nurturing relationships" is a major factor accounting for the low level of coronary heart disease among that population, he says.

Best of all—for his patients—Dr. Sinatra tries to be a good example of what is required to keep one's heart healthy and unpressured. He works hard but he listens to his body so he does not become highly stressed. He takes coQ10, practices the Mediterranean diet, and loves to dance. "I cry when I want to and have my anger—I experience my dark-side, shadow emotions."

He never forgets that becoming ill, whether with high blood pressure or other heart ailments, "is really a form of disease that emerges from the chaotic imbalance of mind, body, and spirit." For a cardiovascular therapy to be completely successful, says Dr. Sinatra, it must heal this "disturbed relationship," addressing heart stress at the metabolic, physiological, psychological, and even spiritual levels.

It's important not to overlook the

crucial role that emotions

can play in the development of high

blood pressure, notes Dr. Sinatra.

"The psychological risk factors

can be just as lethal as the more accepted

physical risk factors," he says.

Unresolved emotions, such as anger,

hostility, and rage, and the way one reacts

to stress, are hidden risk factors

in heart disease that many

cardiologists fail to acknowledge.

Chinese Medicine

HOW IT CAN HELP REVERSE HIGH BLOOD PRESSURE

T RADITIONAL CHINESE medicine (TCM) is a well-established method of health care that combines the use of medicinal herbs, acupuncture, food therapy, massage, and therapeutic exercise. It has proven effective for many conditions, including high blood pressure.

As a result of imbalance in the body, high blood pressure can begin to creep up even in an otherwise seemingly healthy person. If left untreated, it can lead to more serious heart disease. High blood pressure can also develop as a symptom of other conditions, such as adult-onset diabetes and a liver imbalance. In the following section, acupuncturist **Ira J. Golchehreh, Lic.Ac., O.M.D.**, of San Rafael, California, explains how this can happen and how traditional Chinese medicine can reverse it and prevent the development of more serious conditions.

High Blood Pressure on the Way to Diabetes

Many people in the West develop serious health problems, such as heart disease, diabetes, cancer, or arthritis, when they reach middle age. Although these may seem to arise out of nowhere, almost always there is a medical history of many chronic conditions that were never treated correctly.

Based on my experience with acupuncture and Chinese herbs, I can say confidently that serious illness at midlife does not have to happen. With the strategic use of Chinese medicine, for example, you can successfully *prevent* a series of chronic problems from becoming one big acute problem later. The case of Ronald shows this perfectly. When I first met Ronald, 44, he presented the classic symptoms of a lifelong liver imbalance. Technically, in Chinese medicine we call this "hyperactivity of liver yang." It represents a liver whose energy, or "fire," is so overactive, or "yang," and, therefore, so imbalanced, that it creates problems throughout the mind and body.

When I first treated Ronald, I made an emergency house call, as he didn't feel well enough to come to my office. His acute symptom was painful, bright red, and terribly itchy skin lesions on his inner thighs and groin. I knew at once this was a flare-up along his liver meridian. When I learned that he had a job with much pressure and responsibility, I understood that these factors might have precipitated this crisis from the basis of a liver energy imbalance. I also noted that as it was spring and the liver is the organ of this season in Chinese medical thinking, the timing of the flare-up was appropriate.

I applied needles to acupuncture points on the front of Ronald's body to redirect healing energy (or *qi*) to the area of inflammation. I also gave him *Gypsum fibrosum* powder (calcium sulfate) to apply topically (moistened with water) to the lesions and to take internally to "cool down" his system because there was too much "heat" in his liver.

One week later, Ronald came to my office, where I took his complete health history. As a child, he suffered from colitis and constipation, angry outbursts, and nearsightedness. As an adult, Ronald had been bothered with chronic indigestion, bloating, gas, heartburn, multiple food allergies, a recurrent dry cough, night sweats, periodic irritability, and fluctuating body temperature. His complexion was pale, he was overweight, his abdomen was tight and distended, and his breathing was shallow. Ronald's pulse, as we "read" it in Chinese medicine, was fast and taut, especially for his liver.

Ronald's blood sugar level at 150 was high, as normal is 80-120. His body temperature was two degrees below normal; his blood pressure was elevated at 130/89; and the oxygen saturation of his blood was a dangerously low 87% (normal is 95%-97%). In his immediate family, there was a history of diabetes, gallbladder dysfunction, and bloating.

What an Unbalanced Liver Can Do

It was clear to me that Ronald was well on the way towards developing adult-onset diabetes with possible prostate and heart complica-

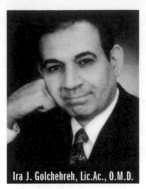

"Many people in the West develop serious health problems, such as heart disease, diabetes, cancer, or arthritis, when they reach middle age. Based on my experience with acupuncture and Chinese herbs, I can say confidently that serious illness at midlife does not have to happen," says Ira J. Golchehreh, Lic.Ac., O.M.D.

Ira J. Golchehreh, Lic.Ac., O.M.D.

tions. One never knows for sure, but he could have been as close as five years from these problems. With Ronald, a single organ—the liver—was clearly the cause of many symptoms. Chinese medicine has a name for the quality of Ronald's liver energy. We call it "rebellious *qi*." The energy of his liver was excessive and too strong. It rose up through his system like a volcano and was subject to periodic eruptions, which he might experience as angry outbursts. His liver was in rebellion, energetically speaking, against his other organs.

The healthy liver is the source of an estimated 13,000 different enzymes and biochemicals which it produces every day. The enzymes in Ronald's liver were wild and hyperactive, exploding throughout the body like sparks from a volcano. Even though he had too many enzymes, his system could not use them to digest his food; hence, he had many digestive problems.

The liver heat dried up his lungs, making them contract and stiffen. That's why his blood-oxygen level was so dangerously low. This, in turn, meant his heart and other organs were becoming oxygen-deprived. The cough was an attempt by his lungs to suck more air into them. Although he exercised regularly and ate a low-fat diet, Ronald was both overweight and undernourished, conditions caused by faulty metabolism, thanks to the liver.

The liver imbalance also upset Ronald's pancreas, which produces insulin to regulate blood-sugar levels, hence, his blood sugar was high. Finally, the overactive liver was depleting Ronald's basic life force, which Chinese medicine says is stored in the kidneys. Three years earlier he had been sick for a month with a bladder infection; this of course is a sign of an underlying kidney imbalance.

When you understand the *root* cause that produces many health

When you understand the *root* cause that produces many health problems in a person, you see that all the signs and symptoms of illness actually make perfect sense. In Ronald's case, they all resulted from a liver imbalance.

problems in a person, you see that all the signs and symptoms of illness actually make perfect sense. In Ronald's case, they all resulted from a liver imbalance that he was probably born with. With this in mind, I developed my treatment plan.

Taming the Volcano

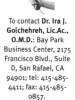

As he arrived for his second treatment, Ronald told me that his cough had become constant. He could not speak without coughing. To help this, I applied six vacuum glass cups to the surface of his back. These would open his lungs, draw toxins out of them and towards the skin surface, and enable him to breathe better. Next, I applied two hydro hot packs to the

To contact **Dr. Ira J. Golchehreh, Lic.Ac., O.M.D.**: Bay Park Business Center, 2175 Francisco Blvd., Suite D, San Rafael, CA 94901; tel: 415-485-4411; fax: 415-485-0857.

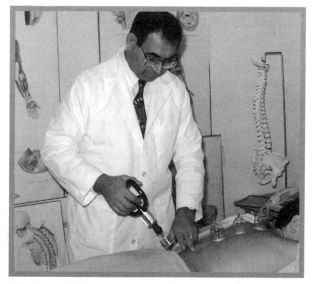

Chinese medicine uses a practice called *cupping* in which vacuum glass cups are applied to the skin's surface, in this case, on the back, to "open" the lungs, draw toxins out of them and towards the skin surface, and to facilitate better breathing.

same points on his back. These are thick hot tubes containing minerals that release heat through the skin to the lungs.

Then I focused two mineral infrared lamps onto the lung and liver areas of his back. These lamps project heat through a filter containing 33 different minerals and nutrients; the skin absorbs the energy of these elements and conducts it inwards. I gave Ronald several capsules of the herb *Ephedra* to ease his cough and further open his lungs. Finally, I applied about 50 needles to points on the Liver, Lung, Spleen, and Stomach acupuncture meridians. Normally I do not use this many needles, but it was important to treat many organs and energy systems at once to start bringing his entire system into harmony.

I told Ronald to take two capsules of *Ephedra* three times daily, for a daily total of 1,800 mg, to help open his lungs so he could breathe more fully and saturate his blood with more oxygen. I gave him another Chinese herb called *Bupleurum* to help disperse excess liver heat, to keep the liver from "exploding" with too much energy, to regulate blood pressure, and to destroy pathogens in his system. He would take one teaspoon of this mixed in water, twice daily.

Next, I gave Ronald CO-197 containing ten Chinese herbs, to be taken three times daily. In addition, I asked him to drink at least $^1/_2$ gallon of pure water every day; this would promote the excretion of toxins from the system through frequent urination.

Finally, I asked him to radically change his diet to one that was high-protein, low-fat and low-carbohydrate, and completely yeast-free. I asked Ronald to eat vegetable soups, whole grains (excepting wheat), lots of protein (preferably chicken and fish as he was allergic to beans), and no fruit, no fresh raw vegetables, nothing yeasted, no coffee, alcohol, salt, sugar, spices, or dairy products of any kind. The purpose of the diet was to give Ronald's liver some breathing space to clean itself out thoroughly after many years of having to deal with foods that upset it. To my relief, Ronald said he realized he needed to completely overhaul his diet and welcomed my guidance.

One week later, Ronald returned for his third treatment. He had kept a journal of all his daily symptoms. This was quite instructive because it showed me how the energy was starting to move around in his body, temporarily producing both physical and emotional symptoms. When I checked his vital signs, I was pleased with the results. His blood sugar had dropped to 120, his oxygen saturation had climbed to 97, and his blood pressure was better at 120/78. He was less bloated and his coughing was about 50% reduced.

This time I treated acupoints on Ronald's front, focusing on the Liver, Spleen, and Pancreas meridians. As before, I used a lot of needles and let him lie on the table for about an hour as they helped to harmonize his organs. This time, I sent Ronald home with a new herbal formula called *Eriobotrya* and *Ophiopogon* Combination, one teaspoon mixed in water, to be taken twice daily.

This blend would help remove the "heat" from the lungs so that they could expand more fully; it would also help to harmonize the energies of the spleen and stomach. I also put Ronald on Resplex, a respiratory formula containing beta carotene, vitamin E, wild cherry bark, horehound, lobelia, pleurisy root, hyssop, and mullein, to be taken three times daily, two capsules each time.

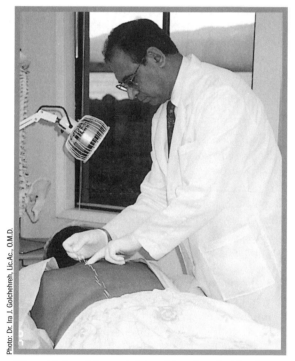

Photo: Dr. Ira J. Golchehreh, Lic.Ac., O.M.D.

Mineral infrared lamps (pictured here) project heat through a filter containing 33 different minerals and nutrients; the skin absorbs the energy of these elements and conducts it inwards.

Out of the Woods After a Month

By the time of the fourth treatment, one month after beginning with Ronald, he was out of the woods as far as his acute problems were concerned. By the way, he had taken only one day off from work during this period, although he slept heavily on the weekends.

When you reset the energy patterns of a major organ, especially the liver, which influences so much else in the body, and after a lifetime of imbalance, it takes many weeks for one's full supply of energy to return. It's like trying to irrigate a parched field for the first time; the water reserves are stretched at first because the ground is so dry. That's why Ronald was exhausted every Saturday. Had he taken two weeks off from work, his total healing time would have been reduced to about five weeks instead of what ended up taking ten weeks.

At this point, Ronald's vital signs were the best yet. His blood sugar was 78, his pulse was much calmer, oxygen saturation was 97%, and blood pressure was a much more balanced 119/88. His cough was only sporadic, probably 80% improved. Ronald's complexion was noticeably rosier, as the higher blood-oxygen content had brought more life, literally, to his face. This time I again treated acupoints that would harmonize the interactions of all his organs. For his fifth treatment, I worked on harmonizing the energies flowing among the liver, lungs, and kidneys by placing needles at points on the front of Ronald's body. Following this treatment, he reported that he felt energized and vibrant.

Two weeks later, Ronald returned for another treatment but his vital signs and pulse indicated he actually did not need one. His blood pressure was even better at 116/81, while the other readings remained stable. I kept him on the *Ephedra*, Resplex, *Eriobotrya* and *Ophiopogon* Combination, and the restricted diet, and added two more herbal formulas. I gave him *Ma Huang Coix* including *Ephedra*, taken at the rate of nine pills daily. I also started him on another *Bupleurum* powder, two teaspoons daily in water.

Excellent in Four Months

One month later, Ronald returned for a checkup and maintenance treatment. After two months on the program, he had lost 20 pounds and looked fit and rosy. His energy had returned to normal, his liver was calm, and he was in good spirits. This time I used the needles to fine-tune the energies of his liver, lungs, and other organ systems.

I was gratified to see how well he had responded to the treatment. There was no doubt the body was healing itself after a lifetime of imbalance. I asked Ronald to remain on the diet for another month to complete the liver's total detoxification. All of his original symptoms were gone. Four months after beginning treatment, Ronald's blood pressure was a healthy 112/78, his oxygen level was 98%, and his liver pulse was calm. Provided he continues with a moderate diet and periodic acupuncture checkups, it is quite likely the symptoms will not return for the rest of his life.

In retrospect, I can see now that Ronald's initial health crisis of inflammation on his thighs and groin was sufficiently acute to get him into treatment for what proved to be a lifetime disorder seated in his liver. This is a good example of how an acute problem today can also be an opportunity to *prevent* something far more serious just around the corner in a person's life. ■

Fundamentals of Traditional Chinese Medicine

TCM has been practiced for over 3,000 years and, at present, one-quarter of the world's population makes use of one or more of its therapies. A complete system of medicine, it has been selected by the World Health Organization for worldwide propagation to meet the health care needs of the twenty-first century.[1]

TCM's approach to health and healing is very different from modern Western medicine. TCM looks for the underlying causes of imbalances and patterns of disharmony in the body, and views each patient as unique. Western medicine generally provides treatment for a specific illness, whereas traditional Chinese medicine addresses how the illness manifests in a particular patient and treats the patient, not just the disease. As Roger Hirsh, O.M.D., L.Ac., Dipl. NCCA, of Beverly Hills, California, explains, "The conventional Western physician focuses predominantly on the pathogenic factor (the disease), rather than the response of the patient to the factor."

The philosophy of traditional Chinese medicine is preventive in nature and views the practice of waiting to treat a disease until the symptoms are full-blown as being similar to "digging a well after one has become thirsty."[2] In line with this, TCM makes a point of educating patients with regard to lifestyle so that they can assist in their own therapeutic process. The TCM practitioner educates the patient about diet, exercise, stress management, rest, and relaxation.

The terms yin and yang are used by the TCM practitioner to describe the opposing physical conditions of the body. These terms

The philosophy of traditional Chinese medicine is preventive in nature and views the practice of waiting to treat a disease until the symptoms are full-blown as being similar to "digging a well after one has become thirsty."

stem from a basic Chinese concept describing the interdependence and relationship of opposites. Much as hot cannot be understood or defined without having experienced cold, yin cannot exist without its opposite yang, and yang cannot exist without yin.

Roger Jahnke, O.M.D., an acupuncturist based in Santa Barbara, California, explains that when applying these concepts to the human body, "Yin refers to the tissue of the organ, while yang refers to its activity. In yin deficiency, the organ does not have enough raw materials to function. In yang deficiency, the organ does not react adequately when needed."

These two conditions are forever connected, though, "in a system of interdependence and interrelatedness," adds Maoshing Ni, D.O.M., Ph.D., L.Ac., president of Yo San University of Traditional Chinese Medicine in Santa Monica, California. For example, says Dr. Ni, a yin deficiency in thyroid hormone levels, the raw material of the thyroid gland, would eventually cause a yang deficiency in the thyroid, as its function becomes impaired by the lack of hormones. Likewise, poor thyroid function, a yang deficiency, would eventually result in a yin deficiency, as the gland's output of hormones decreased.

Traditional Chinese medicine also introduces a major component of the body, *qi* (also referred to as chi), that Western medicine does not even acknowledge. *Qi*, according to Dr. Ni, is difficult to define. "We call it life force. It is all-inclusive of the many types of energy within the body and is essential for life itself," he says. This vital life energy flows through the body following pathways called meridians.

These meridians flow along the surface of the body, and through the internal organs, with each meridian being given the name of the organ through which it flows, such as "Liver," or "Large Intestine." Organs can be accessed for treatment through their specific meridians, and illness can occur when there is a blockage of *qi* in these channels. Therefore it is essential in traditional Chinese medicine to keep the *qi* flowing in order to maintain health. The healthy individual has an abundance of *qi* moving smoothly through the meridians and organs. With this flow, the organs are able to harmoniously support each other's functions.

Five Phase Theory

The interrelationship of the body's organs is another important concept in traditional Chinese medicine. Ten organs are arranged into a system that places each in one of five categories: fire, earth, metal, water, and wood. This system, called the Five Phase Theory, is based on the premise that each organ either nourishes or inhibits the proper functioning of another organ, just as the basic elements act either adversely or beneficially on each other. "The Chinese have, for thousands of years, watched how things worked around them in order to understand why things happen, why things transform from one thing to another," says Dr. Ni. "They've taken this same conceptual model and applied it to the human body and found it really works well."

For example, as fire melts metal, the heart, which is associated with fire, controls the lungs, which are associated with metal. Likewise, as metal cuts wood, the lungs control the

Under traditional Chinese medical treatment, the patient's blood pressure dropped from 180/130 to 130/90 in less than two weeks.

liver; as wood penetrates the earth, the liver controls the spleen; as the earth dams water, the spleen controls the kidneys; and as water quenches fire, the kidneys control the heart.

The organs are also divided up into two groups of yin and yang organs. "The heart, spleen, lungs, kidney, and liver belong to the yin group, because they are what we call more substantial organs, more solid," explains Dr. Ni, "whereas, the yang organs are hollow organs like the small intestine, stomach, large intestine, and bladder, where things just pass through. They're more functional—remember, yang is function, action, and yin is more passive, solid, substantial—that's why they're categorized that way."

ELEMENT	YIN ORGAN	YANG ORGAN
Fire	Heart	Small intestine
Earth	Spleen	Stomach
Metal	Lungs	Large intestine
Water	Kidney	Bladder
Wood	Liver	Gallbladder

According to TCM, essential hypertension is usually due to a problem in the circulation of energy *(qi)* in the body. Treatment is aimed at bringing the energy flow of the body back into balance through a combination of acupuncture and herbs.

The Practice of Traditional Chinese Medicine

In treating a patient, a TCM practitioner first looks for patterns in the details of his or her clinical observations of that patient. This allows the practitioner to discover the disharmony in the system of that individual. Familiar with symptoms that are standard to each disease, the doctor also considers what symptoms or behaviors would be especially telling to the individual patient. For example, some people are very active and constantly moving, even red in the face, yet these appearances may not indicate any malady. On the other hand, it is perfectly normal for others to exhibit slowness and inactivity. It is against this individual landscape that the TCM practitioner attempts to correctly assess the pattern of disharmony when an individual becomes ill.

A pattern may be so commonly associated with a certain treatment that the pattern and treatment carry the same name. But often the doctor must develop a strategy by carefully balancing many details. Stomach ulcers, for instance, may originate in very different patterns of disharmony, although the resulting ulcers may appear identical. Therefore, each type of ulcer may require a very different type of treatment, and the wrong treatment could worsen the condition.

"Yet in Western medicine, ulcers are generally treated with whatever anti-ulcer medication there may be, without differentiating," says Dr. Ni. "What Chinese medicine does is decipher the response of the patient. How is the patient's body reacting to the illness, to the cause of the illness? It's these patterns that we seek to determine and then treat accordingly." Alternatively, people with different symptoms, but the same pattern of disharmony, can often be treated by the same medicines or therapies.

Methods of Diagnosis

A first-time patient, accustomed to Western medicine, may be surprised that TCM diagnosis does not require procedures such as blood tests, X rays, endoscopy (the inspection of the inside of a body cavity by an endoscope), or exploratory surgery. Instead, the TCM practitioner performs the five following, noninvasive methods of investigation:

- Inspection of the complexion, general demeanor, body language, and tongue
- Questioning the patient about symptoms, medical history, diet, lifestyle, history of the present complaint, and any previous or concurrent therapies received
- Listening to the tone and strength of the voice
- Smelling any body excretions, the breath, or the body odor
- Palpation (feeling with the fingers) of the pulse at the radial arteries of both wrists (pulse diagnosis), the abdomen, and the meridians and/or acupuncture points

Through pulse diagnosis, a skilled practitioner can examine the strength or weakness of the *qi* and "blood," which includes lymph and other bodily fluids, and assess how these affect each of the organs, tissues, and layers of the body. The practitioner will also look at the impact of a wide range of personal and environmental factors. Mood influences, activity, sex, food, drugs, weather, and seasons of the year can each affect health and the healing process. "All these factors need to be weighed when making a diagnosis," states Dr. Hirsh, "but the presence of one factor doesn't always warrant a disease outcome."

Dr. Ni explains that what TCM practitioners try to do with all

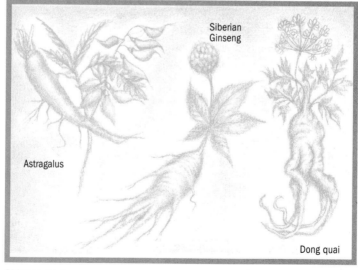

Siberian Ginseng

Astragalus

Dong quai

Chinese herbs

forms of diagnosis is look at illness in the body from the point of view of function. "Too much function or too little function—illness can really be simplified in this way," says Dr. Ni.

Treatments in Traditional Chinese Medicine

Herbs are a primary part of a TCM treatment. A prescription consists of generous piles of ingredients, distributed in paper packets containing one-day or two-day doses. The visually intriguing ingredients— perhaps bark, roots, or oyster shell—come from the vegetable, animal, and mineral kingdoms. The formulas may contain from 6 to 19 different substances and are assembled with great care. These are prescribed to treat the root of the disease and its manifestation, and the formula must also be balanced within itself.

Although the herbs are taken internally as decoctions (herbs boiled in water), TCM doctors also prescribe pills, powders, syrups, tinctures, inhalants, suppositories, enemas, douches, soaks, plasters, poultices, and salves. Specific foods may also be part of the protocol.

Acupuncture is also extensively used in traditional Chinese medicine. Using the meridian system and its thousands of corresponding surface points, acupuncture uses special needles placed strategically into these "acupoints" to help correct and rebalance the flow of energy within the specific meridian, consequently relieving pain and restoring health. Moxibustion, the burning of special "moxa" herbs on or above a specific acupoint, is another technique TCM employs.

Massage and manipulation are integral parts of the modern practice of TCM, including professional remedial massage therapies such as osteopathic and chiropractic adjustments. "There are many different massages in Chinese medicine," says Dr. Ni. "We have one massage called *Tui Na*, which is a combination of acupressure, massage, and manipulation.

"The purpose of massage is not dissimilar to acupuncture, in that the whole goal is to promote the flow of *qi* and to remove blockages, thereby alleviating any imbalances." Dr. Ni adds that massage is most often used in conjunction with other treatment therapies, such as acupuncture. "They are often used together for musculoskeletal problems such as a sprain."

Qigong and other therapeutic exercises are another aspect of TCM, particularly as a means of stress reduction and preventative therapy. Meditative relaxation, calisthenics, internal energy exercises, and the laying on of hands are all incorporated into the overall Chinese medicine approach, along with an emphasis on spiritual meditation.

With early diagnosis and TCM treatment, not only can hypertension be alleviated, but complications including damage to the heart, brain, kidneys, and liver can be prevented.

Conditions Treated by
Traditional Chinese Medicine

Traditional Chinese medicine addresses the full range of human illness. While best known for treating chronic illnesses such as high blood pressure, asthma, allergies, headaches, gallbladder disease, lupus, diabetes, and gynecological disorders, TCM also treats acute, infectious illness. Extensive research is continuously being pursued in a wide range of TCM applications and reported on in scores of medical journals published around the world.[3] Research has shown that TCM can effectively complement modern Western medicine when the two systems are used in concert for acute, chronic, or life-threatening diseases.[4]

According to TCM, high blood pressure is usually due to a problem in the circulation of energy (*qi*) in the body. Diet and long-term emotional distress such as chronic nervousness, anger, and depression can lead to this condition. "Treatment is aimed at bringing the energy flow of the body back into balance through a combination of acupuncture and herbs," says Harvey Kaltsas, Ac. Phys. (FL), D.Ac. (RI), Dipl. Ac. (NCCA), of Sarasota, Florida, former president of the American Association of Acupuncture and Oriental Medicine.

"Secondary hypertension often occurs when the energy reserves become exhausted (called 'kidney yin deficiency' in traditional Chinese medicine), and can also be treated with a combination of acupuncture and herbs to build up and restore one's energy."

With early diagnosis and treatment, not only can hypertension be alleviated, but complications including damage to the heart, brain, kidneys, and liver can be prevented. In addition to acupuncture and herbs, other important elements of treatment include exercises such as qigong, meditation, and a diet high in vegetables and low in fat, sugar, and alcohol.

Mark T. Holmes, O.M.D., L.Ac., director of the Center for Regeneration in Beverly Hills, California, relates two cases in which TCM successfully controlled hypertension. The first case involved a 46-year-old white male attorney with essential hypertension, whose

High Blood Pressure Reversed with Chinese Herbs

D r. Wu, a famous Chinese physician, was visited by a 42-year-old man who had been diagnosed with hypertension and the early stages of coronary heart disease. He complained of throbbing temples and soreness at the top of his head. An examination identified the following elements: red (not pink) tongue, dark yellow urine, constipation, poor appetite, painful teeth and eyes, insomnia, pain on the right side of the body, and excessive dreaming. His pulse was "wiry and sinking." The man was diagnosed with "constrained liver *qi* accompanied by liver fire ascending to disturb the head."

The treatment called for harmonizing the liver, cooling the liver fire, and transforming mucus. Twelve herbs were given as a tea for three days and another combination for nine additional days. With this treatment, the patient's blood pressure dropped from 180/130 to 130/90, well within normal range, and soon all his symptoms disappeared. A final herbal prescription was then given. The patient then took this for a longer period of time to ensure that his blood pressure remained normal.

blood pressure was 160/90. Additional symptoms included impotence, insomnia, red eyes, nervousness, and a decreased desire to exercise.

An inability to relax after work, combined with a nightly habit of drinking two bottles of wine were determined to be causative factors. Laboratory tests revealed elevated liver enzymes. In TCM this is referred to as a "flaring up of liver fire." After seven months of daily herbal intake combined with regular acupuncture treatments, the patient's hypertension was reversed, his incidence of impotency was significantly reduced, and all the other symptoms abated.

Dr. Holmes also successfully treated an 80-year-old woman suffering from secondary hypertension. Her blood pressure was unusually high, around 210/90. With conventional drugs, it dropped moderately to 180/90. Using Chinese herbs combined with bimonthly acupuncture and homeopathic remedies, Dr. Holmes was able to stabilize her blood pressure at 130-140/85. A subsequent Western clinical examination revealed a 20% increase of carotid artery circulation.

Traditional Chinese medicine also introduces a major component of the body, *qi* (also referred to as chi), that Western medicine does not even acknowledge. *Qi*, according to Dr. Ni, is difficult to define. "We call it life force. It is all-inclusive of the many types of energy within the body and is essential for life itself," he says. This vital life energy flows through the body following pathways called meridians.

CHAPTER

12

Lower Your Blood Pressure With Herbs

MANY BOTANICALS and herbs have hypotensive (blood pressure–lowering) properties. These include garlic, ginseng, hawthorn, valerian, maitake and other medicinal mushrooms, and noni, discussed in this chapter. In many cases, the correct use of simple herbs can make a clinically important difference in the status of your blood pressure and make the use of harsh conventional drugs entirely unnecessary.

Garlic (*Allium sativum*)

Garlic is probably the most well-recognized medicinal herb. According to David Hoffmann, B.Sc., M.N.I.M.H., of Sebastopol, California, eating a clove of raw garlic daily will help considerably in preventing or reversing the effects of high blood pressure. While garlic has been used for centuries in traditional cultures throughout the world as a multipurpose medicinal food, in recent decades more than 2,000 clinical studies have validated many of the folk-healing claims for "the stinking rose," as garlic was once called.

Prominent among these substantiated claims is garlic's ability to lower blood pressure, inhibit cholesterol production, promote blood circulation, and discourage clot formation. Yu-Yan Yeh, Ph.D., of the Department of Nutrition at Pennsylvania State University, reviewed extensive multi-laboratory studies on garlic's ability to reduce cardiovascular disease and concluded, "Collectively, the results suggest that garlic may lower the risk for this disease by reducing plasma lipids, lowering blood pressure, and depressing platelet adhesion and aggregation [clotting]."

A scientific panel of the European community has endorsed garlic for its cardiovascular benefits.[1] In Germany, garlic extracts are approved over-the-counter drugs to supplement dietary measures in patients with elevated blood lipid (fat) levels and to avert age-associated vascular changes."[2]

In a Chinese study, 70 patients with clinically diagnosed high blood pressure took garlic oil for several weeks. At the end of the study, 35 registered a "marked" lowering of their blood pressure, while another 14 subjects experienced "moderate" drops. Garlic can not only lower high blood pressure, but apparently elevate low blood pressure as well, leading researchers to propose that its true effect is in *normalizing* blood pressure.

Prominent among the substantiated healing claims of garlic is its ability to lower blood pressure, inhibit cholesterol production, promote blood circulation, and discourage clot formation.

In a study published in *Atherosclerosis*, 20 patients with elevated levels of lipoproteins took garlic for four weeks. At the end of the period, all subjects showed a 10% drop in blood pressure and blood cholesterol levels. Researchers studying a vegetarian community in India found that those who consumed "liberal" amounts of garlic (and onions) had an average of 25% lower cholesterol levels than those who did not.

A study directed by Benjamin H.S. Lau, M.D., Ph.D., of the School of Medicine at Loma Linda University in Loma Linda, California, studied the effect of garlic supplementation on 32 subjects with high cholesterol.[3] During the six-month study, subjects took four capsules daily of liquid garlic extract, after which time cholesterol levels had returned to normal in 65% of the participants. More specifically, levels of HDL cholesterol (believed to protect the heart) rose steadily, while levels of LDL cholesterol (believed to harm the heart) dropped. Garlic appears to produce its cholesterol-lowering effect by slowing down the synthesis of cholesterol by the liver in the first place.

Garlic has also been shown to promote blood circulation, both peripheral (to the hands and feet) and "microcirculation" (into the tiniest capillaries). It can also interrupt the harmful tendency of the

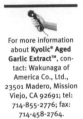

platelets and fibrin in the blood to form clots, a condition associated with heart attacks and stroke. Researchers reported in the *Journal of the American College of Nutrition* (October 1994) the results of a clinical study involving 45 men, 30-70 years old, with high cholesterol levels. Of this group, 66% received "beneficial effects" in these levels and in platelet activity after taking garlic extract (at 700 mg, nine times daily for six months). The result was "cardiovascular risk reduction."

According to Brenda Lynn Petesch, nutritionist with Wakunaga of America Co., Ltd., manufacturers of Kyolic® Aged Garlic Extract™, garlic can prevent the spread of smooth muscle cells in blood vessels that would otherwise further the progression of heart disease. Petesch also notes that a recent Australian study showed that garlic extract "may afford protection against the onset of atherosclerosis [hardening of the arteries]."

Finally, with respect to existing heart conditions, dietary garlic may reduce the risk of having a second heart attack as well as the general risk of dying from heart disease. Over a study period of three years, based on a group of 432 subjects, regular use of garlic reduced the rate of repeat heart attack by 30% in the second year and by 60% in the third year . Researchers proposed that garlic's benefit is cumulative, building with continuous use.[4]

Studies indicate general benefits from almost any type of garlic, be it raw garlic, dried garlic, garlic oil, or a prepared commercial product, such as the odorless or odor-controlled garlic preparations which enable the user to avoid the bad breath associated with garlic consumption.[5] However, garlic liquid extract that has been aged for at least one year appears to produce better results than fresh raw garlic. A Bulgarian study on cats showed that fresh garlic juice produced only a "slight and temporary" decrease, while aged garlic extract produced more significant and sustained drops in blood pressure.

Ginseng (*Panax ginseng*, Oriental ginseng; *Panax quinquefolius*, American ginseng)

Ginseng has an ancient history and has accumulated much folklore about its actions and uses. The genus name *Panax* is derived from the Latin word panacea, meaning "cure-all." Many of the claims that surround ginseng are exaggerated but it is clearly an important remedy, receiving attention from researchers around the world.[6] It is a powerful adaptogen (supporter of the adrenal glands),[7] aiding the body to cope with stress.[8] In addition, ginseng may lower blood cholesterol.[9] If

After eight weeks on hawthorn, the blood pressure of 40 heart patients dropped from an average of 171/115 to 164/110 and their ability to tolerate the heart stress of physical work increased.

ginseng is abused, however, side effects can occur, including headaches, skin problems, and other reactions. For this reason, the proper dosage for the individual should be determined and respected.

Hawthorn (*Crataegus oxyacantha*)

Hawthorn has been used in folk medicine in Europe and China for centuries. Europeans have employed both the edible fruit as well as the leaves and flowers, primarily for their beneficial effects on the cardiovascular system. Hawthorn is one of the primary heart tonics in traditional medicine. Fruit and leaf extracts are known for their cardiotonic, sedative, and hypotensive (blood pressure–lowering) activities.

Hawthorn has been extensively tested on animals and humans and is known to cause: a decrease in blood pressure with exertion; increase in heart muscle contractility (the ability to contract or shorten); increase in blood flow to the heart muscle; decrease in heart rate; and decrease in oxygen use by the myocardium (the middle layer of the walls of the heart).[10] In Germany, hawthorn extracts are used clinically for a number of heart-related conditions, often in conjunction with digoxin, the primary conventional pharmaceutical drug. Hawthorn extracts are approved by the German Ministry of Health for declining heart performance, sensations of pressure or restrictions in the heart area, senile heart in cases where digitalis is not yet required, and mild forms of bradyarrhythmia (slow heartbeat).[11]

"An infusion of hawthorn berries drunk twice daily is a gentle and effective way of helping the body to normalize blood pressure," says David Hoffmann. "The infusion can be strengthened by combining linden flowers or by adding chamomile or valerian, if tension or headaches are present."

In a study conducted by A. Schmidt, M.D., of Cologne, Germany, 40 patients (average age, 60) with high blood pressure and "stable coronary insufficiency" took doses of hawthorn extract at the rate of 200 mg, three times daily, for eight weeks. Before taking the hawthorn, they tired easily and had diminished physical ability, but after eight weeks on hawthorn, these symptoms occurred 42% fewer times. Blood pressure dropped from 171/115 to 164/110 and the patients' ability to tolerate the heart stress of physical work increased.

QUICK DEFINITION

Adaptogens are substances that provide a nonspecific effect on the entire body by increasing resistance to stress and toxins (physical, chemical, or biological) and promoting a balancing or normalizing condition. The key function of adaptogens is support for the adrenal glands, which are located near the kidneys and are activated in response to stress. Chronic stress can overwhelm the adrenals, leading to symptoms including fatigue, reduced immune function, and poor blood sugar metabolism. Adaptogens help reinvigorate and support the adrenals, enabling the body to deal more effectively with stress. In addition to adrenal support, adaptogens enhance central nervous system activity, provide protection for the liver, act as antioxidants, and increase stamina. Herbs that are considered adaptogenic include Asian and Siberian ginseng, *Ashwagandha*, Astragalus, *Codonopsis ("Dangshen")*, and *Schizandra*.

In a related study by German physicians K. Bödigheimer, M.D., and D. Chase, M.D., 36 patients (average age, 61) who had angina, a history of heart attacks and arrhythmia, and who were 20% overweight, took 300 mg daily of hawthorn extract for 28 days. As a result, their cardiovascular health and performance improved, both during the stress of exercise and the rest period.[12]

Siberian Ginseng or Eleuthero (*Eleutherococcus senticosus*)

Siberian ginseng is one of the best adaptogen herbs, increasing the body's ability to resist and endure stress. This herb has a very low toxicity. A wealth of clinical and laboratory research has been conducted on Siberian ginseng in the former Soviet Union. Initial findings from controlled experiments indicate a dramatic reduction of total disease occurrence, especially in diseases related to environmental stress.[13] There is a long list of illnesses that improve with the use of this herb, including chronic gastritis, diabetes, and atherosclerosis (hardening of the arteries).

Valerian (*Valeriana officinalis*)

The odorous root of valerian has been used in European traditional medicine as a stimulant for centuries. In Germany, valerian root and its teas and extracts are approved as over-the-counter medicines for "states of excitation" and "difficulty in falling asleep owing to nervousness."[14] A scientific team representing the European community has reviewed the scientific research on valerian and concluded that it is a safe nighttime sleep aid.

These scientists also found that there are no major adverse reactions associated with the use of valerian and, unlike barbiturates and other conventional drugs used for insomnia, valerian does not have a synergy with alcohol,[15] meaning it is safe to have a drink while taking valerian. Herbalist Christopher Hobbs, L.Ac., founder of the American School of Herbalism, notes that other uses for valerian include application for nervous heart conditions. He recommends a valerian-hops preparation as a daytime sedative, as it will not interfere with or slow one's reflexive responses.[16]

A 73-year-old man saw his blood pressure drop from 170 to 128 after taking four grams of maitake daily for only three weeks. A heavy drinker, 48, dropped his blood pressure from 180 to 130 in only two weeks at the rate of three grams daily of maitake.

Other Useful Botanicals

Maitake Mushroom

Prized for centuries by Japanese herbalists for its ability to strengthen health, Maitake mushroom (which means "dancing mushroom") is now being investigated in Japan and America for its healing abilities in a number of diseases, including hypertension.

Maitake is available in tablet form as Grifron® from: Maitake Products, P.O. Box 1354, Paramus, NJ 07653; tel: 800-747-7418.

In over 30 cases, maitake mushrooms gradually decreased high blood pressure to normal levels.[17] A woman, 61, had taken hypotensive drugs for 20 years but could never get her systolic blood pressure lower than 150; it was usually 190. After taking maitake at five grams daily for 30 days, it went down to 130. A 73-year-old man saw his blood pressure drop from 170 to 128 after taking four grams daily for only three weeks. A diabetic man, 45, reduced his blood glucose from 139 to 80 and his blood pressure from 165 to 132 after only three weeks, taking four grams daily. A heavy drinker, 48, dropped his blood pressure from 180 to 130 in only two weeks of taking three grams daily of maitake.

Reishi Mushroom

Chinese herbal medicine physicians regard the reishi mushroom as an "elixir of immortality." Research confirms that reishi is an effective cardiotonic. In a study of 54 people (average age, 58.6) whose blood pressure was over 140/90 and who were unresponsive to hypertension medication, those taking reishi mushroom extract in tablet form three times a day for four weeks experienced a significant drop in their blood pressure compared to the control group.[18] The blood pressure of all the test subjects fell below 140/90.

Tahitian Noni

Among the lay healers of Tahiti, the reputation of the noni fruit (*Morinda citrifolia*) as a medicinal food ranks high. The plant itself is found throughout French Polynesia and can grow as high as 20 feet,

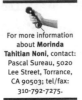

For more information about **Morinda** **Tahitian Noni**, contact: Pascal Sureau, 5020 Lee Street, Torrance, CA 90503; tel/fax: 310-792-7275.

bearing noni fruits the size of potatoes. In Malaysia, it is known as *Mengkudu* and is used for urinary problems, coughs, and painful menstruation, while in the Caribbean, people know it as the Pain Killer Tree. People throughout the region have long used the noni fruit as a dietary staple.

Anecdotal reports suggest that juice from this fruit can be significantly helpful in numerous health conditions, such as hypertension, wounds and infections, ulcers, skin rashes, digestive disorders, colds, influenza, arthritis, and cancer. Mitchell Tate, director of the Center for Lifestyle Disease in St. George, Utah, reports that while researching noni at the University of Honolulu in Hawaii (noni also grows in Hawaii), he found that "a significant amount of research had been done on the plant and that most of it substantiated claims by the Tahitians." One study confirmed the belief that noni helps lower blood pressure.

Research by R.M. Heinicke, Ph.D., at the University of Hawaii, suggests that the active ingredient in noni is xeronine, a digestive enzyme similar to bromelain in pineapple. Dr. Heinicke emphasizes that noni must be consumed on an empty stomach, preferably upon rising in the morning, for the enzyme to become activated by the intestines. Dr. Heinicke believes that, once activated, xeronine helps to repair damaged cells by regulating the rigidity and shape of particular proteins comprising those cells. "Since these proteins have different functions within the cells, this explains how the administration of noni juice causes a wide range of physiological responses," states Dr. Heinicke.

According to Morinda, the product's manufacturer, about 25% of the users of noni experience a noticeable difference after using the drink for three weeks, while 50% notice benefits after three to eight weeks of daily use. Mitchell Tate suggests a daily dosage of two tablespoons for general health maintenance, but three to four tablespoons daily for an existing health condition.

In a study published in *Atherosclerosis*, 20 patients with elevated levels of lipoproteins took garlic for four weeks. At the end of the period, all subjects showed a 10% drop in blood pressure and blood cholesterol levels. Researchers studying a vegetarian community in India found that those who consumed "liberal" amounts of garlic (and onions) had an average of 25% lower cholesterol levels than those who did not.

Alternative Medicine Options

FOR LOWERING HIGH BLOOD PRESSURE

I N A D D I T I O N to the therapies for high blood pressure covered in the preceding chapters and those for general heart health and heart disease discussed in Part One, the following alternative treatment methods can be effective for preventing and reversing high blood pressure.

Aromatherapy

Victor Marcial-Vega, M.D., of Miami, Florida, relates a case of successfully lowering blood pressure using aromatherapy. Martin had dangerously high blood pressure, topping 182/130. After taking his blood pressure and recording this level, Dr. Marcial-Vega asked Martin to gently inhale the aroma of ylang-ylang essential oil after rubbing it on his palms. After breathing its vapor for only five minutes, Martin's blood pressure dropped to 135/80. Dr. Marcial-Vega recommends applying the oil onto the palms, rather than on a cloth, because whatever is not inhaled as aroma is absorbed directly through the skin.

As often as five times a day, Dr. Marcial-Vega himself daubs a few drops of an essential oil on his palms, rubs it in, cups his palms around his nose, and gently inhales.

Before and after patients occupy his office, he mists the air with a blend of various aromas such as lavender, tea tree, eucalyptus, or myrrh (dispersed in water), all of which have strong actions against ambient bacteria, viruses, or fungi. Equal parts of ylang-ylang, orange, or patchouli oils also impart a cleansing atmosphere. When patients arrive and inhale the aromas, they are likely to relax, facilitating their recovery. Dr. Marcial-Vega also recommends a foot bath or full-body soak as an antidote to stress. Take a large Pyrex glass tray, fill it with warm water, dribble in a few drops of lavender oil, and immerse your feet for 20 minutes. Similarly, you can fill a bath and disperse five drops of a single oil or a blend into the water, and soak yourself until you feel relaxed.

Aromatherapy is More than Aroma

Aromatherapy is a unique branch of herbal medicine that utilizes the medicinal properties found in the essential oils of various plants. Through a process of steam distillation or cold-pressing, the volatile constituents of the plant's oil (its essence) are extracted from its flowers, leaves, branches, or roots. According to Dr. (rer. nat.) Kurt Schnaubelt, director of the Pacific Institute of Aromatherapy, the term "aromatherapy" is somewhat misleading, as it can suggest an exclusive role for the aroma in the healing process. "In actuality," says Dr. Schnaubelt, "the oils exert much of their therapeutic effect through their pharmacological properties and their small molecular size, making them one of the few therapeutic agents to easily penetrate bodily tissues."

Aromatherapy has been used to lower blood pressure and is highly effective for bacterial infections of the respiratory system,[1] immune deficiencies such as Epstein-Barr virus (a form of herpes virus believed to be the causative agent in infectious mononucleosis), and numerous skin disorders.[2] The immediate and often profound effect that essential oils have on the central nervous system also makes aromatherapy an excellent method for stress management[3] and therefore of additional benefit in the treatment of hypertension.

History of Aromatherapy

Plants and their essential oils have been used therapeutically from ancient times in countries as diverse as Egypt, Italy, India, and China.[4] In most of the world, plant essences remain popular as therapeutic

CAUTION

Dr. Marcial-Vega cautions however that not every version of ylang-ylang oil will produce this remarkable result in five minutes. You need to use oils that are pure and of the highest quality to achieve these effects. People with low blood pressure should not use ylang-ylang oil in this way because it could further lower their blood pressure. Dr. Marcial-Vega reports using this oil with many people with normal to high blood pressure, without side effects.

For more about aromatherapy applications, contact: Victor Marcial-Vega, M.D., 4037 Poinciana Avenue, Miami, FL 33133; tel: 305-442-1233; fax: 305-445-4504. For information about the aromatherapy oils, contact: Phyto Medicine Company, 6701 Sunset Drive, Suite 100, Miami, FL 33143; tel: 305-662-6396; fax: 305-667-5619.

Research shows that oils such as orange, jasmine, and rose have a tranquilizing effect and work by altering the brain waves into a rhythm that produces calmness and a sense of well-being. In the same way, the so-called stimulating oils—basil, black pepper, rosemary, and cardamom—work by producing a heightened energy response.

agents and are utilized in everything from antiseptic creams and skin ointments to liniments for arthritic pain.

The term aromatherapy was coined in 1937 by the French chemist René-Maurice Gattefossé. While working in his family's perfume laboratory, Dr. Gattefossé burned his hand. He knew lavender was used in medicine for burns and inflammation, and immediately immersed his hand in a container of pure lavender oil he had on his workbench. When the burn quickly lost its redness and began to heal, he was impressed enough by the oil's regenerative ability to begin researching the curative powers of other essential oils. This marked the beginning of the modern-day science of aromatherapy for the treatment of common ailments. In the United States, the popularity of aromatherapy

Limbic system of the brain

Olfactory neurons

Olfactory bulb

Nasal cavity

Airborne odor molecules

Aromas affect the *limbic system*, which is connected to the part of the brain that controls heart rate, blood pressure, and stress levels.

has grown rapidly over the last ten years, fueled by the increasing demand for nontoxic restorative therapies.

How Aromatherapy Works

According to Dr. Schnaubelt, "The chemical makeup of essential oils gives them a host of desirable pharmacological properties ranging from antibacterial, antiviral, and antispasmodic to use as diuretics (promoting production and excretion of urine), vasodilators (widening blood vessels), and vasoconstrictors (narrowing blood vessels). Essential oils act on the adrenal glands, ovaries, and the thyroid and can energize or pacify, detoxify, and facilitate the digestive process." The oils' therapeutic properties also make them effective for treating infection, interacting with the various branches of the nervous system, modifying immune response, and harmonizing moods and emotions.

Aromatic molecules that interact with the top of the nasal cavity give off signals that are modified by various biological processes before traveling to the limbic system, the emotional switchboard of the brain.[5] There they create impressions associated with previous experiences and emotions.

After breathing ylang-ylang oil vapor for only five minutes, Martin's blood pressure dropped from 182/130 to 135/80.

The limbic system is directly connected to those parts of the brain that control heart rate, blood pressure, breathing, memory, stress levels, and hormone balance. As scientists have learned, oil fragrances may be one of the fastest ways to achieve physiological or psychological effects.

John Steele, Ph.D., of Sherman Oaks, California, and Robert Tisserand, of London, England, leading researchers in the field of aromatherapy, have studied the effects on brain-wave patterns when essential oils are inhaled or smelled. Their findings show that oils such as orange, jasmine, and rose have a tranquilizing effect and work by altering the brain waves into a rhythm that produces calmness and a sense of well-being. In the same way, the so-called stimulating oils—basil, black pepper, rosemary, and cardamom—work by producing a heightened energy response.[6]

Inhaling the fragrance of certain essential oils can help clear sinuses or free congestion in the chest, as well as alter the neurochemistry of the brain to produce changes in mental and emotional behavior. Even aromas too subtle to be consciously detected can have significant effects on central nervous system activity, sometimes to the point of cutting in half the amount of time needed to perform a visual search task.[7]

Conditions Benefited by Aromatherapy

The value of aromatherapy in the treatment of infectious diseases has gained increased attention in recent years. Its use for this purpose is widespread in France, where a system of aromatherapeutic medicine has been developed.[8] French physicians routinely prescribe aromatherapy preparations, and French pharmacies stock essential oils alongside the more conventional drugs. In England, aromatherapy is used mainly for stress-related health issues. Hospital nursing staffs administer essential-oil massage to relieve stress and pain and to induce sleep.[9] English hospitals also use a variety of vaporized essential oils (including lemon, lavender, and lemongrass) to help combat the transmission of airborne infectious diseases.[10] Essential oils are also used topically on wound sites to counter infection.

Essential oils like citronella and *Eucalyptus citriodora* can be diffused in the air or rubbed on the wrists, solar plexus, and temples for quick and effective relaxation. Mandarin is a fragrance favored by children, and its calming qualities can slow hyperactivity. Lavender oil added to the bath or sprayed on the bed sheets reduces tension and enhances relaxation.[11] Roman chamomile (*Anthemis nobilis*) is also recommended to calm an upset mind or body. A drop rubbed on the solar plexus can bring rapid relief of mental or physical stress.

CAUTION

In their pure state, certain oils, such as clove and cinnamon, can cause irritation or skinburn. These oils call for careful and expert application. It is recommended that they be diluted with a less irritating essential oil before being applied to the skin. Essential oils can cause a toxic reaction if ingested. Consult a physician before taking any oils internally.

For more information about **aromaSpa™** aromatic steam capsule, contact: Variel Health International, 9618 Variel Avenue, Chatsworth, CA 91311; tel: 818-407-4717; fax: 818-407-0738. The single-seater "Serene" unit sells for about $1500; the two-seater "Gemini" model sells for about $2300.

Aromatherapy Spa: Detoxify, Relax Muscles, and Enhance Immunity

Physicians have long known of the many therapeutic benefits of steam heat, also known as hyperthermia or heat stress detoxification. Similarly, the benefits of aromatherapy—the inhalation of the vapors of essential plant oils—are widely recognized among alternative practitioners. Now, Variel Health International has combined both modalities in the form of the aromaSpa™ aromatic steam capsule, suitable for home use as a portable health spa.

The unit stands 5'6", weighs about 68 pounds, may be easily disassembled, and plugs into any standard 115-volt socket. Its walls and sliding door are made of transparent polycarbonate, used to make airplane windows. The steam generator and aroma diffuser are located on the floor of the unit. Any of at least 250 aromatherapy oils may be used, singly or in combination, to support muscle relaxation, detoxification, and immune system stimulation, or for eliminating fatigue, lifting mood, revitalizing skin, or general rejuvenation.

Other self-care benefits include general mind and body relaxation, stress reduction, energizing, emotional cleansing, and "customized personal pampering," depending on the aromatherapy formula used, says Variel's Cathy Dammann.

In the self-contained aromatherapy and steam heat diffuser, soothing mists carrying aromatic molecules envelop the entire body surface for maximum absorption and benefit.

The aromaSpa uses one quart of distilled water (preferable to chlorinated and fluoridated tap water) for a 40-minute steam heat session, and inside temperatures can reach 115°-120° within about 10 minutes. These temperatures are necessary, as hyperthermia provides its benefits by temporarily raising the body temperature to between 101° and 103° and inducing perspiration. Clinical information suggests that steam heat may have therapeutic advantages over the dry heat associated with most saunas, says Dammann.

The aromaSpa was tested in 1994 by Jerry Schindler, Ph.D., director

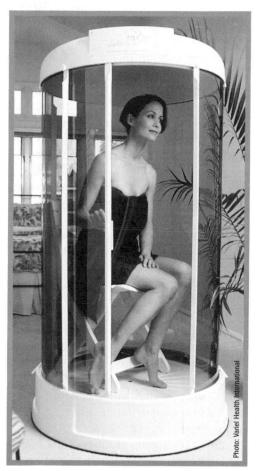

Photo: Variel Health International

Steam heat therapy using aromatherapy essences may increase blood circulation and heighten immune response by stimulating white blood cell production.

of the Sports Health Science Human Performance Lab at Life College School of Chiropractic in Marietta, Georgia. Dr. Schindler reported that the unit was effective in decreasing the risk of everyday and athletic injuries, primarily by increasing muscle flexibility, blood flow, and oxygen delivery to the muscles. Dr. Schindler demonstrated these benefits by way of thermographic studies (which register nerve sense pathways) comparing the left and right sides of a test subject's body. Individuals whose thermographic readings are asymmetrical (indicating imbalances and sensory interference) are prone to injury, says Dr. Schindler. Symmetrical patterns were achieved after 30 minutes in the aromaSpa.

According to Dammann, aroma steam therapy can also reduce lactic acid buildup in muscles following exercise, thereby preventing soreness. The approach may be effective in reducing cellulite (lumpy fat areas in the skin), especially when used with rosemary, sandalwood, juniper, geranium, or lemon essential oils. These can produce detoxifying and water-draining effects in only 10 minutes, compared to standard hot body wraps, which require 60 minutes, says Dammann.

Steam heat therapy may increase blood circulation and heighten immune response by stimulating white blood cell production, Dammann says. The aromaSpa is now being used experimentally by patients with chronic fatigue syndrome, she reports. According to Zand Gard, M.D., "the only detoxification program that has proven successful in removing fat-stored toxins from the body is hyperthermia." The use of the essential oils of clove, cinnamon, melissa, and lavender has been clinically shown to benefit bronchial conditions as effectively as antibiotics, especially when delivered by steam heat, Dammann says.

How to Use Aromatherapy

Aromatherapy uses essential oils to affect the body in several ways. The benefits of essential oils can be obtained through inhalation, external application, or ingestion.

■ Through a diffusor: Diffusors disperse microparticles of the essential oil into the air. They can be used to achieve beneficial results in respiratory conditions, or to simply change the air with the mood-lifting or calming qualities of the fragrance.

■ External application: Oils are readily absorbed through the skin. Convenient applications are baths, massages, hot and cold compresses, or a simple topical application of diluted oils.[12] Essential oils in a hot bath can stimulate the skin, induce relaxation, and energize the body. According to Debra Nuzzi St. Claire, M.H., an aromatherapist and herbalist from Boulder, Colorado, using certain essential oils, such as rosemary, in the bath can stimulate the elimination of toxins through the skin. In massage, the oils can be worked into the skin and, depending on the oil and the massage technique, can either calm or stimulate an individual. When used in compresses, essential oils soothe minor aches and pains, reduce swelling, and treat sprains.

■ Floral waters: These can be sprayed into the air or sprayed on skin that is too sensitive to the touch.

■ Internal application: For certain conditions (such as organ dysfunction/disorder), it can be advantageous to take oils internally. It is essential to receive proper medical guidance for internal use of oils. However, such professional guidance is difficult to obtain in the United States.

Purchasing Oils

Aromatherapy is ideally suited for home use. While it is true that irresponsible or ignorant use of essential oils may pose certain risks, these risks are small compared to the potential gain. Typical problems are caused by excessive use of potentially irritating or allergenic oils such as clove, cinnamon, oregano, or savory, but with proper knowledge these pitfalls are easily avoided.

Most health food stores now carry essential oils, and many even carry "starter kits" with selections of the most widely used essential oils. However, selecting essential oils from the many different offerings in the marketplace can be confusing. Vast differences in price exist for what seems to be the same oil. Inquiries are often met with the universal assurance that the oil is absolutely pure and natural. This is not always the case. Many suppliers do not verify the purity of the oils they distribute. When purchasing essential oils, it is important to take note of their purity, quality, and price.

"Pure essential oils are expensive," according to Dr. Schnaubelt. "Often 1,000 pounds of plant are needed to produce one pound of essence. This process involves manpower to cultivate and harvest the plant, and the energy cost for distillation. Because of the variations in these factors, the prices of essential oils can differ. If every oil in a line carries the same price tag, this is a sure sign of large-scale homogenization and adulteration for the production of sheer fragrance oils as opposed to essential oils.

"Essential oils should be called 'essential oils'. If names are used that sound evasive, such as 'pure botanical perfume' or 'pure fragrance essence,' this is an indication that the supplier is aware that the oils are

The greatest successes in controlling hypertension are with patients who combine biofeedback training with other forms of relaxation, visualization, exercise, and a low-salt diet.

not true essential oils," adds Dr. Schnaubelt. Oil essences are most commonly produced to create fragrances and to process food. The quality requirements of these oils are substantially lower than of those used for aromatherapy. Companies that concern themselves solely with aromatherapy will go to great lengths to ensure purity.

While pure, natural essential oils may seem expensive, the smallest amounts will go far, and this makes them cost-effective. In contrast, the effectiveness of lower-grade oils, or oils that are diluted, drastically diminishes over time due to a loss of their essential properties.

The best way to purchase essential oils for aromatherapy applications is from a supplier who specializes in essential aromatherapy oils.

Ayurvedic Medicine

Ayurvedic medicine treats hypertension according to metabolic type. According to Virender Sodhi, M.D. (Ayurveda), N.D., director of the American School of Ayurvedic Sciences in Bellevue, Washington, hypertension is found most often in *pitta* and *kapha* types and is usually due to a combination of genetics and lifestyle. Patients of Dr. Sodhi are put on a diet low in sodium, cholesterol, and triglycerides (the latter cause the blood to become viscous and therefore raise blood pressure).

Yogic breathing exercises help to relax the body and stimulate the cardiovascular system, effectively reducing hypertension, says Dr. Sodhi. "Breathing first with one nostril, then the other for ten to 15 minutes, two to three times a day is highly effective in lowering blood pressure. I have patients try this in the office, and after ten minutes, their blood pressure drops considerably," he adds.

Herbs also play an important role in treating hypertension. Herbs are usually used in combinations, depending on the patient's individual needs, and are often combined with rose water and minerals such as calcium, magnesium, silicon, and zinc.

According to Dr. Sodhi, the following herbs are indicated for hypertension: *Convolvulus pluricaulis* has a calming effect, reduces anxiety and anger, and lowers serum cholesterol while increasing high-density lipoproteins (this

For information about **Ayurvedic health products**, contact: Maharish Ayurvedic Products International, P.O. Box 49667, Colorado Springs, CO 80949-9667; tel: 719-260-5500 or 800-255-8332; fax: 719-260-7400.

helps to improve circulation and lower blood pressure). *Ashwaganda* also has a calming effect and helps to reduce stress and thus blood pressure. Coral in rose water is an excellent tonic for the heart, as it contains calcium and magnesium, which are usually deficient in hypertensives.

Biofeedback

The idea that a person can learn to modify his or her own vital functions is relatively new. Before the 1960s, most scientists believed that autonomic functions, such as heart rate and pulse, digestion, blood pressure, brain waves, and muscle behavior, could not be voluntarily controlled. Recently, biofeedback, along with other methods of self-regulation such as guided imagery, progressive relaxation, and meditation, has found widespread acceptance among physiologists and psychologists alike.

Biofeedback training is a method of learning how to consciously regulate normally unconscious bodily functions (such as heart rate, blood pressure, and breathing) in order to improve overall health. It refers to any process that measures and reports back immediate information about the biological system of the person being monitored so he or she can learn to consciously influence that system.

How Biofeedback Works

Instrumented biofeedback was pioneered by O. Hobart Mowrer in 1938, when he used an alarm system triggered by urine to stop bed-wetting in children. But it was not until the late 1960s, when Barbara Brown, Ph.D., of the Veterans Administration Hospital in Sepulveda, California, and Elmer Green, Ph.D., and Alyce Green of the Menninger Foundation in Topeka, Kansas, used EEG biofeedback to observe and record the altered states/self-regulation of yogis, that biofeedback began to attract widespread attention.

A person seeking to regulate his or her heart rate trains with a biofeedback device set up to transmit one blinking light or one audible beep per heartbeat. By learning to alter the rate of the flashes and beeps, the subject is subtly programmed to control the heart rate. "The self-regulation skills acquired through

Ayurveda is the traditional medicine of India, based on many centuries of empirical use. Its name means "end of the Vedas" (which were India's sacred scripts), implying that a holistic medicine may be founded on spiritual principles. Ayurveda describes three metabolic, constitutional, and body types (*doshas*), in association with the basic elements of Nature— *vata, pitta,* and *kapha*—and uses them as the basis for prescribing individualized formulas of herbs, diet, massage, and detoxification techniques.

Rauwolfia and its extract, reserpine, are particularly useful in helping to regulate blood pressure. Care must be taken when prescribing rauwolfia and reserpine, however, because they can depress the central nervous system, and should not be given to patients suffering from depression.

By teaching self-regulation skills, biofeedback can allow patients to take more control of their health and help prevent disorders that can result in costly medical procedures.

biofeedback training are retained by the individual even after the feedback device is dispensed with," explains Patricia Norris, Ph.D., biofeedback specialist in private practice and former clinical director of the Biofeedback and Psychophysiology Clinic at the Center for Applied Psychophysiology at the Menninger Clinic in Topeka, Kansas. "In fact, with practice, biofeedback skills continue to improve. It is like taking tennis lessons. If you stop taking the lessons but continue playing, your game will improve. With biofeedback, it works the same way. The more you practice, the better you get."

The effects of biofeedback can be measured in a variety of ways: monitoring skin temperature (ST) influenced by blood flow beneath the skin; monitoring galvanic skin response (GSR), the electrical conductivity of the skin; observing muscle tension with an electromyogram (EMG); tracking heart rate with an electrocardiogram (EKG); and using an electroencephalogram (EEG) to monitor brain wave activity.

For biofeedback, electrodes are placed on the patient's skin (a simple, painless process). The patient is then instructed to use various techniques such as meditation, relaxation, and visualization to effect the desired response (muscle relaxation, lowered heart rate, or lowered temperature). The biofeedback device reports the patient's progress by a change in the speed of the beeps or flashes.

Normal, healthy, "relaxed" readings include fairly warm skin, low sweat gland activity (this keeps the skin's conductivity low), and a slow, even heart rate. Biofeedback technologies utilize computers to provide a rapid and detailed analysis of activities within the complex human system. Biofeedback practitioners interpret changes in these readings to help the patient learn to stabilize erratic and unhealthy biological functions.

Conditions Benefited by Biofeedback Training

Biofeedback training has a vast range of applications for health and prevention, particularly in cases where psychological factors play a role. Heart dysfunctions, loss of control due to brain or nerve damage, sleep disorders, hyperactivity in children, postural problems, back pain, and cerebral palsy have all shown improvement when patients undergo biofeedback training. Severe structural problems like broken bones and slipped discs are among the only conditions that don't respond to biofeedback.

One of the most common uses for biofeedback training is the treatment of stress and stress-related disorders, including hypertension, insomnia, migraines, asthma, gastrointestinal disorders, and muscular dysfunction. Teaching people self-regulation and relaxation through biofeedback helps lower blood pressure.[13] The greatest successes in controlling hypertension are with patients who combine biofeedback training with other forms of relaxation, visualization, exercise, and a low-salt diet. Through biofeedback, people become aware of their innate ability to regulate themselves and influence their health.

Your Heart Rate Can Tell You How Well a Medicine Works

Biofeedback and the monitoring of your heart rate can be used to obtain important information besides the health of your heart.

Physicians at The Royal Center of Advanced Medicine in Henderson, Nevada, report that a test called Heart Rate Variability (HRV), which has been in testing and development for several decades, is now available as a dependable means of showing how the nervous system responds to high-dilution medicines, typically homeopathic remedies. According to Daniel F. Royal, D.O., of The Royal Center of Advanced Medicine and Medi-Tec Systems, Inc., which distributes HRV technology, HRV testing can be used to monitor the way a patient's autonomic nervous system responds to any medical therapy. As such, it has the capacity to objectively demonstrate and thus *prove* the effectiveness of a given remedy, says Dr. Royal.

"As a diagnostic device, HRV could also supply the alternative medical community with a common testing procedure by which different approaches could be uniformly evaluated and compared," states Dr. Royal. HRV also has a treatment function: frequency information, originally obtained by HRV from the patient's nervous system, is returned (a biofeedback function) to the patient through light and sound waves generated in accordance with the specific rhythm of the heart. Over a 24-minute period, the time between human heartbeats varies somewhat; when measured, this variability in heart rate provides useful information about the state of the autonomic nervous system, which regulates about 87% of the body's functions.

Specifically, HRV is a computerized graph showing the shape of the pulse wave of the left versus the right carotid artery. The approach is called "noncognitive" biofeedback because it works without the conscious participation or awareness (cognition) of the patient; the HRV device talks

For more information about **HRV** equipment and training, contact: F. Fuller Royal, M.D., Medi-Tec Systems, Inc., 3663 Pecos McLeod, Las Vegas, NV 89121; tel: 702-732-1400; fax: 702-732-9661; website: www.nevadaclinic.com. For Daniel Royal, D.O., contact: The Royal Center of Advanced Medicine, 38 Diplomat Ct., Henderson, NV 89014; tel: 702-433-8800; fax: 702-269-6395.

directly with the subject's nervous system. When the heart rate shifts, these changes are routed, by computer, into audiovisual signals (light flashes and intermittent sounds); the patient becomes aware of these through headphones and a TV screen, and this triggers the autonomic nervous system to rebalance itself.

HRV testing can indicate an imbalance even when the patient reports feeling well, because an imbalance in the autonomic nervous system will eventually produce physical symptoms. On the other hand, if a patient reports still feeling sick, but the HRV shows improvement, this indicates that the treatment is still working at the level of the nervous system.

A statistical analysis of 12 years of Israeli clinical experience with HRV, used in 30,000 sessions, indicates that about 66% of the positive improvements from HRV sessions take place suddenly and dramatically, as if through major nervous system shifts, explains Dr. Royal. The Israeli study also suggested that over 50 common health problems (such as autism, hyperactivity, insomnia, chronic digestive complaints, psoriasis, stress, and poor circulation) were traceable to an inefficient nervous and regulatory system.

The advantage of HRV is speed and specificity. It normally takes about 72 hours for the autonomic nervous system to respond to a biofeedback stimulus, explains Dr. Royal; homeopathic remedies produce a much faster response. When this response occurs, it effects changes in several aspects of the nervous system and the heart rate. HRV can measure these subtle but important changes immediately after ingestion of the homeopathic remedy. HRV also improves communication between left and right brain hemispheres.

The minimum course of treatment is one weekly HRV session for 12 weeks. Each session is recorded on videocassettes that the patient watches privately at home twice weekly with a 48-hour gap in between each viewing. In effect, rewatching the video of the lights, sounds, and graph images helps the patient's autonomic nervous system reset itself in accordance with the more healthy pattern, says Dr. Royal.

For example, a woman, 56, had suffered with goiter for 30 years. After one dose of homeopathic *Iodum* 200C, the HRV registered an immediate positive effect; then, 24 hours later, Dr. Royal gave her a follow-up single dose of

QUICK DEFINITION

Standard anatomy describes two components to the nervous system. The **central nervous system** (CNS) comprises the spinal cord, containing millions of nerve fibers, and the brain, while the **peripheral nervous system** (PNS) is the network of nerves, estimated to extend 93,000 miles inside the body. The PNS is the sensory motor branch that pertains to the five senses and is how sensory information from the outside world gets translated into muscle movements.

The **autonomic nervous system** (ANS) involves elements of both the CNS and PNS, is controlled by the brain's hypothalamus gland, and pertains to the automatic regulation of all body processes, such as breathing, digestion, and heart rate. It can be likened to the body's automatic pilot, keeping you alive without your being aware of it or participating in its activities. Neural therapy focuses its injections of anesthetics into body structures whose nerve supply is linked with the autonomic nervous system.

homeopathic *Nux Vomica* 30C. Three months later, she reported she was feeling better; after 6 months, her improvement continues, states Dr. Royal. "HRV testing provides objective information which, in turn, enables the physician to choose the most effective therapeutic regimen for each patient as well as monitor the response to treatment," states Dr. Royal. This can include the patient's response to nutritional supplements, dental amalgam removals, chiropractic adjustments, and acupuncture treatments, for example.

Detoxification

Detoxification is the body's natural process of eliminating internal toxins, and is accomplished by the various systems and organs of the body, including the liver, kidneys, intestines, and skin, with toxins eliminated through urine, feces, and perspiration. Everyone has a specific level of tolerance to toxicity that cannot be exceeded if good health is to be maintained; if the system becomes overwhelmed, various symptoms can occur, including hypertension.

William Lee Cowden, M.D., puts hypertensive patients through a detoxification regimen consisting of daily saunas, homeopathic remedies, and a vegetarian diet supplemented with cayenne (*Capsicum annuum*) and garlic. "Cayenne mixed with vegetable juices or lemon juice is excellent for lowering blood pressure," says Dr. Cowden. He adds that after a few days of treatment, alternating cayenne/vegetable juice with cayenne/lemon juice, patients are often able to come off medication, because this regime helps to cleanse the body of toxins that may be causing the high blood pressure.

Dr. Cowden notes that individuals with hypertension often suffer from a liver insufficiency, in which the liver does not properly clear steroid hormones (sex hormones and hormones of the adrenal glands as well as other toxic substances) from the blood. Saunas and a vegetarian diet can help to restore liver function and lower blood pressure. (Patients with more severe hypertension should be medically supervised in their use of saunas.)

A toxic lymphatic system can also contribute to hypertension. Dr. Cowden suggests deep breathing exercises and dry brushing of the skin for three weeks, ten minutes daily. For this, brush the entire body using a dry brush with soft, natural vegetable fiber bristles. Move the brush toward the middle of the collarbone on each side of the body, as important lymph drainage sites are located here. Brush gently at first (some body parts are more sensitive than others) and build up

Research has shown that potassium supplementation can help reduce a patient's reliance on blood pressure medication or diuretic drugs.

to vigorous brushing. Dry brushing helps the skin detoxify, stimlates lymph drainage, and, by applying friction to acupuncture points on the skin, invigorates the entire nervous system.

Another way to stimulate the flow of lymph and to clear the lymph system of toxins is to use a small trampoline or rebounder for 20 minutes a day, says Dr. Cowden. One of rebounding's special benefits is its ability to improve flow in the lymphatic system. This is the body's primary system for collecting and eliminating wastes and toxins. "The lymphatic system is the metabolic garbage can of the body," says Morton Walker, D.P.M., in *Jumping for Health* (1989). "It rids the body of toxins, fatigue substances, dead cells, cancer cells, nitrogenous wastes, trapped protein, fatty globules, pathogenic bacteria, infectious viruses, foreign substances, heavy metals, and other assorted junk the cells cast off."

Stagnant or inadequate lymph flow is associated with the onset of many symptoms and illnesses, including bursitis in the shoulders, bunions, joint stiffness or soft tissue spasms, dry flaking skin, bad breath, body odors, lethargy, depression, and cancer. The lymph system lacks a pump such as the heart to move the fluid around. Instead, the lymphatic system must rely on physical movement and gravity to keep waste products from building up in the lymph glands and tissues. Aerobic exercise, and rebounding in particular, helps to keep the lymph flowing.

So, it is vital that the lymph fluids continue to flow in order to eliminate waste from the body. Lymph flow is dependent on muscle con-

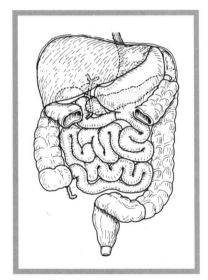

The intestines, when stretched out, are over 25 feet long. In fact, if the inner surface of the small intestines was smooth and flat rather than convoluted, they would stretch for 2¼ miles or completely cover an area the size of a tennis court. Once the bowel is toxic, it creates toxicity for the entire body and an inability to absorb the nutrients necessary for healing.

tractions and body movements, massage and other compression of the tissues, and gravity. Rebounding specifically stimulates the flow of lymph fluid. The change in gravitational forces experienced during rebounding allows for greater blood flow, which in turn increases the amount and movement of interstitial fluids, flushing the cells of waste products.

"The lymphatic [flow] becomes very active during exercise but sluggish under resting conditions," states Arthur C. Guyton, M.D., chairman of the Department of Physiology and Biophysics at the University of Mississippi School of Medicine and author of *Basic Human Physiology*. "During exercise, the rate of lymph flow can increase to as high as 3 to 14 times normal because of the increased activity." The lymph ducts expand during rebounding, leading to a greater flow (by as much as 14 times) of these toxins out through the lymphatic system. Or, as Dr. Walker says, rebounding stimulates "an optimum drainage of the lymphatic circulation."

Dr. Cowden reports a case of a woman who was severely hypertensive, with blood pressure of 240/140. She had tried every prescription hypertensive drug and had adverse reactions to all of the medications. When she came to his office, Dr. Cowden found that, due to years of poor dietary habits and an unhealthy lifestyle, her system was highly toxic. He put her on a detoxification program that included a vegetarian diet, fasts of vegetable juice and lemon juice with garlic and cayenne, supplements of oral magnesium, saunas, simple stress-reduc-

For information on **rebounders** and books and videos about rebounding exercise, check at your local fitness and sporting goods store, or contact: Best of Health (Needak® brand), Unit #1758 W.E. Mall 8770-170st, Edmonton, Alberta T5T-4J2, Canada; tel: 800-207-2249 or 403-487-7898; fax: 403-444-1048. A typical rebounder price is around $300.

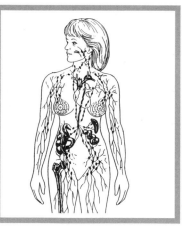

The lymphatic system consists of numerous lymph nodes. These are clusters of immune tissue that work as filters or "inspection stations" for detecting foreign and potentially harmful substances from the lymph. Acting like spongy filter bags, they are part of the lymphatic system, which is the body's master "drain." Cells inside the nodes examine the lymph fluid, as collected from body tissues, for foreign matter. While the body has many dozens of lymph nodes, they are mostly clustered in the neck, armpits, chest, groin, and abdomen. Lymph fluid (1-2 quarts) accounts for about 1% of body weight.

A study of 21 patients with hypertension found that daily supplementation with a combination of antioxidants and zinc lowered blood pressure from 165/89 to 160/85.5 in eight weeks.

tion techniques, and cranial electrotherapy stimulation. Within two weeks her blood pressure went down to a safe 140/80. She went off her hypertension medications, and her blood pressure continued to remain in that safe range during her follow-up visits over the next six months.

Nutritional Supplements

In addition to the supplements listed for general heart health (see Chapter 5), nonchloride potassium salts, calcium, and magnesium can help reduce hypertension. Other beneficial supplements include the antioxidant vitamins A, C, and E, niacin (vitamin B3), bioflavonoids (particularly rutin), and the amino acid taurine.[14]

Antioxidants and Zinc

Research has found that antioxidants are linked to an increase in nitric oxide activity.[15] Nitric oxide helps to open blood vessels, which in turn helps to lower blood pressure. Zinc activates SOD (superoxide dismutase, an antioxidant enzyme). A study of 21 patients with hypertension found that daily supplementation with a combination of antioxidants and zinc (500 mg of vitamin C, 50,000 IU of beta carotene, 600 IU of vitamin E, and 80 mg of zinc) lowered blood pressure from 165/89 to 160/85.5 in eight weeks.[16]

CAUTION

High dosages of vitamin E are not recommended for people with hypertension, rheumatic heart disease, or ischemic heart disease except under close medical supervision.

Calcium

A daily dosage of 1,000 mg of calcium has been shown to lower blood pressure in hypertensives.[17] Calcium can lower high blood pressure for both the contracting (systolic) and expanding (diastolic) phases of the heartbeat. When eight patients with high blood pressure took 1.4 g of calcium every day for 18 weeks, their blood pressure was significantly decreased.[18]

Many hypertensives have a lower daily calcium intake than people with normal blood pressure, so calcium-rich foods, including nuts and leafy green vegetables such as watercress and kale, are advisable as part of the diet.[19]

Magnesium

In one study, magnesium supplementation lowered blood pressure in 19 of 20 hypertensives, compared to none out of four in the control group.[20] Dietary magnesium is found in nuts (almonds, cashews, pecans), rice, bananas, potatoes, wheat germ, kidney and lima beans, soy products, and molasses.

Sodium and Potassium

As mentioned in Chapter 5, research has shown that potassium supplementation can help reduce a patient's reliance on blood pressure medication or diuretic drugs.[21] In order to reduce blood pressure, sodium intake must be restricted at the same time potassium intake is increased.[22] Individuals with high blood pressure should be aware of "hidden" salt in processed foods. Although their salt intake is comparable, vegetarians generally have less hypertension and cardiovascular disease than non-vegetarians do because their diets contain more potassium, complex carbohydrates, polyunsaturated fat, fiber, calcium, magnesium, and vitamins A and C.[23]

According to Dr. Cowden, regular consumption of potassium-rich fruits (such as avocados, bananas, cantaloupe, honeydew melon, grapefruit, nectarines, and oranges) and vegetables (such as asparagus, broccoli, cabbage, cauliflower, green peas, potatoes, and squash) can lower high blood pressure. Steaming rather than boiling vegetables helps prevent vital nutrient loss.

Additional Alternative Therapies

Self-Care

The following therapies for the treatment and prevention of hypertension can be undertaken at home under appropriate professional supervision:

- Fasting
- Yoga
- Hydrotherapy: Constitutional hydrotherapy—apply two to five times weekly.
- Juice Therapy: Celery, beet, and carrot or cucumber, spinach, and parsley. Add a little raw garlic to vegetable juices. Or, run a clove of garlic through a juicer, followed by enough carrots to make eight ounces of juice. Drink once per day.

Professional Care

The following therapies can only be provided by a qualified health professional:

- Acupuncture
- Chelation Therapy
- Environmental Medicine
- Hypnotherapy
- Orthomolecular Medicine
- Osteopathy
- Bodywork: acupressure, reflexology, *shiatsu*, massage, Rolfing, Feldenkrais, Alexander technique, therapeutic touch
- Magnetic Field Therapy: Recent studies from Russia show that magnetic treatments reduce blood pressure in certain patients with hypertension.[24]
- Cranial Electrical Stimulation: William Lee Cowden, M.D., uses cranial electrical stimulation to treat hypertensive patients, reporting that it can lower blood pressure and alleviate panic attacks within 30 to 40 minutes of treatment.

William Lee Cowden, M.D., puts
hypertensive patients through a
detoxification regimen consisting of daily
saunas, homeopathic remedies, and a
vegetarian diet supplemented with cayenne
(*Capsicum annuum*) and garlic.
He says that after a few days
of treatment, alternating cayenne/
vegetable juice with cayenne/lemon juice,
patients are often able to come off
medication, because this regime helps
to cleanse the body
of toxins that may be causing the
high blood pressure.

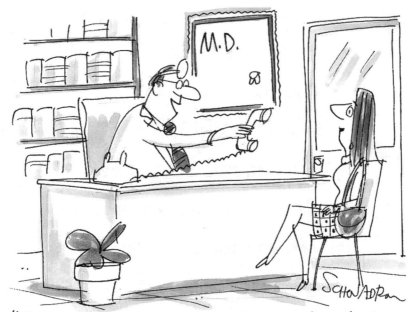

"I NOW OFFER NUTRITIONAL COUNSELING. HERE'S A RECORDING OF MY MOM'S RECIPE FOR CHICKEN SOUP."

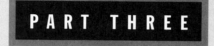

PART THREE

Stroke

CHAPTER 14

What Causes Stroke?

STROKE (or cerebrovascular accident) is the sudden disturbance of blood flow to the brain as a result of a clogged or burst artery. It is the third leading cause of death in the U.S. and the leading cause of adult disability, with an estimated annual medical cost of $30 billion. Approximately 500,000 Americans suffer a stroke each year. That's 200 out of every 100,000 people and the percentage is higher among men and the elderly. However, women who suffer a stroke die from it more often than men do.[1]

About 30% of strokes are fatal. In 1994, 154,350 people in the U.S. died from this "brain attack."[2] Among women 45-64 years old, stroke is the number two killer, causing more deaths in that age group than breast cancer.[3]

> **In the U.S., there are about 1.7 million stroke survivors at any given moment, and 75% of them are 55-84 years old.**

In the U.S., there are about 1.7 million stroke survivors at any given moment, and 75% of them are 55-84 years old. Only about 10% of stroke survivors are fit enough to return to work without a disability; 40% have a mild disability, 40% are severely disabled, and 10% must be hospitalized.

By interrupting the flow of blood to a region of the brain, a stroke starves the brain cells of oxygen, thereby producing tissue death. Stroke symptoms may develop within a few minutes to over several days and can include loss of speech, physical movement, or eyesight, depending on the area of the brain affected. Headaches, dizziness, confusion, and difficulty swallowing are also associated symptoms.

Many people who become paralyzed by a stroke learn to walk again. However, lost intellectual functioning tends not to be recovered as fully. When the symptoms from a stroke last for 24 hours or less, followed by full recovery of lost functions, the episode is called a transient ischemic attack (TIA). TIAs are warning signals and the person who suffers such an attack would be well advised to begin taking some of the steps toward heart health detailed in this book.

What Causes a Stroke?

Arteriosclerosis (thickening and hardening of the lining of the arteries) is a major risk factor associated with stroke. Atherosclerosis (the most common form of arteriosclerosis; due to deposits of plaque composed of fatty substances on arterial walls) of the cerebral arteries can decrease blood flow to the brain and increase the likelihood of stroke.

Stroke caused by diminished blood supply to the brain is called an ischemic stroke and represents about 70% of all cases. In addition to

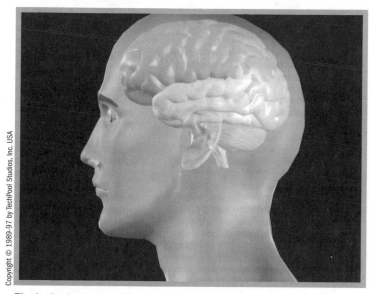

Copyright © 1989-97 by TechPool Studios, Inc. USA

The brain. **A stroke, which involves the sudden disturbance of blood flow to brain tissues, can be described as a "heart attack" in the brain. Most commonly, an artery, blocked by a blood clot, interrupts the flow of blood and oxygen to a region of the brain, producing tissue death by starving the brain cells of oxygen.**

The Five Warning Signs of Stroke

Many people can recite the seven warning signs of cancer, but do you know how to recognize when you've had or are having a stroke? Being aware of these five warning signs could save your life and reduce the damage inflicted by a stroke. Seek medical assistance immediately upon noticing one or more of these signs:

1. Numbness, weakness, or paralysis of the face, arm, or leg on one side of the body

2. Sudden blurring or loss of vision in one or both eyes

3. Difficulty speaking or comprehending simple statements

4. Unexplainable dizziness, loss of balance, or loss of coordination, especially when experienced with one of the other four signs

5. Sudden severe headache with no apparent cause—described by those who have suffered it as "the worst headache of your life"[4]

artery blockage produced by arteriosclerosis, blood flow to the brain can be impeded by a blood clot which, if the blockage is extensive enough, will result in a stroke. A blood clot that forms in an artery and is attached to the arterial wall is called a thrombus. A thrombus in itself is not life-threatening. In fact, it is lifesaving when it forms as the result of hemorrhage. But when it occurs in a narrow artery and blocks blood flow, a thrombus becomes dangerous. This condition is called thrombosis.

When a blood clot travels in the bloodstream from another part of the body, it is called an embolus. An embolus can also be a foreign object or an air or gas bubble traveling in the bloodstream. An embolus in the head, usually having arrived from the heart or from arteries of the neck, can produce a stroke.

Another cause of stroke is a blood vessel that ruptures (hemorrhage). Blood spills into the brain, not only damaging the brain cells directly, but producing further damage to brain tissue due to lack of oxygen when the blood supply is interrupted. This is known as a hemorrhagic stroke and can result from injury to the head or a burst aneurysm (bulging of a blood vessel due to disease in the arterial wall).

Who is Likely to Have a Stroke?

Once you have suffered one stroke or TIA, you are in the higher risk category. Inherited disorders, birth defects, and certain rare blood diseases are also linked to the occurrence of strokes.[5] Blood platelet stickiness, associated with a raised level of red blood cells (polycythemia) or with low levels of nutrients, such as vitamin B6, that prevent stickiness,

A study of 116,759 women, 30-55 years old, found that overweight women had a higher risk of ischemic stroke; extremely obese women more than doubled their stroke risk as compared to lean women; and those who had gained more than 24 pounds between the ages of 18 and 42 had almost twice the risk.

is another risk factor. In addition, the following increase your risk of having a stroke:

- smoking
- being over the age of 55
- high cholesterol
- a recent heart attack
- lack of exercise
- excessive consumption of alcohol
- diabetes
- history of a damaged heart valve
- obesity
- irregular heartbeat (atrial fibrillation)
- hypertension
- carotid artery disease
- overuse of decongestants[6]

A study of 116,759 women, 30-55 years old, found that overweight women had a higher risk of ischemic stroke; extremely obese women more than doubled their stroke risk as compared to lean women; and those who had gained more than 24 pounds between the ages of 18 and 42 had almost twice the risk.[7]

Various components in the blood have also been linked with an increased risk of stroke. These include lipoproteins, homocysteine, and fibrinogens.

Lipoproteins—Multiple studies have demonstrated the connection between lipoproteins (fat-carrying proteins) and stroke. Lipoproteins occur in two principal forms. Low-density lipoproteins (LDLs) are combination molecules of proteins and fats, particularly cholesterol. LDLs circulate in the blood and act as the primary carriers of cholesterol to the cells of the body. An elevated level of LDLs, the so-called bad cholesterol, is a contributing factor in causing atherosclerosis (plaque deposits on the inner walls of the arteries). A diet high in saturated fats can lead to an increase in the level of LDLs in the blood.

An excess of homocysteine, which increases the risk of stroke, is linked with deficiencies of folic acid and vitamins B12 and B6. Researchers state that elevated homocysteine levels can be reduced fairly easily with supplementation of these nutrients.

Low Iron is Better When It Comes to Stroke

One factor in how well or poorly a person fares after a stroke is the iron level in the blood. A study of 67 patients found that those with a poor outcome had elevated iron levels within the 24 hours following an ischemic stroke, while those with a good outcome did not.[11]

For more about **homocysteine**, see Chapter 1: What Causes Heart Disease?, pp. 33-37.

High-density lipoproteins (HDLs) are also fat-protein molecules in the blood, but contain a larger amount of protein and less fat than LDLs. HDLs are able to absorb cholesterol and related compounds in the blood and transport them to the liver for elimination. HDL, the so-called good cholesterol, may also be able to take cholesterol from plaque deposits on the artery walls, thus helping to reverse the process of atherosclerosis. A higher ratio of HDL to LDL cholesterol in the blood is associated with a reduced risk of cardiovascular disease.

The Copenhagen Heart Study of 693 stroke victims found that levels of triglyceride (a lipid or fat) were positively associated with risk of a nonhemorrhagic stroke; this means the higher your levels, the greater your risk. The study also showed a negative relationship between HDL cholesterol and nonhemorrhagic stroke risk; the more HDLs you have in your blood, the lower your risk.[8]

Another study found lipoprotein (a) levels to be a "critical risk factor" in ischemic stroke[9] and a third group of researchers demonstrated that a high lipoprotein (a) blood level was associated with a more than 20 times greater risk of cerebrovascular disease.[10] Lipoprotein (a) is a form of cholesterol.

Homocysteine—Homocysteine, an amino acid, is a normal by-product of protein metabolism; specifically, of the amino acid methionine, which is found in red meat, milk, and milk products and which does not create a problem when present in small amounts. Methionine is converted in the body to homocysteine, which is normally then converted to the harmless amino acid, cystathionine. But in individuals deficient in the enzyme necessary to convert homocysteine to cystathionine, homocysteine will be abnormally high. "Protein intoxication" starts damaging the cells and tissues of arteries, setting in motion the many processes that lead to loss of elasticity, hardening and calcification, narrowing of the lumen, and formation of blood clots within arteries. Homocysteine can, when allowed to accumulate to toxic levels, degenerate arteries and produce heart disease. The homocysteine theory suggests that heart disease is attributed to abnormal processing of protein in the body because of deficiencies of B vitamins in the diet.

An elevated blood level of homocysteine puts a person at risk for stroke, as it does for cardiovascular disease in general. In 107 cases of stroke in men, 40-59 years old, homocysteine levels were significantly higher than in the control group.[12]

In another study, patients with elevated homocysteine levels had two to three times the risk of recurrent thrombosis (blood clot blockage) in the veins.[13] An excess of homocysteine is also linked to deficiencies of folic acid and vitamins B12 and B6. On the positive side, researchers state that elevated homocysteine levels can be reduced fairly easily with supplementation of these nutrients.[14]

Bypass Surgery Can Cause a Stroke

A study reported in the *New England Journal of Medicine* reveals that the risk of suffering a stroke or other brain damage as a result of coronary artery bypass surgery is as much as ten times higher than previously thought. Of those who had bypass surgery, more than 6% had to have brain surgery afterward to address brain injury caused by the operation. This adds up to 25,000 patients in the U.S. and 50,000 worldwide. These numbers do not include all those patients who did not require further surgery but suffered strokes or other mental impairment, including difficulty remembering or thinking clearly.[15]

Fibrinogens—A high level of fibrinogens (protein in the blood that is converted into fibrin, which is vital for blood clotting) is considered by some researchers to be a far stronger stroke risk factor than cholesterol.[16] They suggest that this is because the higher levels may make the blood more sluggish and trigger plaque formation as well. One study of 140 stroke patients found that those with the higher degrees of artery blockage had higher levels of fibrinogens. The area of stroke damage in the brain was also significantly related to the fibrinogen level; in other words, higher levels of fibrinogens were associated with a larger area of damage.[17] Research has also found that elevated fibrinogen increases the risk in stroke survivors of a second stroke, heart attack, or other cardiovascular event.[18]

Hormones—Hormones are the chemical messengers of the endocrine system that impose order through an intricate communication system among the body's estimated 50 trillion cells. Examples include the "male" sex hormone (testosterone), the "female" sex hormones (estrogen and progesterone), melatonin (pineal), growth hormone (pituitary), and DHEA (adrenal).

The incidence and severity of stroke appear to be linked with hormones. For example, women under 50 who take oral contraceptives increase their risk of stroke. One study found, however, that low-estrogen oral contraceptives do not result in greater risk.[19] On the other hand, testosterone seems to have a protective effect. Men with decreased testosterone levels who had a stroke suffered greater damage and were more likely to die from the stroke than men with higher testosterone levels.[20]

Homocysteine can, when allowed
to accumulate to toxic levels,
degenerate arteries
and produce heart disease. The
homocysteine theory suggests
that heart disease is
attributed to abnormal
processing of protein in the body
because of deficiencies
of B vitamins in the diet.

Self-Care Essentials for Stroke

AS WITH HEART disease and high blood pressure, attention to diet, exercise, and lifestyle is essential in preventing the conditions that lead to stroke and in helping the body to recover if a stroke has occurred. Many of the recommendations in these areas for heart disease (see Chapter 2) and high blood pressure (see Chapter 9) apply to stroke as well, but the following are a few additional considerations.

Diet

A whole foods diet composed of whole grains, raw nuts and seeds, and plenty of fresh fruits and vegetables (all organically raised and pesticide-free) is recommended. Yellow and green fruits and vegetables, including broccoli, sprouts, and kelp, are particularly helpful. An emphasis on garlic, onions, and vitamin B6 is advisable, because all three tend to prevent platelets from sticking together. Fats (unprocessed only) should be limited to 10% to 15% of your total diet. Deep-fried foods, animal fats, and semi-solid fats should be avoided. Foods that are natural plant sources of estrogens, such as soybeans and peanuts, are also best to avoid, along with alcoholic beverages and especially alcoholic binges (four drinks or more in a short period of time).

Numerous studies have shown that eating fish, especially freshwater fish, can enhance blood circulation and reduce the risk of stroke. According to the *Harvard Heart Letter* (October 1994), moderate fish consumption leads to mild, beneficial blood "thinning," which helps prevent strokes. A study of 552 men, from 50 to 69

Increasing fruit and vegetable intake by three servings per day decreased the risk of having a stroke by 25%, and by 50% for hemorrhagic stroke in particular.

years old, found that eating at least one serving of fish a week is associated with less risk of stroke. Consuming too much fish, on the other hand, can be detrimental to health. Men who ate more than 35 g of fish daily had the highest stroke rates and more deaths from stroke than men who ate less fish.[1]

A second study of 4,410 whites and 782 blacks, 45 to 75 years old and with no stroke history, found that eating fish more than once a week cuts stroke risk in half for white and black women and black men. This study found no stroke protection for white men as a result of eating fish, but the kind of fish consumed was not studied and that may have had an effect on the results.[2]

The reason why fish intake reduces stroke risk may be because certain kinds of fish are high in alpha-linolenic acid (ALA), an omega-3 fatty acid. Remember, essential fatty acids contribute to heart health. One study increased the ALA intake of 96 stroke victims compared to 96 controls. Each 0.13% increase in the ALA level in the blood was associated with a 37% reduction in stroke risk. The study concluded that getting more omega-3 fatty acids in your diet from any source (fish, soybeans, walnuts, or leafy green vegetables) can help prevent stroke.

Eating more fruits and vegetables can also contribute to reducing your stroke risk. In one study of 832 middle-aged men, increasing fruit and vegetable intake by three servings per day decreased the risk of having a stroke by 25%, and by 50% for hemorrhagic stroke in particular.[3] This effect may be due to the concentration of flavonoids in fruits and vegetables. Flavonoids are plant pigments that are known to inhibit platelet clustering, a contributing factor in stroke.

According to one study, carrots and spinach may be especially useful in stroke prevention. The 87,000 female nurses who ate five or more servings of carrots per week had a 68% reduced risk of stroke compared to women eating one serving or less per month. The risk among those

QUICK DEFINITION

Omega-3 and omega-6 oils are the two principal types of essential fatty acids, which are unsaturated fats required in the diet. The digits "3" and "6" refer to differences in the oil's chemical structure with respect to its chain of carbon atoms and where they are bonded. A balance of these oils in the diet is required for good health. The primary omega-3 oil is called alpha-linolenic acid (ALA) and is found in flaxseed (58%), canola, pumpkin and walnut, and soybeans. Fish oils, such as salmon, cod, and mackerel, contain the other important omega-3 oils, DHA (docosahexaenoic acid) and EPA (eicosapentaenoic acid). Omega-3 oils help reduce the risk of heart disease. Linoleic acid or cis-linoleic acid is the main omega-6 oil and is found in most plant and vegetable oils, including safflower (73%), corn, peanut, and sesame. The most therapeutic form of omega-6 oil is gamma-linolenic acid (GLA), found in evening primrose, black currant, and borage oils. Once in the body, omega-6 is converted to prostaglandins, hormone-like substances that regulate many metabolic functions, particularly inflammatory processes.

Eating at least one serving of fish a week is associated with less risk of stroke.

who ate a daily serving of spinach was 43% lower.[4]

As mentioned in Chapter 2, eating onions and apples and drinking black tea can reduce the risk of cardiovascular disease. This holds true for stroke as well. The common denominator which onions, apples, and black tea share is quercetin, a dietary flavonoid. Quercetin helps prevent oxidation of LDL cholesterol, which in turn helps prevent atherosclerosis. One study of 552 men, 50 to 69 years old, found that higher intake of dietary flavonoids, mainly quercetin, was linked to lower incidence of stroke. For example, those men who drank more than 4.7 cups of black tea daily had 69% less risk of stroke than those who drank under 2.6 cups.[5]

Exercise

Exercise makes a significant contribution to both the prevention and treatment of stroke. Scientists found that in 906 men and women, 57-82 years old, who regularly had moderate to heavy exercise in the form of fast walking or calisthenics, there was a 63% reduction in the risk of stroke. Light exercise resulted in a 57% reduced chance of stroke, compared to inactivity. Nearly any form of physical activity can significantly reduce the risk,[6] but high levels of activity do not provide any more protection than medium levels.[7]

Another study produced similar results. Among 7,700 men, between 40 and 59 years old, with a history of heart disease, moderate exercise reduced the risk of stroke and heart attack by more than 50%. The exercises included bicycling, walking, running, playing golf or tennis, and gardening or doing other household jobs.[8]

Surprisingly, exercise in youth carries over to middle age in reducing stroke risk. A comparison between 125 men and women, 35-74 years old, who had suffered a first stroke, and 198 controls revealed that those who had exercised vigorously from the age of 15 to 25 reduced their risk of stroke by two-thirds over those who had not.[9] The exercises included swimming, bicycling, running, playing tennis or squash, and digging. In addition, the protection against stroke increased with the number of years the person exercised. For example, exercising between 15 and 40 brought the risk down to slightly over one-fifth the risk of those who were less active.

The study also demonstrated, however, that starting exercise later in life can still help in prevention. Those who had recently been exercising vigorously had two-fifths the risk of stroke than their less-active counterparts, and those who had taken at least a mile walk sometime in the previous month had two-thirds less chance of suffering a stroke than those who had not exerted themselves even that much.

The benefits of exercise as treatment for stroke are also evident. Aerobic exercise after suffering a stroke has been found to improve physical function (especially oxygen consumption), reduce cardiovascular risk, control blood pressure, prevent muscle atrophy, and boost self-confidence.[10]

Lifestyle

Probably the single greatest stroke risk factor among lifestyle habits is cigarette smoking. Research has clearly demonstrated the link. One study of 7,264 men, followed over 12 years, found that current smokers had a four times greater risk of stroke than those who had never smoked. Previous smokers had an increased risk as well, but it was lower than for those who were still smoking.

Probably the single greatest stroke risk factor among lifestyle habits is cigarette smoking.

In addition, contrary to what many might think, switching from cigarettes to a pipe or cigar made little difference in the risk level. Those who had been heavy cigarette smokers and quit were still twice as likely to have a stroke as those who had never smoked. However, ceasing to smoke had clear benefits, especially for those who smoked less than 20 cigarettes a day. For these men, their risk of stroke five years after quitting was comparable to that of those who had never smoked.[11]

Similarly, a study of 117,006 female nurses, between 30 and 55 years old, showed that the risk of stroke was over two-and-a-half times greater among current smokers, compared to those who had never smoked. The risk among former smokers was only slightly elevated and this difference for the most part disappeared after two to four years without smoking. This study found that the benefits of quitting were not dependent on the number of cigarettes the person previously smoked daily.

Finally, it appears you are at risk of a stroke if you are younger than 45, have migraines, and smoke cigarettes, according to research reported in the *British Medical Journal* (July 31, 1993). French doctors found in a study of 212 women that those under the age of 45 with a previous history of migraines had a significantly higher risk factor for stroke. If they smoked cigarettes, the risk was even higher. However, men of all ages and women older than 45 were not more likely to have a stroke if they had migraines.

Eleven Steps to Prevent Stroke

David A. Steenblock, M.S., D.O., of Mission Viejo, California, a specialist in alternative treatments (especially hyperbaric oxygen) for stroke, offers the following recommendations for stroke prevention:

1. Avoid tobacco smoke and alcohol.
2. Don't use amphetamines, cocaine, or other illicit drugs, as these can be harmful to the heart.
3. After age 50, have your carotid arteries checked every five years for atherosclerosis.
4. Monitor your blood pressure (normal=120/70).
5. Exercise daily.
6. Eat fresh, nonprocessed vegetables.
7. Eat a high-fiber diet.
8. Avoid fats, cholesterol, and sugar and keep your weight down to help prevent diabetes, which affects the heart.
9. Take magnesium, calcium, vitamins E and C, and bioflavonoids.
10. If you are a woman over 35, avoid birth control pills.
11. Quickly correct any medical problems that develop.

Two Ways to Check Your Heart Status—Here are two physician-delivered noninvasive ways of checking your heart status: Doppler Ultrasound and Diagnostic Thermography.

Doppler Ultrasound—This test uses a flowmeter to measure blood flow and transmits the information by sound frequency. Some of the sound waves emitted by the flowmeter are reflected back by the red blood cells; the difference in pitch between sound waves sent and received is indicative (and proportional to) the speed of blood flow. The flowmeter can be incorporated into a standard stethoscope, so that information about blood flow in selected veins and arteries may be obtained. The device can detect very rapid changes in flow as well as steady flow rates.

Diagnostic Thermography—This approach provides

For more information about **Diagnostic Thermography**, contact: Therma-Scan™ Inc., 26711 Woodward Avenue, Suite 203, Huntington Professional Building-South, Huntington Woods, MI 48070; tel: 810-544-7500.

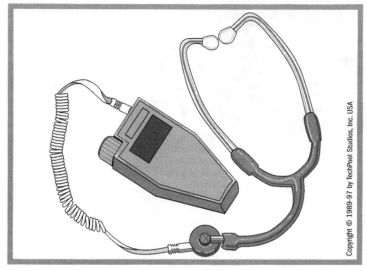

The Doppler Ultrasound test uses a *flowmeter* to measure blood flow and transmits the information by sound frequency.

---

a noninvasive cerebrovascular analysis. The Therma-Scan™ device measures infrared energy emissions from targeted areas of the body, including the heart. These emissions are the result of emanations of physiologic processes such as the flow of blood and nutrients. If this flow is deficient in a particular body area, such as the heart, the temperature value for that area will be abnormal and the diagnostic thermography read-out will indicate this in terms of different colors. Patterns of abnormal cooling (in blood vessels, as measured by the device) correlate directly with a diminished blood flow in that blood vessel.

CHAPTER

16

Oxygen Therapy

HOW IT CAN HELP STROKE RECOVERY

THE MAJORITY of stroke victims in the U.S. spend many months working with physical therapists, sometimes recovering only minimal bodily function. Unfortunately, most are unaware that there is a far more effective alternative. It is called hyperbaric oxygen therapy (HBOT), and the results of treatment for stroke using this technique are dramatic.

Hyperbaric oxygen therapy has long been used on divers, but its application to stroke treatment is relatively recent. Researchers, particularly in Germany, recognized that the loss of functioning of an arm or leg after a stroke is similar to the symptoms of the "bends," a sometimes **Hyperbaric oxygen therapy may be the single most effective technique, conventional or alternative, for reversing the damage caused by a stroke.** fatal affliction deep-sea divers get from ascending too quickly to the surface. Restoring the balance of nitrogen and oxygen in the blood via a hyperbaric oxygen chamber cured divers of the bends, and physicians suspected that victims of stroke or heart attack might be helped in the same way.

Their conjecture has proven correct and, today, hyperbaric oxygen therapy may be the single most effective technique, conventional or alternative, for reversing the damage caused by a stroke. Every emergency room in the United States should have a hyperbaric oxygen chamber, and every physician should be trained in its use, says David A. Steenblock, M.S., D.O., of Mission Viejo, California, who is well qualified to make this kind of sweeping statement. He is one of the country's leading practitioners in the therapeutic use of oxygen under pressure to dramatically reduce the effects of stroke and brain injury.

While drug companies continue to search for a "cure" for acute stroke, an effective way to restore a damaged brain to healthy function already exists: oxygen. "If you can get more oxygen to the brain within the first 24 hours of having a stroke, you can often stop most of the damage and salvage a great deal of brain tissue, eliminating 70% to 80% of the damage," Dr. Steenblock says. "Treating the patient by getting more oxygen to the brain during the first three weeks after the stroke makes it still possible to minimize the damage." In fact, Dr. Steenblock has produced unexpected positive outcomes when treating people as long as 15 years after their stroke.

Since 1971, over 1,000 cases demonstrating a 40%-100% rate of improvement for stroke victims receiving oxygen under pressure have been reported in scientific journals. Given the facts about positive outcomes, Dr. Steenblock encourages U.S. physicians to consider the merits of this approach as revealed in the following cases.

Moving Again After Right-Side Paralysis—Barbara, 62, had a stroke that completely paralyzed her right arm and left her severely bent over, limping, with pain in her right leg, and unable to control her urination. She had physical therapy and took conventional prescription medications, but nothing helped her. Barbara remained in this condition for 42 months before seeing Dr. Steenblock.

Over the course of 12 weeks, he started Barbara on a series of 60 treatments in a hyperbaric oxygen chamber (hyperbaric means pure oxygen under pressure). Oxygen is delivered to the body at an atmospheric pressure 1.5 to 1.75 times stronger than what we normally experience. During the treatment, Barbara wore an oxygen mask and laid down inside a sealed chamber that resembles a miniature submarine.

Barbara breathed pure oxygen for an hour. The higher

QUICK DEFINITION

Hyperbaric oxygen therapy refers to pure oxygen delivered for 30 to 60 minutes to patients inside sealed chambers with high pressure (hence "hyperbaric" as in high barometric pressure), usually at 2.5 times higher than the atmospheric pressure at sea level. A monoplace chamber accommodates a single patient who absorbs the concentrated oxygen through the skin as well as through inhalation. A multiplace chamber services several people at once; patients wear oxygen masks.

According to Dr. Steenblock, if you can get more oxygen to the brain within the first 24 hours of having a stroke, you can often eliminate 70% to 80% of the damage.

For more on **chelation therapy,** see Chapter 3: Scrubbing the Arteries Naturally, pp. 70-92.

Due to its wide application for a number of conditions, oxygen therapy can save money in long-term health costs.

Barbara's Stroke Recovery Prescription

- N-acetyl carnitine: ¼ tsp, 2X daily, increasing to ½ tsp in water, 3X daily
- Cytidine disphosphate choline: 2 capsules, daily (A.M.)
- N-acetyl cysteine: 2 capsules, 3X daily
- Glycine: ¼ tsp, 2X daily, increasing to ½ tsp in water, 3X daily
- Super KMH (72 trace minerals, 18 herbs): 1 tsp, 2X daily
- Vitamin E: 400 IU, 3X daily
- Lipoic acid (an essential fatty acid): 1 capsule, 3X daily
- L-carnitine: 50 mg, daily
- Calcium magnesium potassium: 1 tablet, 3X daily
- Brewer's yeast: 2 tablets, 3X daily
- Aqua Flora (a homeopathic remedy for *Candida*): 2 tbsp, daily
- Calcium: 1,200 mg, daily
- Magnesium: 1,200 mg, daily
- Co-enzyme B complex: 1 capsule, daily
- Free Radical Quenchers: 2 capsules, 2X daily
- Zinc picolinate: 1 tablet, daily
- Low-fat, low-cholesterol diet
- Lescol (Fluvastatin, a conventional drug for lowering cholesterol)

atmospheric pressure inside the chamber literally forced more oxygen into her blood. In fact, hyperbaric oxygen can deliver eight to nine times more oxygen to the capillaries compared to breathing normal air, says Dr. Steenblock. "With 100% oxygen under pressure, oxygen is dissolved into the red blood cells and into body and brain fluids."

The goal is to get as much oxygen into the brain as possible. This helps to revive oxygen-starved brain tissue that was damaged but not entirely destroyed by the stroke, Dr. Steenblock explains. The principle holds true for traumatic brain injury as well, such as people sustain from accidents. Some of the brain tissue is irreversibly destroyed, as brain cells deprived of oxygen usually die within ten minutes, but a larger portion is potentially revivable.

A stroke produces most of its damage through swelling of and injury to surrounding brain tissue, yet this tissue lies dormant, not dead but not active either, surviving on as little as 15% to 20% of its normal oxygen supply. If you can restore blood flow and flood this area with oxygen, there is a strong likelihood of restoring these "hibernating" brain cells to function, five or even ten years after a stroke, says Dr. Steenblock.

For more information about OPC-95 (for licensed practitioners only), contact: Jarrow Formulas, 1824 South Robertson Boulevard, Los Angeles, CA 90035; tel: 800-726-0886 or 310-204-6936; fax: 310-204-2520. To contact Dr. Steenblock: Health Restoration Medical Center, David Steenblock, D.O., Medical Director, 26381 Crown Valley Parkway, Suite 130, Mission Viejo, CA 92691; tel: 714-367-8870; fax: 714-367-9779. For a useful reference work: K.K. Jain, M.D., *Textbook of Hyperbaric Medicine*, 2nd Edition (1996), Hogrefe & Huber Publications, P.O. Box 2487, Kirkland, WA 98023; tel: 206-820-1500; fax: 206-823-8324.

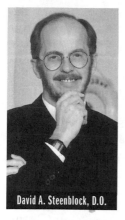

David A. Steenblock, D.O.

A stroke produces most of its damage through swelling of and damage to surrounding brain tissue, yet this tissue lies dormant. If you can restore blood flow and flood this area with oxygen, there is a strong likelihood of restoring these "hibernating" brain cells to function, five or even ten years after a stroke, says Dr. Steenblock.

Dr. Steenblock also gave Barbara a two-month course of chelation therapy, consisting of 23 infusions, to improve her general circulation. Her carotid artery, which is the main artery that passes through the neck, supplying blood to the brain, was about 50% blocked; in addition, Barbara had high blood pressure and atherosclerosis (arteries lined and clogged with deposits)—conditions that contributed strongly to her stroke, says Dr. Steenblock. Barbara also received about two hours of physical therapy five days a week and went on a nutritional supplementation program.

After one month of treatment, Barbara showed clear signs of improvement. Her walking improved noticeably and, instead of shuffling, she could raise her right heel off the ground and move with a smoother gait. Her posture was more erect. Barbara was able to open and close her right hand, and use it to grip and squeeze objects. She could also raise her arm to her chest level.

Hyperbaric oxygen, by restoring proper circulation to damaged brain tissues, can also stimulate the growth of new blood vessels and the repair

---

David's Stroke Recovery Prescription

- N-acetyl-carnitine: ½ tsp, 2X daily
- Cytidine choline: 1 capsule, 2X daily
- N-acetylcysteine: ½ tsp, 2X daily
- Melatonin: as needed for sleep
- Chlorella: 5 tablets, 2X daily
- OPC-95 (grape seed): 2X daily
- Juice Plus+™: Orchard Blend, 2X daily; Garden Blend, 2X daily
- Ginger root: 2 tablets, daily
- Pycnogenol: 10 tablets, daily
- Psyllium root powder: 2X, daily
- Goldenseal root: 2X, daily
- DHEA (hormone): 100 mg, daily

of damaged ones, but this takes time, Dr. Steenblock explains. "It may take upwards of two years of this therapy for all these cells to regrow, reconnect, and start to function again. But you're going to keep on seeing improvement."

A Quadriplegic Regains His Ability to Move—One day while getting up from a sofa in the lounge at chiropractic school, David, 25, fell over, unconscious. He had sustained a hemorrhagic stroke (caused by a burst aneurysm) that left him a quadriplegic. He could move only his eyelids and occasionally one eye. He ate by way of a stomach tube. He had to have everything done for him and was transported on an electric cart. David also suffered from a chronic cough and recurrent pneumonia. By the time David came to Dr. Steenblock, he had endured eight years of physical therapy and numerous other therapies, all of which failed to improve his condition.

Dr. Steenblock started David on a two-month series of daily hyperbaric oxygen treatments. At the end of two months, David began regaining neck strength and right-side motion. He could stand, with support straps or parallel bars, for up to an hour and for three minutes without any assistance. Feeling started to return on his right side. He could sit up in his wheelchair and hold his head erect. His constant drooling started to diminish and his swallowing became easier. His eyes were able to track objects normally and his facial muscles filled out. For the first time in eight years, David was able to feed himself.

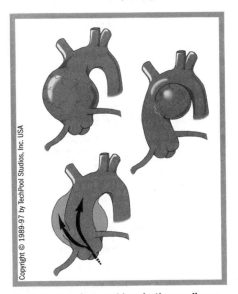

An *aneurysm* is a problem in the cardiovascular system in which a sac is formed by the expansion of a wall in an artery, vein, or the heart; it is usually filled with fluid or clotted blood. The most common site for an aneurysm is the aorta. Aneurysms are usually associated with atherosclerosis (hardening of the arteries from plaque deposits); however, trauma and injury may also cause them. Over time, an aneurysm tends to increase in size and pose the danger of rupture. A ruptured aneurysm is usually accompanied by severe pain and blood loss, followed by shock; symptoms may resemble those associated with a stroke.

Since 1971, over 1,000 cases demonstrating a 40%-100% rate of improvement for stroke victims receiving oxygen under pressure have been reported in scientific journals.

David also received regular physical therapy, biofeedback, and a nutritional prescription (see sidebar). After four months on this program, David regained full hearing in his right ear; since childhood, he had had only 70% of hearing capacity in that ear. "He's gradually getting better, and his voice is starting to come back, but it's a slow process when somebody has that level of damage," says Dr. Steenblock.

David works out regularly with weights and is able to lift about 100 pounds with his legs and 60 pounds with his arms. "And his brain is fine," adds Dr. Steenblock.

Out of the Wheelchair in Just Fifteen Treatments—Ten years prior to seeking treatment with Dr. Steenblock, Sonya had suffered a stroke that left her confined to a wheelchair and unable to take care of herself. After consulting 22 doctors for her paralysis and severe pain, she was no better and despairing. Dr. Steenblock gave Sonya ten treatments with hyperbaric oxygen. At nine times the level provided to her body's capillaries by breathing normal air, the oxygen began to revive brain tissue that hadn't functioned since the stroke. Her pain subsided. After another five treatments, Sonya was able to walk again and begin taking care of herself.

All About HBOT

Hyperbaric oxygen therapy dates back to the beginning of this century, although its modern use in the United States dates only to the formation of the Undersea Medical Society in 1967. HBOT may be administered in individual oxygen chambers that consist of acrylic tubes about seven feet long and 25 inches in diameter. The patient lies on a stretcher that slides into the tube. The entry is sealed and the tube is pressurized with pure oxygen for 30 to 120 minutes.

The increased pressure makes it possible to breathe oxygen at a concentration higher than that allowed by any

QUICK DEFINITION

Oxygen therapies involve the use of oxygen and can be used in various forms to promote healing and to destroy pathogens in the body. Oxygen-based therapies treat a variety of conditions, including cancer, infections, circulatory problems, chronic fatigue syndrome, arthritis, allergies, and multiple sclerosis. There are 2 principal types of oxygen therapy, classified according to the chemical process involved. *Oxygenation* is the process of enriching the oxygen content of the blood or tissues. One oxygenation therapy is called hyperbaric oxygen therapy, which introduces oxygen to the body in a pressurized chamber. Oxygenation employed under strictly controlled conditions can have positive therapeutic effects. The second type of oxygen therapy is called *oxidation*, which is a chemical reaction occurring when electrons (electrically-charged particles; frequently, but not always, oxygen) are transferred from one molecule to another. Although uncontrolled oxidation can be destructive—as is the case when free radicals are produced in excess—it can also be therapeutic when carefully used on weak and devitalized cells as the targets.

other means. After treatment, the chamber is depressurized slowly with the patient resting inside. Most of the hyperbaric facilities in the United States are either part of, or affiliated with, American hospitals or the military.

Multiplace chambers can accommodate many patients at once and the oxygen is delivered by mask. These chambers allow nurses and technical personnel to attend to patients during the treatment. An added advantage of multiplace chambers is that a patient can be removed immediately if problems arise, whereas in individual chambers, the patient cannot be removed until the entire chamber is depressurized.

Conditions Benefited by Hyperbaric Oxygen Therapy

The use of oxygen under pressure to treat serious health conditions including stroke is medically well-established, though not yet widely used in this country. There are only 300 hyperbaric oxygen chambers in the U.S., while in Russia, for example, there are 2,000. HBOT is primarily used in the U.S. for traumas such as crash injuries, burns, wounds, gangrene, carbon monoxide poisoning, bed sores, stasis (the stagnation of the normal flow of fluids), radiation

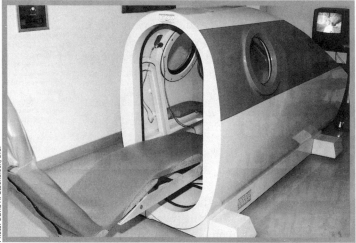

Photo: David A. Steenblock, D.O.

HBOT may be administered in individual oxygen chambers that consist of acrylic tubes about seven feet long and 25 inches in diameter. The patient lies on a stretcher which slides into the tube. The entry is sealed and the tube that is pressurized with pure oxygen for 30 to 120 minutes.

In West Germany, HBOT has been used extensively to treat stroke victims, and government sponsorship of HBOT has reduced aftercare costs for stroke victims by 71%.

necrosis (death of an area of tissue or bone surrounded by healthy parts), and skin grafting that doesn't take. Some microsurgical procedures for the repair and restoration of severed limbs are made possible only by the use of HBOT during the surgery.

⚠CAUTION⚠
Hyperbaric oxygen therapy may cause problems for those with a history of middle-ear infection, emphysema, or spontaneous pneumonia, due to the pressure it requires.

"In West Germany, HBOT has been used extensively to treat stroke victims, and government sponsorship of HBOT has reduced aftercare costs for stroke victims by 71%," reports David Hughes, Ph.D., of the Hyperbaric Oxygen Institute in San Bernardino, California. A landmark 1971 study showed that hyperbaric oxygen treatment of 40 stroke patients produced moderate to significant improvement in 80% of patients.

"In France," says Dr. Hughes, "HBOT is employed for peripheral vascular and arterial problems, and in Russia, it is used in drug and alcohol detoxification. In Japan, the medical establishment boasts that no citizen is ever more than half an hour away from a hyperbaric chamber." In Great Britain, more than 25,000 multiple sclerosis patients have benefited from HBOT.[1] HBOT is gaining acceptance and is utilized by both alternative and conventional physicians. Its broad spectrum of applications gives it enormous potential for more widespread therapeutic use and accessibility.

Oxygen Therapy

Hyperbaric oxygen therapy is one in a wide range of therapies utilizing oxygen in various forms to promote healing and destroy pathogens (disease-producing microorganisms and toxins) in the body. These therapies are grouped according to the type of chemical process involved: the addition of oxygen to the blood or tissues is called "oxygenation," and "oxidation" is the reaction of splitting off electrons (electrically-charged particles) from any chemical molecule. Oxidation may or may not involve oxygen (oxidation refers to the chemical reaction and not to oxygen itself).

Hyperbaric oxygen therapy utilizes the oxygenation process. Hydrogen peroxide therapy, on the other hand, uses the process of oxidation. Ozone therapy utilizes both of these chemical processes.

The Suppression of Hyperbaric Oxygen Therapy: State Raids Dr. Steenblock's Clinic

During the Communist era, political dissidents were routinely arrested, subjected to mock trials, imprisoned, and often murdered in the remote Gulag Archipelago of the Soviet Union. Thanks to the Food and Drug Administration (FDA), conventional medicine trade groups, state medical boards, and the big drug companies, America has its own "Gulag" for doctors who deviate from the enforced norms and who practice alternative medicine. What the Soviet Union accomplished through state-imposed tyranny, American medicine accomplishes through licensing, regulations, and the FDA—the suppression of your freedom of choice in medical care.

Our American Gulag ruins alternative doctors through suppression, harassment, indictments, licensure revocation, and bankruptcy. David A. Steenblock, D.O., M.S., is one physician who has endured this political intimidation. Here is his story:

Dr. Steenblock was forced into bankruptcy in September 1995 when state medical authorities confiscated six FDA-approved hyperbaric oxygen machines, worth $600,000, which he used to treat patients who had had strokes and heart attacks. No patient complaints were registered, but 30 very ill patients were forced to wait two months for treatment, and one died the day after being grilled by state medical authorities. The embargo was lifted in November 1995 and the clinic struggles on.

Research is needed on the effects of hyperbaric oxygen therapy for the treatment of early complications of stroke. This type of therapy could prove revolutionary by preventing permanent damage to stroke patients and could be a great money saver.

Although various oxygen therapies have been employed in Europe for many years for a wide range of conditions, in the United States most remain controversial and are currently unapproved by the FDA (Food and Drug Administration). Legality of oxygen therapies varies from state to state.

How Oxygenation Therapy Works

All human cells, tissues, and organs need oxygen to function. Oxygenation saturates the body with oxygen in the form of gas, sometimes at high pressure (hyperbaric), increasing the total amount of available oxygen in the body. Insufficient oxygenation may promote the growth of pathogens, whereas excessive oxygenation may damage normal tissues. Oxygenation employed under strictly controlled conditions can have very positive therapeutic effects.

Otto Warburg, former Director of the Max Planck Institute for

Cell Physiology in Germany and a two-time Nobel laureate, proposed that a lack of oxygen at the cellular level may be the prime cause of cancer, and that oxygen therapy could be an effective treatment for it.[2] He showed that normal cells in tissue culture, when deprived of oxygen, become cancer cells, and that oxygen can kill cancer cells in tissue cultures.

Oxygen therapy may be professionally administered in many ways: orally, rectally, vaginally, intravenously (into a vein), intra-arterially (into an artery), through inhalation, or by absorption through the skin. High concentrations of oxygen gas can also be given orally through masks or tubes, via oxygen tents, or within pressurized hyperbaric chambers. Oxygen may also be injected subcutaneously (beneath the skin). Ionized oxygen, both positively and negatively charged, is administered by inhalation or dissolved in drinking or bath water.

How Oxidation Therapy Works

The word oxidation refers to a chemical reaction whereby electrons are transferred from one molecule to another. Oxygen molecules are frequently, but not always, involved in these reactions. The molecules that "donate" electrons are said to be oxidized, whereas the molecules that accept electrons are called oxidants.

Oxidation therapy needs to be administered under clinical supervision, since uncontrolled oxidation may be destructive to the body.

A healthy state of oxidative balance is necessary for optimal function of the body, but when the body is exposed to repeated environmental stresses, its oxidative function is weakened. When oxidation is partially blocked by toxicity in the body or by pathological (disease-causing) organisms, oxidation therapy may help by "jump-starting" the body's oxidative processes and returning them to normal,[3] according to Charles Farr, M.D., Ph.D., of Oklahoma City, Oklahoma.

When properly administered, oxidation therapy selectively destroys pathogenic (disease-producing) bacteria, viruses, and other invading microbial organisms, and deactivates toxic substances without injury to healthy tissues or cells.[4] For example, if diluted hydrogen peroxide is placed on a wound, the normal cells thrive while the pathogens die.

Oxidation therapy must be administered under clinical supervision, since uncontrolled oxidation may be destructive to the body. Oxidation therapy may be given intravenously, orally, rectal-

According to Dr. Farr, arteriosclerosis and strokes may also benefit from hydrogen peroxide therapy. Infusing highly diluted *medical-grade* 35% hydrogen peroxide into the bloodstream brings oxygen to the tissues (as does hyperbaric oxygen therapy), which is what produces beneficial results in the case of stroke.

There are few side effects with hydrogen peroxide therapy. In rare cases, a problem involving inflammation of veins at the site of injection will occur. Hydrogen peroxide should not be taken orally, as it causes nausea and vomiting, and rectal administration can lead to inflammation of the lower intestinal tract. Other side effects observed include temporary faintness, fatigue, headaches, and chest pain. Most problems stem from an inappropriate administration route, administration above patient tolerance, the mixing of oxidative chemicals with other substances, or using oxidative chemicals in too great a concentration, reports Dr. Farr.

ly by enema, vaginally, or transcutaneously (absorbed through the skin).

Hydrogen Peroxide Therapy

Hydrogen peroxide is a liquid with the molecular structure of two atoms of hydrogen and two atoms of oxygen (H_2O_2). Because it is less stable than water (H_2O), hydrogen peroxide readily enters into oxidative reactions, ultimately becoming oxygen in water. It was Dr. Farr who, in 1984, first characterized the oxidative effects of hydrogen peroxide in humans.[5] Today, the use of hydrogen peroxide for its oxidative effects has spread to over 38 countries, and remains one of the least expensive, yet effective, oxidation therapies.

Oxidation administered through hydrogen peroxide therapy regulates tissue repair, cellular respiration, growth, immune functions, the energy system, most hormone systems, and the production of cytokines (chemical messengers that are involved in the regulation of almost every system in the body). Oxidation therapy can also work as a defense system, directly destroying invading bacteria, viruses, yeast, and parasites, according to Dr. Farr.

Conditions Benefited by Hydrogen Peroxide Therapy

Dr. Farr uses hydrogen peroxide for a variety of health problems, including AIDS, arthritis, cancer, candidiasis, chronic fatigue syndrome, depression, lupus erythematosus (a chronic inflammatory disease with symptoms including arthritis, fatigue, and skin lesions), emphysema, multiple sclerosis, varicose veins, and fractures.

According to Dr. Farr, arteriosclerosis and strokes may also benefit from hydrogen peroxide therapy.[6] Infusing highly diluted *medical-grade* 35% hydrogen peroxide into the bloodstream brings oxygen to the tissues (as does hyperbaric oxygen therapy), which is what produces beneficial results in the case of stroke. Concerning arteriosclerosis, hydrogen peroxide has been shown to dissolve fats (lipids) from the arterial walls.[7]

Ozone Therapy

Ozone therapy relies on the process of oxidation as well as oxygenation. Approximately one-fifth of the air humans breathe is comprised of two atoms of oxygen (O_2). Ozone (O_3) contains three oxygen atoms and is a less stable form of molecular oxygen. Due to this added molecule, ozone is more reactive than oxygen and readily enters into reactions to oxidize other chemicals. During oxidation in the body, the extra oxygen molecule in ozone breaks away, leaving a normal O_2 molecule. This increases the oxygen content of the blood or tissues. For this reason, ozone therapy is a combination of both oxygenation therapy and oxidation therapy.

Research is needed into the many conditions oxygen therapy can benefit. Because oxygen therapy can help the body repair itself, it is an ideal treatment to integrate into a comprehensive health care system.

Ozone is a common substance in nature, but can also be a source of air pollution when produced by man-made combustion. Medical-grade ozone is made from pure oxygen. Used therapeutically, ozone increases local oxygen supply to lesions, improves and accelerates wound healing, deactivates viruses and bacteria, and increases local tissue temperature, thus enhancing local metabolic processes, according to Gerard Sunnen, M.D., of New York City.

Ozone therapy can be used to treat arterial circulatory disturbances and to dissolve atherosclerotic plaque. Typically, intra-arterial injection (injection into an artery) is the method employed for this type of treatment.

Since the FDA has not approved the practice of ozone therapy in the United States, it is difficult to get data on its use. For fear of FDA reprisals, many physicians use ozone therapy without calling attention to themselves. However, numerous patient anecdotes are available.

Like many oxygen therapies, ozone therapy is widely employed and practiced in Europe, but still not readily available in the United States. According to Dr. Sunnen, prospective patients and doctors in America must await two further animal studies before the FDA sanctions a phase-one clinical trial with humans, and ultimately approves the therapeutic use of ozone.

The Future of Oxygen Therapy

The main stumbling blocks for all oxygen therapies, according to Dr. Hughes, are the FDA, health insurance companies, and the entrenched medical establishment. "The problem is that most areas of conventional medicine in this country are driven by the pharmaceutical companies," he says. "The incentive is always to sell pills, and you can't sell oxygen pills. This tends to hold it back, especially since a very large percentage of the research that's done at universities is funded by pharmaceutical companies."

Despite this fact, as Dr. Farr points out, the medical profession is becoming more receptive to oxygen therapy's potential benefits. For example, 10 to 12 years ago there were only eight locations in America for the use of hyperbaric oxygen. Now, according to Dr. Hughes, there are 28, and that number is increasing all the time. "More and more people are becoming familiar with HBOT, and we're getting more and more requests from the medical profession about what other conditions it can help."

"Treating the patient by getting more oxygen to the brain during the first three weeks after the stroke makes it still possible to minimize the damage," says David A. Steenblock, M.S., D.O. In fact, Dr. Steenblock has produced unexpected positive outcomes when treating people as long as 15 years after their stroke.

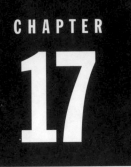
More Options for Treating Stroke

ANY OF THE THERAPIES discussed in Part One (Heart Disease) and Part Two (High Blood Pressure) are applicable to stroke as well. The following additional alternative medicine techniques have proven particularly useful in preventing or treating stroke.

Lasers

Margaret A. Naeser, Ph.D., associate research professor of neurology at Boston University School of Medicine and a licensed acupuncturist in Massachusetts, has conducted research on the use of low-energy lasers (20 milliwatt red-to-infrared laser light) in the treatment of paralysis from stroke. Five of her six subjects showed improvement, and patients with mild to moderate paralysis responded better than those with severe paralysis, according to Dr. Naeser. The improvements were observed even when treatments were begun three or four years after the stroke.

Neuropathways EEG Imaging

California therapist Margaret Ayers has been researching brain biofeedback for 20 years, a study that led her to invent a new form of therapeutic neurofeedback she calls Neuropathways EEG Imaging™. Ayers' brain research has shown that Neuropathways EEG Imaging

Research has shown that Neuropathways EEG Imaging may be an effective adjunct in the treatment of numerous serious brain disorders and injuries, including stroke.

may be an effective adjunct in the treatment of numerous serious brain disorders and injuries, including stroke, oxygen deprivation (anoxia), epileptic seizures, depression, and closed head injury, among others.

The device used in this technique displays the shape and electrical strength of a patient's brain waves on a computer screen and enables a person to interact, in real time, with the brain-wave pattern. Ayers has brought five patients out of Level Two coma using this device. (Level Two means the patient is unable to respond to sound, verbal commands, light, touch, or pressure.) Although a coma is not exactly like a stroke, some of the damage to the brain that can produce a coma is similar to the damage suffered in some strokes. The following examples will give you an idea of how the treatment works and how it could be used to regain movement and skills impaired by stroke.

Collin, 21, had spent two years in a coma following a motorcycle accident. He came out of his coma after two 1-hour treatments, states Ayers. Peter, 30, had been in a coma for three months following eight brain surgeries to remove a baseball-sized tumor. After a 60-minute session, in which Peter's brain was trained to make small responses to electrical stimulation, he snapped out of his coma, opened his eyes, and kissed his wife. After four more one-hour sessions, spaced one month apart, Peter was able to speak, eat, and move one side of his body.

A study Ayers conducted in 1987 with 250 individuals with closed head injuries (concussions), showed that long-term brain wave abnormalities resulting from the injury could be improved within six treatments, and entirely corrected within 24 sessions.

The brain constantly emits electrical impulses, registered as waves, that indicate the state of health and activity of the brain. In Neuropathways EEG Imaging, gold-plated cup electrodes are placed on certain areas of the head, corresponding to the brain regions whose waves the patient wishes to bring into balance. In effect, the brain is trained—this is the neuro (brain cells) feedback function—to replace abnormal waves with normal rhythmic patterns, explains

For more about **biofeedback,** see Chapter 13: Alternative Medicine Options for Lowering High Blood Pressure, pp. 217-221.

Biofeedback training is a method of learning how to consciously regulate normally unconscious bodily functions (such as heart rate, blood pressure, and breathing). It uses a monitoring device to measure and report back immediate information about the heart rate, for example, transmitting one blinking light or beep per heartbeat. The person being monitored learns techniques such as meditation, relaxation, and visualization to slow their heart rate and then uses the flashes or beeps to check their progress and make adjustments accordingly.

Ayers. The brain is encouraged to recognize the normal, healthy brain waves as the computer produces audio and visual reinforcements when these desired waves are achieved.

According to Ayers, once the brain learns how to change its beat, the new wave patterns are permanent. Mastering neurofeedback is a lot like learning to ride a bicycle; once learned, it's a skill never forgotten. Demonstrated benefits include improvements in short-term memory, concentration, speech, motor skills, energy level, sleep regularity, and emotional balance.[1]

Nutritional Supplements

The nutritional supplements discussed here are specific to stroke and may be considered along with the supplements recommended for maintaining general heart and circulatory health. As mentioned previously, excess homocysteine in the blood has been linked to stroke and is also associated with deficiencies of folic acid and vitamins B12 and B6. Therefore, supplementation with these nutrients may be advisable. Since low blood levels of the antioxidant vitamins C and E and beta carotene have also been linked to stroke,[2] supplementation can be preventive. As always, it is best to consult a health practitioner for assistance in designing the optimum supplement program for your individual biochemistry and health status.

As part of a stroke prevention regimen, coenzyme Q10, lipoic acid (especially if you are diabetic and eat lots of sweets or drink fruit juices), selenium, chromium GTF, and magnesium are also useful, reports David A. Steenblock, M.S., D.O. Vitamin B complex, *Ginkgo biloba*, and superoxide dismutase (SOD, an antioxidant enzyme) can be beneficial as well. In addition, vitamin E and essential fatty acids are important nutritional components for stroke prevention and recovery.

Vitamin E
According to Dr. Steenblock, vitamin E has been shown to reduce the damage from a stroke or transient ischemic attack. If you are at risk of a stroke, supplementing with this vitamin may therefore be a wise precaution.

When consumed in doses higher than 1,200 IU daily, vitamin E can have anticoagulant effects. This means it will increase your tendency to have a hemorrhagic stroke; especially if you have high blood pressure, do not have atherosclerosis (cholesterol deposits on the arterial walls) or arteriosclerosis (hardened arteries, reduced blood flow), and are female, frail, or have dry and brittle ("friable") blood vessels.

On the other hand, if you are of a stout build and have significant atherosclerosis or diabetes, or both, you probably would do well with higher doses of vitamin E, in the range of 1,200 to 2,000 IU daily, says Dr. Steenblock. At this dosage, the vitamin can act as a blood thinner (preventing blood clots) and may also decrease or stop atherosclerosis by stopping the spread of certain cells. Additionally, it can slow down or even prevent the production of harmful free radicals in the arterial walls. This is very important for diabetics since it stops a process in which sugars become attached to proteins when the blood sugar level is too high. These "sugar-proteins" are thought to be one of the main mechanisms of aging and atherosclerosis.

A daily dose of 400 to 800 IU of mixed tocopherols should be good for almost everyone, states Dr. Steenblock. These are various fat-soluble compounds with vitamin E antioxidant activity. Reliance on only one antioxidant (to neutralize free radicals) for stroke prevention is incorrect, he says. As always, he cautions, consult with your own qualified health professional before commencing any treatment.

Essential Fatty Acids

Research has shown that supplementation with EPA (eicosapentaenoic acid, an omega-3 essential fatty acid) from fish oil significantly reduces fibrinogen,[3] high levels of which can contribute to stroke.

William Lee Cowden, M.D., has noticed that if patients can be treated within the first 12 hours after a stroke with a combination of essential fatty acids, a high antioxidant intake, and either hyperbaric oxygen therapy or ozone therapy (see Chapter 16), a dramatic regression of symptoms of stroke can occur. Patients regain sensation, strength, and mental clarity, as well as motor and sensory skills and orientation. In his treatment, Dr. Cowden uses the antioxidants vitamin E, beta carotene, ascorbyl palmitate (a fat-soluble form of vitamin C), and pycnogenol (a fat-soluble antioxidant found in grape seeds and pine bark), along with the essential fatty acids EPA and DHA (docosahexaenoic acid, from fish oil) to help prevent damage to the fatty-acid membranes in brain cells.

QUICK DEFINITION

A **free radical** is an unstable molecule with an unpaired electron that steals an electron from another molecule and produces harmful effects. Free radicals are formed when molecules within cells react with oxygen (oxidize) as part of normal metabolic processes. Free radicals then begin to break down cells, especially if there are not enough free-radical quenching nutrients, such as vitamins C and E, in the cell. While free radicals are normal products of metabolism, uncontrolled free-radical production plays a major role in the development of degenerative disease, including cancer and heart disease. Free radicals harmfully alter important molecules, such as proteins, enzymes, fats, even DNA. Other sources of free radicals include pesticides, industrial pollutants, smoking, alcohol, viruses, most infections, allergies, stress, even certain foods and excessive exercise.

Additional Alternative Therapies

Self-Care

The following therapies can be undertaken at home under appropriate professional supervision:

- Flower Remedies
- Guided Imagery
- Massage
- Meditation
- Qigong
- Yoga
- Aromatherapy: For muscular paralysis, use lavender—Rub the spinal column and paralyzed area with a mixture of one quart of rubbing alcohol and one ounce each of essence of lavender, essence of rosemary, and essence of basil.
- Herbs: To improve circulation to extremities—elder flowers, hyssop, rosemary, yarrow. To nourish the nervous system—damiana, lavender, rosemary, Siberian ginseng. Consult a trained herbalist.
- Hydrotherapy: Constitutional hydrotherapy—apply two to five times weekly.
- Swimming to restore strength
- Reflexology: tip of big toe (opposite side from paralysis), other toes, reflexes to affected areas

Professional Care

The following therapies should only be provided by a qualified health professional:

- Chelation Therapy
- Hypnotherapy
- Light Therapy
- Magnetic Field Therapy
- Naturopathic Medicine
- Osteopathy
- Sound Therapy
- Traditional Chinese Medicine
- Reconstructive Therapy
- Bodywork: Feldenkrais
- Vision Therapy: Vision therapy may be an important ingredient in rehabilitation. Victims suffer impairment in aim, focus, and eye movement, as well as visual-field and perceptual defects. Without

William Lee Cowden, M.D., has noticed that if patients can be treated within the first 12 hours after a stroke with a combination of essential fatty acids, a high antioxidant intake, and either hyperbaric oxygen therapy or ozone therapy, a dramatic regression of symptoms of stroke can occur.

evaluation by a behavioral optometrist, these can be overlooked and recovery hindered. Therapy includes awareness training, visual/motor exercises, and lenses and prisms. Gross and fine movement control, hand-eye coordination, attention, memory, and learning skills improve dramatically.

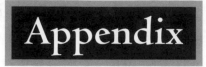

Appendix

Where to Find Help

For additional information and referrals concerning treatment for heart disease, hypertension, and stroke, contact the following organizations:

American Academy of Environmental Medicine
P.O. Box 1001-8001
New Hope, Pennsylvania 18938
(215) 862-4544
(215) 862-4583 (Fax)
The academy offers extensive training for physicians interested in learning more about environmental medicine. For information on physicians practicing environmental medicine send a self-addressed, stamped envelope along with your request.

American Holistic Medical Association
4101 Lake Boone Trail, Suite 201
Raleigh, North Carolina 27607
(919) 787-5181
A professional organization for holistic practitioners, the AHMA offers information and services for its members and lobbies for holistic issues. It also provides referrals for the public; requests must be in writing.

Aromatherapy

The Pacific Institute of Aromatherapy
P.O. Box 6723
San Rafael, California 94903
(415) 479-9121
(415) 479-0119 (Fax)
The Pacific Institute of Aromatherapy offers courses to individuals and companies interested in learning about, or becoming certified in, the practice of aromatherapy. Call for a brochure and course listing.

Aromatherapy Seminars
117 N. Robertson Blvd.
Los Angeles, California 90048
(800) 677-2368

(310) 276-1191
(310) 276-1156 (Fax)
Provides programs to become a certified aromatherapist, locally or through a correspondence course. They offer specialty classes for those already certified and have available videotapes, audiotapes and blending materials.

Lotus Light
P.O. Box 1008
Silver Lake, Wisconsin 53170
(414) 889-8501
(414) 889-8591 (Fax)
Provides mail order distribution of aromatherapy videotapes, books, and materials.

Ayurvedic Medicine

American School of Ayurvedic Sciences
2115 112th Avenue NE
Bellevue, Washington 98004
(206) 453-8022
This college provides medical training for physicians and health care practitioners, as well as individual courses for lay people. Dr. Virender Sodhi's Ayurvedic, Naturopathic Medical Clinic is also located at this address.

Ayurvedic Institute
11311 Menaul NE
Albuquerque, New Mexico 87112
(505) 291-9698
(505) 294-7572 (Fax)
The institute, directed by Dr. Vasant Lad, trains people from all walks of life in most of the aspects of Ayurveda.

The College of Maharishi Ayur-Veda Medical Center
P.O. Box 282
Fairfield, Iowa 52556
(515) 472-8477
The center provides referrals to health centers which offer methods of prevention and treatment of a broad range of illnesses. They also

train practitioners and provide information to the lay public.

Biofeedback

Association for Applied Psychophysiology and Biofeedback
10200 West 44th Avenue, Suite 304
Wheat Ridge, Colorado 80033
(303) 422-8436
(303) 422-8894 (Fax)
Provides names and phone numbers of chapters in your state (formerly Biofeedback Society of America).

Biofeedback Certification Institute of America
10200 West 44th Avenue, Suite 304
Wheat Ridge, Colorado 80033
(303) 420-2902
Runs the major certification program for biofeedback practitioners and provides information about certified local practitioners.

Tools for Exploration
47 Paul Drive
San Rafael, California 94903
(415) 499-9050
(415) 499-9047 (Fax)
Carries home biofeedback devices. Call for catalog.

Biological Dentistry

American Academy of Biological Dentistry
P.O. Box 856
Carmel Valley, California 93924
(408) 659-5385
(408) 659-2417 (Fax)
The purpose of the AABD is to promote biological dental medicine, which uses nontoxic diagnostic and therapeutic approaches in the field of clinical dentistry. They publish a quarterly journal, *Focus*, and hold regular seminars on biological diagnosis and therapy.

The Safe Water Coalition
5615 West Lyons Court
Spokane, Washington 99208
(509) 328-6704
The purpose of this organization is to educate legislators and the public on the hazards of fluoridation.

Chelation Therapy

American College of Advancement in Medicine
P.O. Box 3427
Laguna Hills, California 92654
(714) 583-7666
ACAM seeks to establish certification and standards of practice for chelation therapy. It provides training and education, and sponsors semiannual conferences for physicians and scientists. It provides referrals and informational material, including a directory listing of all physicians worldwide who have been trained in preventive medicine as well as in the ACAM protocol. The directory is updated monthly. The organization also provides a copy of the ACAM protocol for chelation to the public. For more information, send a stamped, self-addressed envelope along with your request.

The Rheumatoid Disease Foundation
5106 Old Harding Road
Franklin, Tennessee 37064
(615) 646-1030
This nonprofit, charitable organization has a listing of physicians who perform chelation therapy. Send a legal-size, stamped, self-addressed envelope, along with a donation, when requesting information.

Herbal Medicine

American Botanical Council
P.O. Box 201660
Austin, Texas 78720
(800) 373-7105
Nonprofit research and education organization. Publishes *HerbalGram* magazine, booklets on herbs, and reprints of scientific articles.

The American Herbalists Guild
P.O. Box 746555
Arvada, Colorado 80006
(303) 423-8800
(303) 402-1564 (Fax)
The Guild, with members ranging from clinical practitioners to ethnobotanists, has become an important influence in the reemergence of medical herbalism in the United States. A directory of schools and teachers is available.

Herb Research Foundation
1007 Pearl Street, Suite 200
Boulder, Colorado 80302
(303) 449-2265
(303) 449-2265 (Fax)
Co-publishes *HerbalGram* with ABC. Provides research materials for consumers, pharmacists, physicians, scientists, and industry.

Magnetic Field Therapy

Bio-Electro-Magnetics Institute
2490 West Moana Lane
Reno, Nevada 89509-3936
(702) 827-9099
A private, nonprofit organization established to provide research, education, support, and technical assistance in matters relating to bioelectromagnetics. A national clearinghouse for information relating to both health risks from power line magnetic fields and the health benefits from magnetic therapy.

Enviro-Tech Products
17171 Southeast 29th Street
Choctaw, Oklahoma 73020
(405) 390-3499
(405) 390-8934 (Fax)
This service includes self-help information, information for physicians, and information and guidance for research projects under the Institutional Review Board of the Bio-Electro-Magnetics Institute of Reno, Nevada.

Dr. Wolfgang Ludwig
Silcherstrasse 21
Horb A.N.1, Germany
011-49-7451-8648 (Fax)
For information regarding German instruments utilizing magnetic energy and pulsing frequencies, such as Endomet and Magnetron.

Prometheus Italia SrL
Centro Commerciale, VR-EST
Viale del Lavoro 45
I-36037, S. Martino B.A. (VR), Italy
This company produces magnetic blankets according to Dr. Ludwig's design.

Nutritional Supplements

American College of Advancement in Medicine
P.O. Box 3427

Laguna Hills, California 92654
(714) 583-7666
ACAM provides a directory listing of physicians worldwide who have been trained in nutritional and preventative medicine. The directory also provides an extensive list of books and articles on nutritional supplementation.

Oxygen Therapy

The American College of Hyperbaric Medicine
Ocean Medical Center
4001 Ocean Drive, Suite 105
Lauderdale-by-the-Sea, Florida 33308
(954) 771-4000
(954) 776-0670 (Fax)
A group of physicians dedicated to the clinical aspects of hyperbaric medicine. Their purpose is to foster ethical growth and development of the science and practice of hyperbaric oxygen therapy. Promotes research and education.

International Bio-oxidative Medicine Foundation
P.O. Box 891954
Oklahoma City, Oklahoma 73189
(405) 478-IBOM Ext. 4266
(405) 623-7320 (Fax)
The foundation publishes and distributes a newsletter as well as scientific research data. Supports educational programs that highlight current research and the therapeutic use of oxidative therapies. Encourages basic and clinical research. Membership available.

International Ozone Association
31 Strawberry Hill Avenue
Stamford, Connecticut 06902
(203) 348-3542
A professional scientific organization disseminating information on use and production of ozone through meetings, synopses, and world congresses. Publishes books and journals on ozone.

Medical Society for Ozone Therapy
Klagen Furtestrasse 4
D. 7000 Stuttgart 30, Germany
An excellent informational resource for the public and professionals. Addresses the differences between free ozone and medical ozone. The Society can explain how medical ozone is used to treat diseases, provide treat-

ment applications, and explain where and
why medical ozone is used.

Medizone International, Inc.
123 East 54th Street
New York, New York 10022
(212) 421-0303
Developers of ozone-based blood purification
systems and treatments for diseases caused
by lipid-enveloped viruses, including AIDS,
hepatitis B, and herpes.

**Carolina Center for Alternative
and Nutritional Medicine**
4505 Fair Meadow Lane, Suite 111
Raleigh, North Carolina 27607
(800) 473-9812 (U.S. and Canada)
(407) 967-6466 (outside North America)
Outpatient facility which focuses on metabolic and intestinal detoxification. Comprehensive and synergistic treatment regimens for
each patient are developed utilizing therapies
such as colon hydrotherapy, intravenous therapies (including ozone), and external ozone
hydrotherapy. Supportive elements such as
acupuncture and lymphatic massage, as well
as techniques to address the psychologi-
cal/emotional components of health and illness are also part of the program.

Traditional Chinese
Medicine

American Association of Oriental Medicine
433 Front Street
Catasauqua, Pennsylvania 18032
(610) 266-1433
(610) 264-2768 (Fax)
The association (formerly AAAOM) is a
national professional trade organization of
acupuncturists who meet acceptable standards of competency and can provide you
with the names and locations of local members. Referrals by written request only.

Endnotes

Chapter I
What Causes Heart Disease?

1 Privitera, James R., M.D. *Clots: Life's Biggest Killer* Unpublished manuscript. Covina, CA (1992).

2 American Heart Association Internet web site http://www.amhrt.org/hs96/has.html.

3 CASS Principal Investigators and Associates. "Myocardial Infarction and Mortality in the Coronary Artery Surgery Study (CASS) Randomized Trial." *New England Journal of Medicine* 310:12 (March 1984), 750-758.

4 McTaggart, Lynn. *What Doctors Don't Tell You* (San Francisco: Thorsons/HarperCollins, 1996). For her newsletter, *What Doctors Don't Tell You*: 4 Wallace Road, London, N12PG, England.

5 "Study Suggests Common Heart Test May Harm Patients." Internet: CNN Interactive Heath Page (September 16, 1996).

6 Robbins, S. L., R. S. Cotran, and V. Kumar, eds. *Pathological Basis of Disease* (New York: W.B. Saunders, 1984).

7 This report is based solely on product labeling as published by PDR®. Copyright © 1993 by Medical Economics Data, a division of Medical Economics Company, Inc. All rights reserved. There is no affiliation between Medical Economics Company, Inc., and Future Medicine Publishing, Inc.

8 Jaffe, D., et al. "Coronary Arteries in Newborn Children: Intimal Variations in Longitudinal Sections and Their Relationships to Clinical and Experimental Data." *Acta Paediatrica Scandinavica Suppl.* 219 (1971), 3-28.

9 Rath, Matthias, M.D. *Eradicating Heart Disease* (San Francisco: Health Now, 1993). Available from: Health Now, 387 Ivy Street, San Francisco, CA 94102; tel 800-624-2442.

10 Ibid.

11 Kostner, G. M., et al. "The Interaction of Human Plasma Low Density Lipoproteins with Glycosamino-Glycans: Influence of the Chemical Composition." *Lipids* 20:1 (January 1985), 24-28.

12 Passwater, Richard. *Supernutrition for Healthy Hearts* (New York: Dial Press, 1977); Gordon, T., et al. *American Journal of Medicine* 62 (1977), 707-714; Williams, P. et al. *The Lancet*

1 (1979), 72-75.

13 Gruberg, E. R., and S.A. Raymond. *Beyond Cholesterol: Vitamin B6, Arteriosclerosis, and Your Heart* (New York: St. Martin's Press, 1981), 34-35.

14 *British Heart Journal* 29:337 (1967).

15 Kostner, G. M., et al. "HMG CoA Reductase Inhibitors Lower LDL Cholesterol Without Reducing Lp(a) Levels." *Circulation* 80:5 (1989), 1313-1319.

16 Strandberg, T. E., et al. "Long-term Mortality after 5-year Multi-Factorial Primary Prevention of Cardiovascular Diseases in Middle-Aged Men." *Journal of the American Medical Association* 266:9 (September 1991),1225-1229.

17 Folkers, K., et al. "Lovastatin Decreases Coenzyme-Q Levels in Humans." *Proceedings of the National Academy of Sciences of the USA* 87:22 (November 1990), 8931-8934.

18 Public Citizen Health Research Group. *Health Letter* (April 1994).

19 Morris, R. D., et al. "Chlorination, Chlorination Byproducts, and Cancer: A Meta-Analysis." *American Journal of Public Health* 82:7 (July 1992), 955-963.

20 Morin, R. J., and S.K. Peng. "The Role of Cholesterol Oxidation Products in the Pathogenesis of Atherosclerosis." *Annals of Clinical and Laboratory Science* 19:4 (July/August 1989), 225-237.

21 Hattersley, J. G. "Acquired Atherosclerosis: Theories of Causation, Novel Therapies." *Journal of Orthomolecular Medicine* 6:2 (1991), 83-98.

22 Morin, R. J., and S.K. Peng. "The Role of Cholesterol Oxidation Products in the Pathogenesis of Atherosclerosis." *Annals of Clinical and Laboratory Science* 19:4 (July/August 1989), 225-237.

23 McCully, K. S. "Homocysteine Theory of Arteriosclerosis: Development and Current Status." *Atherosclerosis Reviews* 11 (1983), 157-246.

24 Morris, R. D., et al. "Chlorination, Chlorination Byproducts, and Cancer: A Meta-Analysis." *American Journal of Public Health* 82:7 (July 1992), 955-963; Yiamouiannis, J. *Fluoride: The Aging Factor: How to Recognize and Avoid the*

Devastating Effects of Fluoride (Delaware, OH: Health Action Press, 1986).

25 McCully, K. S. "Homocysteine Theory of Arteriosclerosis: Development and Current Status." *Atherosclerosis Reviews* 11 (1983), 157-246.

26 Morin, R. J., and S.K. Peng. "The Role of Cholesterol Oxidation Products in the Pathogenesis of Atherosclerosis." *Annals of Clinical and Laboratory Science* 19:4 (July/August 1989), 225-237.

27 Malinow, M. R. "Risk for Arterial Occlusive Disease: Is Hyperhomocysteinemia an Innocent Bystander?" *Canadian Journal of Cardiology* 17 (1989), x-xi; Stampfer, M. J., et al. "A Prospective Study of Plasma Homocysteine and Risk of Myocardial Infarction in U.S. Physicians." *Journal of the American Medical Association* 268:7 (August 1992), 877-881.

28 Barnes, Broda O., M.D., and Lawrence Galton. *Hypothyroidism: The Unsuspected Illness* (New York: Harper & Row, 1976).

29 Peng, S. K. and C.B. Taylor. "Cholesterol Autooxidation, Health and Arteriosclerosis." *World Reviews of Nutrition and Diet* 44 (1984), 117-154.

30 McCully, Kilmer S., M.D. *The Homocysteine Revolution: Medicine for the New Millennium* (New Canaan, CT: Keats Publishing, 1997).

31 Nehler, Mark, M.D., et al., "Homocysteinemia as a Risk Factor for Atherosclerosis: A Review." *Cardiovascular Pathology* 6 (1997), 1-9.

32 Queen, H.L. *Chronic Mercury Toxicity: New Hope Against an Endemic Disease* (Colorado Springs, CO: Queen and Company, 1988).

Chapter 2

Caring for Yourself: Use Diet, Exercise, and Lifestyle Changes to Improve Your Heart Fitness

1 *Circulation* 89:94 (January 1994).

2 *Science* 264:532 (April 22, 1994).

3 *American Journal of Clinical Nutrition* 59:861 (April 1994); *Medical Journal of Australia* 156:Suppl. (May 4, 1992), S9-S16.

4 Schwartz, Elizabeth. "Misunderstood Soy May Lower Cholesterol." Internet: CNN Interactive Fitness & Heath Page (August 2, 1996).

5 "Veggies Fight Heart Disease, Cancer, Study Finds," Internet: Reuters via Individual, Inc. (June 20, 1997).

6 Ornish, Dean, M.D. *Dr. Dean Ornish's Program for Reversing Heart Disease* (New York: Ballantine, 1990).

7 Ibid.

8 "Chocolate May Help Reduce Heart Disease, Study Suggests." Internet: CNN Interactive Heath Page (September 20, 1996).

9 *The Lancet* 344:8933 (November 1994), 1356.

10 Hertog, M.G., et al. "Antioxidant Flavonols and Coronary Heart Disease Risk." *The Lancet* 349:699 (1997).

11 Nash, David T. "Grapeseed Oil Increases High Density Lipoprotein Cholesterol Levels in Dyslipidemic Subjects with Initially Low Levels." *Arteriosclerosis* 10:6 (Nov/Dec 1990). Nash, David T. et al. "Grapeseed Oil, A Natural Agent Which Raises Serum HDL Levels." *Journal of the American College of Cardiology* (March 1993). Huttunen, Jussi K., et al. "The Helsinki Heart Study: Central Findings and Clinical Implications." *Annals of Medicine* 23 (1991), 155-159. Feldman, Henry A. et al. "Impotence and Its Medical and Psychosocial Correlates: Results of the Massachusetts Male Aging Study." *Journal of Urology* 151 (January 1994), 54-61. Humer, Valentin. "Grapeseed Oil: The Champagne of Cooking Oils." *Healthy & Natural Journal* 2:3 (1995), 74-76. Kamen, Betty, Ph.D., "Natural Nutrition: Grapeseed Oil." *Let's Live* 62:12 (December 1994).

12 *American College of Cardiology*, March 14-18, 1993.

13 "Special Report: Olive Oil." *UC Berkeley Wellness Letter* (June 1995), 6. Sinatra, Stephen T., M.D. *Optimum Health: A Natural Lifesaving Prescription for Your Body and Mind* (New York: Bantam Books, 1997). Visioli, Francesco, et al. "Low Density Lipoprotein Oxidation is Inhibited In Vitro by Olive Oil Constituents." *Atherosclerosis* 117 (1995), 25-32. Staninger, Hildegarde L.A., Ph.D. *Olive Oil: Its Medicinal Uses for a Healthier You.* Monograph, (1996). Sharhil, Ltd., International Institute of Medical Toxicology, 2699 Lee Road, Suite 303, Winter Park, FL 32789; tel: 407-628-3399; fax: 407-628-1061.

14 Key, Timothy J.A., et al. "Dietary Habits and Mortality in 11,000 Vegetarians and Health Conscious People: Results of a 17-Year Follow Up." *British Medical Journal* 313 (1996), 775-779.

15 Gruber, E. R., and S.A. Raymond. *Beyond Cholesterol: Vitamin B6, Arteriosclerosis, and Your Heart* (New York: St.Martin's Press, 1981).

16 Ornish, Dean, M.D., et al. "Can Lifestyle Changes Reverse Coronary Heart Disease? The Lifestyle Heart Trial." *The Lancet* 336:8708 (July 1990), 129-133.

17 Halsey, Eugenia. "Researchers Pinpoint Link Between Smoking and Heart Disease." Internet: CNN Interactive Main Food & Heath Page (May 3, 1996).

18 Ciampa, Linda. "Study: Passive Smoke and Even Greater Risk." Internet: CNN Interactive Heath Page (May 19, 1997).

19 Halsey, Eugenia. "Researchers Pinpoint Link Between Smoking and Heart Disease." Internet: CNN Interactive Main Food & Heath Page (May 3, 1996).

20 Hinman, Al. "Studies Show Wine, Beer and Grape Juice Help Prevent Heart Disease." Internet: CNN Interactive Fitness and Health Page (March 18, 1997).

21 Ibid.

22 Stuttaford, Thomas, M.D. "Exercise is at the Heart of the Matter." The Times (April 17, 1997).

23 Kahn, Jason. "Study Says Reduced Exercise, Not Age, Hurts Heart." Medical Tribune News Service (April 18, 1996).

24 Verrill, David E., and Paul M. Ribisl. "Resistive Exercise Training and Cardiac Rehabilitation." Sports Medicine 21:5 (May 1996), 347-383.

25 Woolf-May, Kathryn, et al. "Effects of an 18-Week Walking Programme on Cardiac Function in Previously Sedentary or Relatively Inactive Adults." British Journal of Sports Medicine 31 (1997), 48-53.

26 Journal of the American Medical Association 275:18 (May 8, 1996).

27 Lomama, E., et al. "Rehabilitation of Aged Patients with Bicycle Ergometer after Coronary Surgery." Archives des Maladies du Coeur et des Vaisseaux 89:11 (1996), 1351-1355.

28 Meyer, Katharina, Ph.D. "Effects of Short-Term Exercise Training and Activity Restriction on Functional Capacity in Patients with Severe Chronic Congestive Heart Failure." American Journal of Cardiology 78 (November 1, 1996), 1017-1022.

29 Rafoth, Richard, M.D. Bicycling Fuel (Osceola, WI: Bicycle Books, 1988); Robertson, Gary. "Exercise Goes High-Tech." Richmond Times-Dispatch (February 6, 1997).

Chapter 3

Scrubbing the Arteries Naturally: How Chelation Therapy Can Help Prevent and Treat Heart Disease

1 Farr, C. H., M.D., R. White, and M. Schachter, M.D. "Chronological History of EDTA Chelation Therapy." Presented to the American College of Advancement in Medicine, Houston, TX (May 1993).

2 Olszewer, E., and J. Carter. "EDTA Chelation Therapy: A Retrospective Study of 2,870 Patients." Journal of Advancement in Medicine Special Issue 2:1-2 (1989), 209.

3 McDonagh, E., C. Rudolph, and E. Cheraskin. "An Oculocerebrovasculometric Analysis of the Improvement in Arterial Stenosis Following EDTA Chelation Therapy." Journal of Advancement in Medicine Special Issue 2:1-2 (1989), 155.

4 Chappell, L. Terry, M.D., and John P. Stahl, Ph.D. Questions from the Heart (Charlottesville, VA: Hampton Roads Publishing, 1996).

5 Olszewer, E., and J. Carter. "EDTA Chelation Therapy: A Retrospective Study of 2,870 Patients." Journal of Advancement in Medicine Special Issue 2:1-2 (1989), 183.

6 Walker, M., and G. Gordon. The Chelation Answer: How to Prevent Hardening of the Arteries and Rejuvenate Your Cardiovascular System (New York: M. Evans and Company, 1982).

7 Olszewer, E., and J.P. Carter. "EDTA Chelation Therapy in Chronic Degenerative Disease." Medical Hypotheses 27:1 (September 1988), 41-49.

8 Cranton, E. M., M.D. "Protocol of the American College of Advancement in Medicine for the Safe and Effective Administration of Intravenous EDTA Chelation Therapy." Journal of Advancement in Medicine Special Issue 2:1-2 (1989), 269-305.

9 Walker, M. Chelation Therapy (Stamford, CT: New Way of Life, 1984).

10 Olszewer, E., and J. Carter. "EDTA Chelation Therapy: A Retrospective Study of 2,870 Patients." Journal of Advancement in Medicine Special Issue 2:1-2 (1989), 197-211.

11 Ibid.

12 McDonagh, E. W., C. J. Rudolph, and E. Cheraskin, M.D. "An Oculocerebrovasculometric Analysis of the Improvement in Arterial Stenosis Following EDTA Chelation Therapy." Journal of Advancement in Medicine Special Issue 2:1-2 (1989), 155-166.

13 Alsleben, H. R., M.D., and W. E. Shute, M.D. How to Survive the New Health Catastrophes (Anaheim, CA: Survival Publications, 1973).

14 McDonagh, E. W., C. J. Rudolph, and E. Cheraskin, M.D. "An Oculocerebrovasculometric Analysis of the Improvement in Arterial Stenosis Following EDTA Chelation Therapy." Journal of Advancement in Medicine Special Issue 2:1-2 (1989), 155-166.

15 Casdorph, H. R., M.D. "EDTA Chelation Therapy: Efficacy in Brain Disorders." *Journal of Advancement in Medicine* Special Issue 2:1-2 (1989), 131-153.

16 Alsleben, H. R., M.D., and W. E. Shute, M.D. *How to Survive the New Health Catastrophes* (Anaheim, CA: Survival Publications, 1973).

17 Blumer, W., M.D., and E. M. Cranton, M.D. "Ninety Percent Reduction in Cancer Mortality After Chelation Therapy with EDTA." *Journal of Advancement in Medicine* Special Issue 2:1-2 (1989), 183.

18 Alsleben, H. R., M.D., and W. E. Shute, M.D. *How to Survive the New Health Catastrophes* (Anaheim, CA: Survival Publications, 1973).

19 Ibid.

20 Chappel, T. L., M.D. "Preliminary Findings From the Media Analysis Study of EDTA Chelation Therapy." Presented to the American College of Advancement in Medicine, Houston, TX (May 5-9, 1993).

21 Walker, M., and G. Gordon. *The Chelation Answer* (New York: M. Evans and Company, 1982), 175.

22 Tu, Jack V., et al. "Use of Cardiac Procedures and Outcomes in Elderly Patients with Myocardial Infarction in the United States and Canada." *New England Journal of Medicine* 336:21 (May 22, 1997).

23 Maugh, T.H. "Invasive Heart Attack Treatment Questioned." *Los Angeles Times (*March 20, 1997).

24 Whitaker, Julian, M.D., "Heart Surgery Does More Harm Than Good." *Dr. Julian Whitaker's Health & Healing* 7:5 (May 1997), 1-3.

25 Strauts, Z., M.D. "Correspondence Re: Berkeley Wellness Letter and Chelation Therapy." *Townsend Letter for Doctors* 106 (May 1992), 382-383.

Chapter 4

The Dental Connection: Problems With Your Teeth Can Affect Your Heart— and How to Reverse Them

1 Neuner, O. "The Diagnosis and Therapy of Focal and Field Disorders." *Raum & Zeit* 2:4 (1991), 38-42.

2 Price, W. A. *Dental Infections Volume 1: Oral and Systemic* (Cleveland, OH: Benton Publishing, 1973).

3 Strauss, F. G., and D. W. Eggleston. "IgA Nephropathy Associated with Dental Nickel

Alloy Sensitization." *American Journal of Nephrology* 5 (1985), 395-397.

4 "Dental Mercury Hygiene: Summary of Recommendations in 1990." *Journal of the American Dental Association* 122 (August 1991), 112.

5 "Dental Amalgam: A Scientific Review and Recommended Public Health Service Strategy for Research, Education and Regulation." *Final Report of the Subcommittee on Risk Management of the Committee to Coordinate Environmental Health and Related Programs* (Washington: U.S. Public Health Service, 1993).

6 "Dental Mercury Hygiene: Summary of Recommendations in 1990." *Journal of the American Dental Association* 122 (August 1991), 112.

7 Melillo, W. "How Safe is Mercury in Dentistry?" *The Washington Post Weekly Journal of Medicine, Science and Society* (September 1991), 4.

8 World Health Organization. *Environmental Health Criteria for Inorganic Mercury* 118 (Geneva: World Health Organization, 1991).

9 Hahn, L. J., et al. "Dental 'Silver' Tooth Fillings: A Source of Mercury Exposure Revealed by Whole-Body Image Scan and Tissue Analysis." *FASEB Journal* 3 (1989), 2641-2646; Hahn, L. J., et al. "Whole-Body Imaging of the Distribution of Mercury Released from Dental Fillings into Monkey Tissues." *FASEB Journal* 4 (1990), 3256-3260.

10 Vimy, M. J., et al. "Maternal-Fetal Distribution of Mercury Released from Dental Amalgam Fillings." *American Physiological Society* 258 (1990), R939-R945.

11 For the key research on mercury dental amalgam toxicity, consult: Lorscheider, Fritz, et al. "Mercury Exposure from 'Silver' Tooth Fillings: Emerging Evidence Questions a Traditional Dental Paradigm," *FASEB Journal* 9 (1995), 504-508. Huggins, Hal, D.D.S. *Coors Study: A Landmark in Dental Research,* a video, P.O. Box 49145, Colorado Springs, CO 80949; tel: 719-522-0566; fax: 719-548-8220; website: http://www.hugnet.com. Lichtenberg, H. "Mercury Vapor in the Oral Cavity in Relation to the Number of Amalgam Surfaces and the Classic Symptoms of Chronic Mercury Poisoning." *Journal of Orthomolecular Medicine* 11:2 (Second Quarter 1996), 87-94. See all issues of *Heavy Metal Bulletin: International Forum Focusing on Immuno-Toxic Effects of*

Dental Fillings and Related Disorders (Lilla Aspuddvs. 10, S-12649 Hägersten, Stockholm, Sweden; tel & fax: 46-8-184086; $65 U.S./3 issues). Richardson, G. Mark, Ph.D. *Assessment of Mercury Exposure and Risks from Dental Amalgam* (Medical Devices Bureau, Environmental Health Directorate, Health Canada, August 18, 1995).

12 Ziff, S. "Consolidated Symptom Analysis of 1,569 Patients." *Bio-Probe Newsletter* 9:2 (March 1993), 7-8.

13 Grandjean, P., M.D. "Reference Intervals for Trace Elements in Blood: Significance of Risk Factors." *Scandinavian Journal of Clinical and Laboratory Investigation* 2 (June 1992), 321-337; Schiele, R., et al. *Studies on the Mercury Content in Brain and Kidney Related to Number and Condition of Amalgam Fillings* (Nurnberg, West Germany: Institution of Occupational and Social Medicine, University Erlangen, 1984); Boyd, N. D., et al. "Mercury from Dental 'Silver' Tooth Fillings Impairs Sheep Kidney Function." *American Physiological Society* 261 (1991), R1010-R1014.

Chapter 5

Nutritional Supplements: How They Can Benefit Your Heart

1 Street, D. A., et al. "A Population-Based Case Control Study of the Association of Serum Antioxidants and Myocardial Infarction." *American Journal of Epidemiology* 131 (1991), 719-720.

2 Harvard Physicians Study. Ongoing.

3 Berge, K. G., and P. L. Canner. "Coronary Drug Project: Experience with Niacin. Coronary Drug Project Research Group." *European Journal of Clinical Pharmacology* 40:Suppl.1 (1991), S49-S51; Luria, M. H. "Effect of Low-Dose Niacin on High-Density Lipoprotein Cholesterol and Total Cholesterol/High-Density Lipoprotein Ratio." *Archives of Internal Medicine* 148:11 (November 1988), 2493-2495.

4 Canner, P. L., et al. "Fifteen Year Mortality in Coronary Drug Project Patients; Long-Term Benefit with Niacin." *Journal of the American College of Cardiology* 8:6 (December 1986), 1245-1255.

5 Hattersley, J. G. "Heart Attacks and Strokes." *Townsend Letter for Doctors* 104 (February/March 1992).

6 Berge, K. G., and P. L. Canner. "Coronary Drug Project: Experience with Niacin. Coronary Drug Project Research Group." *European Journal of*

Clinical Pharmacology* 40:Suppl.1 (1991), S49-S51.

7 Olszewski, A. J., et al. "Reduction of Plasma Lipid and Homocysteine Levels by Pyridoxine, Folate, Cobalamin, Choline, Riboflavin, and Troxerutin in Atherosclerosis." *Atherosclerosis* 75:1 (January 1989), 1-6.

8 Mudd, S. H., et al. "The Natural History of Homocystinuria Due to Cystathionine Beta-Synthose Deficiency." *American Journal of Human Genetics* 37:1 (January 1985), 1-31.

9 Editorial. "Is Vitamin B6 an Antithrombotic Agent?" *The Lancet* 1:8233 (June 1981),1299-1300.

10 Suzman, M. M. "Effect of Pyridoxine and Low Animal Protein Diet in Coronary Artery Disease." *Circulation* Suppl. IV-254 (October 1973), Abstracts of the 46th Scientific Sessions.

11 Ibid.

12 McCully, K. S. "Homocysteine Theory of Arteriosclerosis: Development and Current Status." *Atherosclerosis Reviews* 11 (1983), 157-246.

13 Ibid.

14 Brattstrom, L., et al. "Higher Total Plasma Homocysteine Due to Cystathionine Beta-Synthase Deficiency." *Metabolism: Clinical and Experimental* 37:2 (February 1988), 175-178.

15 Ibid.

16 Olszewski, A. J., et al. "Reduction of Plasma Lipid and Homocysteine Levels by Pyridoxine, Folate, Cobalamin, Choline, Riboflavin, and Troxerutin in Atherosclerosis." *Atherosclerosis* 75:1 (January 1989),1-6.

17 Brattstrom, L., et al. "Impaired Homocysteine Metabolism in Early-Onset Cerebral and Peripheral Occlusive Artery Disease. Effects of Pyridoxine and Folic Acid Treatment." *Atherosclerosis* 81:1 (1990), 51-60; Olszewski, A. J., et al. "Reduction of Plasma Lipid and Homocysteine Levels by Pyridoxine, Folate, Cobalamin, Choline, Riboflavin, and Troxerutin in Atherosclerosis." *Atherosclerosis* 75:1 (January 1989), 1-6.

18 Rimm, E., et al. "Vitamin E Consumption and the Risk of Coronary Heart Disease in Men." *New England Journal of Medicine* 328:20 (May 1993), 1450-1456; Stampfer, M. J., et al. "Vitamin E Consumption and the Risk of Coronary Heart Disease in Women." *New England Journal of Medicine* 328:20 (May 1993), 1444-1449.

19 McCully, K. S. "Homocysteine Metabolism in Scurvy, Growth, and Arteriosclerosis." *Nature*

231:5302 (June 1971), 391-392.

20 Rath, M., and L. Pauling. "Hypothesis: Lipoprotein(a) is a Surrogate for Ascorbate." *Proceedings of the National Academy of Sciences of the U.S.A.* 87:16 (August 1990), 6204-6207.

21 Ginter, E. R., et al. "Vitamin C in the Control of Hypercholesterolemia in Man." *International Journal for Vitamin and Nutrition Research* 23:Suppl. (1982), 137-152.

22 Rath, M., and L. Pauling. "Solution to the Puzzle of Human Cardiovascular Disease: Its Primary Cause is Ascorbate Deficiency Leading to the Deposition of Lipoprotein(a) and Fibrinogen/Fibrin in the Vascular Wall." *Journal of Orthomolecular Medicine* 6 (1991), 125-134.

23 Rath, M., and L. Pauling. "Hypothesis: Lipoprotein(a) is a Surrogate for Ascorbate." *Proceedings of the National Academy of Sciences of the U.S.A.* 87:16 (August 1990), 6204-6207.

24 Rath, M., and L. Pauling. "Solution to the Puzzle of Human Cardiovascular Disease: Its Primary Cause is Ascorbate Deficiency Leading to the Deposition of Lipoprotein(a) and Fibrinogen/Fibrin in the Vascular Wall." *Journal of Orthomolecular Medicine* 6 (1991), 125-134.

25 Enstrom, J. E., et al. "Vitamin C Intake and Mortality Among a Sample of the United States Population." *Epidemiology* 3 (1992), 194-202.

26 Sahyoun, Nadine R., et al. "Carotenoids, Vitamins C and E and Mortality in an Elderly Population." *American Journal of Epidemiology* 144:5 (September 1, 1996), 501-511.

27 Jialal, I., and S. M. Grundy. "Effect of Dietary Supplementation with Alpha-Tocopherol on the Oxidative Modification of Low Density Lipoprotein." *Journal of Lipid Research* 33:6 (June 1992), 899-906; Steiner, M. "Influence of Vitamin E on Platelet Function in Humans." *Journal of the American College of Nutrition* 10:5 (October 1991), 466-473.

28 Boscoboinik, D., et al. "Alpha-Tocopherol (Vitamin E) Regulates Vascular Smooth Muscle Cell Proliferation and Protein Kinase C Activity." *Archives of Biochemistry and Biophysics* 286:1 (April 1991), 264-269; Hennig, B., et al. "Protective Effects of Vitamin E in Age-Related Endothelial Cell Injury." *International Journal of Vitamin and Nutrition Research* 59 (1989), 273-279.

29 Rimm, E., et al. "Vitamin E Consumption and the Risk of Coronary Heart Disease in Men." *New England Journal of Medicine* 328:20 (May 1993), 1450-1456; Stampfer, M. J., et al. "Vitamin E Consumption and the Risk of Coronary Heart Disease in Women." *New England Journal of Medicine* 328:20 (May 1993), 1444-1449.

30 Stampfer, M., et al. "Vitamin E and Heart Disease Incidence in the Nurses Health Study." American Heart Association Annual Meeting. New Orleans, LA (November 18, 1992).

31 Rimm, E., et al. "Vitamin E and Heart Disease Incidence in the Health Professionals Study." American Heart Association Annual Meeting, New Orleans, LA (November 18, 1992).

32 Kushi, L.H., et al. "Dietary Antioxidant Vitamins and Death from Coronary Heart Disease in Postmenopausal Women" *New England Journal of Medicine* 334:18 (May 2, 1996), 1156-1162.

33 Gey, K. F., et al. "Inverse Correlation Between Plasma Vitamin E and Mortality from Ischemic Heart Disease in Cross-Cultural Epidemiology." *American Journal of Clinical Nutrition* 53:Suppl. 1 (January 1991), 326S-334S.

34 Stephens, Nigel G., et al. "Randomized Controlled Trial of Vitamin E in Patients with Coronary Artery Disease: Cambridge Heart Antioxidant Study (CHAOS)." *The Lancet* (March 23, 1996), 781-786.

35 Jialal, I., et al. "The Effect of Alpha-Tocopherol Supplementation on LDL Oxidation: A Dose-Response Study." *Arteriosclerosis, Thrombosis, and Vascular Biology* 15 (1995), 190-198.

36 *The Diet-Heart Newsletter* 7:1 (Winter 1994), 2.

37 Karanja, N., et al. "Plasma Lipids and Hypertension: Response to Calcium Supplementation." *American Journal of Clinical Nutrition* 45:1 (January 1987), 60-65.

38 Leifsson, Bjorn G., M.D., and Bo Ahren. "Serum Calcium and Survival in a Large Health Screening Program." *Journal of Clinical Endocrinology and Metabolism* 81:6 (1996), 2149-2153.

39 Simonoff, M, et al. "Low Plasma Chromium in Patients with Coronary Artery and Heart Diseases." *Biological Trace Elements Research* 6:5 (October 1984), 431-439; Newman, H. A., et al. "Serum Chromium and Angiographically Determined Coronary Artery Disease." *Clinical Chemistry* 24:4 (April 1978), 541-544.

40 Press, R. I., et al. "The Effect of Chromium Picolinate on Serum Cholesterol and Apolipoprotein Fractions in Human Subjects."

Western Journal of Medicine 152:1 (January 1990), 41-45.

41 Urberg, M., et al. "Hypercholesterolemic Effects of Nicotinic Acid and Chromium Supplementation." *Journal of Family Practice* 27:6 (December 1988), 603-606.

42 Wood, D. A., et al. "Adipose Tissue and Platelet Fatty Acids and Coronary Heart Disease in Scottish Men." *The Lancet* 2:8395 (July 1984), 117-121.

43 Ferneandes, J.S., et al. "Therapeutic Effect of a Magnesium Salt in Patients Suffering from Mitral Valvular Prolapse and Latent Tentany." *Magnesium* 4 (1985), 283-290.

44 Lichodziejewsa, B., et al. "Clinical Symptoms of Mitral Valve Prolapse Are Related to Hypomagnesemia and Attenuated by Magnesium Supplementation." *American Journal of Cardiology* 79 (1997), 768-772.

45 Seelig, M. S., and H. A. Heggtveit. "Magnesium Interrelationships in Ischemic Heart Disease: A Review." *American Journal of Clinical Nutrition* 27:1 (January 1974), 59-79; Davis, W. H., et al. "Monotherapy with Magnesium Increases Abnormally Low Density Lipoprotein Cholesterol: A Clinical Assay." *Current Therapeutic Research* 36:2 (August 1984), 341.

46 *Northeast Center for Environmental Medicine Health Letter* (Fall 1992).

47 Salonen, J. T., et al. "Interactions of Serum Copper, Selenium and Low Density Lipoprotein Cholesterol in Atherogenesis." *British Medical Journal* 302:6779 (March 1991), 756-760.

48 Stead, N. W., et al. "Effect of Selenium Supplementation on Selenium Balance in the Dependent Elderly." *American Journal of the Medical Sciences* 290:6 (December 1985), 228-233.

49 Koifman, Bella, M.D. "Improvement of Cardiac Performance by Intravenous Infusion of L-Arginine in Patients with Moderate Congestive Heart Failure." *Journal of the American College of Cardiology* 26:5 (November 1, 1995), 1251-1256.

50 Singh, R. B. "A Randomized, Double-Blind, Placebo-Controlled Trial of L-Carnitine in Suspected Acute Myocardial Infarction." *Postgraduate Medical Journal* (1995).

51 Iliceto, Sabino, M.D. "Effects of L-Carnitine Administration on Left Ventricular Remodeling after Acute Anterior Myocardial Infarction." *American Journal of Cardiology* 26:2 (1995), 380-387.

52 Kneki, Paul. "Flavonoid Intake and Coronary Mortality in Finland: A Cohort Study." *British Medical Journal* 312 (1996), 478-481.

53 Hanaki, Y., S. Sugiyama, and T. Ozawa. "Ratio of Low-Density Lipoprotein Cholesterol to Ubiquinone as a Coronary Risk Factor." *New England Journal of Medicine* 325:11 (September 1991), 814-815; Frei, B., et al. "Ubiquinol-10 Is an Effective Lipid-Soluble Antioxidant at Physiological Concentrations." *Proceedings of the National Academy of Sciences of the U.S.A.* 87:12 (1990), 4879-4883.

54 *The Energy Times* (January/February 1995), 12, 56; *Cancer Communication Newsletter* 1:1 (February 1995), 11; Information provided by Michael B. Schacter, M.D. *Dr. Jonathan Wright's Nutrition & Healing Newsletter* 1:1 (August 1994), 3-4.

55 *New England Journal of Medicine* 312 (1985), 1250-1259.

56 *Atherosclerosis* 63 (1987), 137-143; *Hypertension* 4:Suppl. (1982), iii-34.

57 Olszewski, A. J., and K. S. McCully. "Fish Oil Decreases Serum Homocysteine in Hyperlipemic Men." *Coronary Artery Disease* 4 (1993), 53-60.

58 Kromhout, D., et al. "The Inverse Relation Between Fish Consumption and 20-Year Mortality From Coronary Heart Disease." *New England Journal of Medicine* 312:19 (May 1985), 1205-1209.

59 Renaud, S., and A. Nordy. "'Small is Beautiful': Alpha-Linoleic Acid and Eicosapentaenoic Acid in Man." *The Lancet* 1:8334 (May 1983), 1169.

60 Rosenbaum, M. E., M.D., and D. Bosco. *Super Fitness Beyond Vitamins: The Bible of Super Supplements* (New York: New American Library, 1987).

61 Crayhon, Robert. *Health Benefits of FOS* (New Canaan, CT: Keats Publishing, 1995).

62 Pao, E. M., and S. Mickle. "Problem Nutrients in the United States." *Food Technology* (September 1981), 58-79.

63 "Dietary Intake Source Data: U.S. 1976-1980." Data from the *National Health Survey Series 11* #231. (DHHS Publication (PHS) 8361, March 1983).

64 Yankelovich, Clancy, and Schulman. "Survey for Nutritional Health Alliance 1992." *Whole Foods Magazine* 16:3 (March 1993), 55.

Chapter 6
How Herbs Can Aid Your Heart

1 Herb Trade Association. Definition of "Herb." (Austin, TX: Herb Trade Association, 1977).

2 Henry, C. J., and B. Emery. "Effect of Spiced Food on Metabolic Rate. Human Nutrition." *Clinical Nutrition* 40:2 (March 1986), 165-168.

3 Glatzel, H. "Blood Circulation Effectiveness of Natural Spices." *Medizinische Klinik* 62:51 (December 1967), 1987-1989. (Published in German).

4 Barrie, S. A., J. V. Wright, M.D., and J. E. Pizzorno. "Effect of Garlic Oil on Platelet Aggregation, Serum Lipids and Blood Pressure in Humans." *Journal of Orthomolecular Medicine* 2:1 (1987), 15-21.

5 Shoji, N., et al. "Cardiotonic Principles of Ginger (Zingiber officinale Roscoe)." *Journal of Pharmaceutical Sciences* 71:10 (October 1982), 1174-1175.

6 Srivastava, K. C. "Effects of Aqueous Extracts of Onion, Garlic and Ginger on Platelet Aggregation and Metabolism of Arachidonic Acid in the Blood Vascular System." *Prostaglandins Leukotrienes and Medicine* 13 (1984), 227-235.

7 Foster, S. *Ginkgo. Botanical Series 304* (Austin, TX: American Botanical Council, 1991).

8 Kleijnen, J., and P. Knipschild. "*Ginkgo biloba.*" *The Lancet* 340:8828 (November 1992), 1136-1139.

9 Braquet, P., ed. *Ginkgolides—Chemistry, Biology, Pharmacology and Clinical Perspectives,* Volume 1 (Barcelona, Spain: J. Prous Science Publishers, 1988) and Volume 2 (1989); Fungfeld, E. W., ed. *Rokan: Ginkgo biloba* (New York: Springer-Verlag, 1988).

10 *Arzneimittel-Forschung* 43:9 (September 1993), 978.

11 Weiss, R. F. *Herbal Medicine* (Gothenburg, Sweden: A. B. Arcanum, 1988).

12 Walker, Morton, D.P.M. "Antimicrobial Attributes of Olive Leaf Extract." *Townsend Letter for Doctors & Patients* (July 1996), 80-85; Renis, Harold E. "In Vitro Antiviral Activity of Calcium Elenolate." *Antimicrobial Agents and Chemotherapy-1969* (1970), 167-171; Juven, B., et al. "Studies on the Mechanism of the Antimicrobial Action of Oleuropein." *Journal of Applied Bacteriology* 35 (1972), 559-567; Konlee, Mark. "The Olive Leaf: A Sign from Above?" *Positive Health News* 11 (May 1996) [from: Keep Hope Alive, P.O. Box 27041, West Allis, WI 53227; tel: 414-548-4344].

13 Ficarra, Paola, and Rita Ficarra. "HPLC Analysis of Oleuropein and Some Flavonoids in Leaf and Bud of *Olea Europea L.*" *Il Farmaco* 46:6 (1991), 803-815.

14 Visioli, Francesco, and Claudio Gaili. "Oleuropein Protects Low Density Lipoprotein from Oxidation." *Life Sciences* 55:24 (1994), 1965-1971.

15 Farnsworth, N. R., et. al. "Medicinal Plants in Therapy." *Bulletin of the World Health Organization* 63:6 (1985), 965-981; reprinted in *Classic Botanical Reprint* 212 (Austin, Texas: American Botanical Council).

16 Ibid.

17 "New Health and Medical Findings from Around the World." *Life Extension Magazine* 14:12 (December 1994), 99-103.

Chapter 7
Other Alternatives for Heart Health

1 Becker, R. O., M.D. *Cross Currents: The Promise of Electromedicine, The Perils of Electropollution* (Los Angeles: Jeremy P. Tarcher, 1990).

2 Davis, A. R., and W. C. Rawls. *Magnetism and Its Effects on the Living System* (New York: Exposition Press, 1974).

3 Becker, R. O., M.D. *Cross Currents: The Promise of Electromedicine, The Perils of Electropollution* (Los Angeles: Jeremy P. Tarcher, 1990), 187.

4 Nakagawa, K., M.D. "Magnetic Field Deficiency Syndrome and Magnetic Treatment." *Japan Medical Journal* 2745 (December 1976).

5 Philpott, William H., M.D. *Diabetes Mellitus: A Reversible Disease* (an unpublished monograph).

6 Philpott, W., and S. Taplin. *Biomagnetic Handbook* (Choctaw, OK: Enviro-Tech Products, 1990).

7 Farr, C. H. *The Therapeutic Use of Intravenous Hydrogen Peroxide* Monograph. (Oklahoma City, OK: Genesis Medical Center, 1987).

8 Ibid.

9 Chung, H. Y. "Treatment of 103 Cases of Coronary Diseases with *Ilex pubescens.*" *Chinese Medical Journal* 1 (1973), 64.

Chapter 8
What Causes High Blood Pressure?

1 American Heart Association Internet web site: http://www.amhrt.org/hs96/hbps.html.

2 Havlik, R. J., et al. "Weight and Hypertension." *Annals of Internal Medicine* 98:5 pt. 2 (May 1983), 855-859.

3 Egan, K. J., et al. "The Impact of Psychological Distress on the Control of Hypertension." *Journal of Human Stress* 9:4 (December 1983), 4-10.

4 Gruchow, H. W., et al. "Alcohol, Nutrient Intake, and Hypertension in U.S. Adults." *Journal of the American Medical Association* 253:11 (March

1985), 1567-1570.

5 Pizzorno, J. E., and M. T. Murray, eds. "Hypertension." *A Textbook of Natural Medicine* (Seattle, WA: John Bastyr Publications, 1988).

6 Chow, H. Y., et al. "Cardiovascular Effects of Gardenia Florida L. (*Gardenise Fructus*) Extract." *American Journal of Chinese Medicine* 4:1 (1976), 47-51; Brewer, G. J. "Molecular Mechanisms of Zinc Action on Cells." *Agents and Actions* 8:Suppl. (1981), 37-49; Bennett, A. E., et al. "Sugar Consumption and Cigarette Smoking." *The Lancet* 1 (May 1970), 1011-1014; Kershbaum, A., et al. "Effects of Smoking and Nicotine on Adrenocortical Secretion." *Journal of the American Medical Association* 203:4 (January 1968), 275-278; Fortmann, S. P., et al. "The Association of Blood Pressure and Dietary Alcohol: Differences by Age, Sex and Estrogen Use." *American Journal of Epidemiology* 118:4 (October 1983), 497-507.

7 Pizzorno, J. E., and M. T. Murray, eds. "Hypertension." *A Textbook of Natural Medicine* (Seattle, WA: John Bastyr Publications, 1988).

8 He, J., et al. "Effect of Migration on Blood Pressure: The Yi People Study." *Epidemiology* 2:2 (March 1991), 88-97; Poulter, N. R., et al. "The Kenyan Luo Migration Study: Observations on the Initiation of a Rise in Blood Pressure." *British Medical Journal* 300:6730 (April 1990), 967-972; Salmond, C. E., et al. "Blood Pressure Patterns and Migration: A 14-Year Cohort Study of Adult Tokelauans." *American Journal of Epidemiology* 130:1 (July 1989), 37-52.

9 Meneely, G. R., and H. D. Battarbee. "High Sodium-Low Potassium Environment and Hypertension." *American Journal of Cardiology* 38:6 (November 1976), 768-785; Resnick, L. M., et al. "Intracellular Free Magnesium in Erythrocytes of Essential Hypertension: Relationship to Blood Pressure and Serum Divalent Cations." *Proceedings of the National Academy of Sciences of the U.S.A.* 81:20 (October 1984), 6511-6515.

10 Lang, T., et al. "Relation Between Coffee Drinking and Blood Pressure: Analysis of 6,321 Subjects in the Paris Region." *American Journal of Cardiology* 52:10 (December 1983), 1238-1242.

11 Fortmann, S. P., et al. "The Association of Blood Pressure and Dietary Alcohol: Differences by Age, Sex and Estrogen Use." *American Journal of Epidemiology* 118:4 (October 1983), 497-507; Gruchow, H. W., et al. "Alcohol, Nutrient Intake, and Hypertension in U.S. Adults." *Journal of the American Medical Association* 253:11 (March 1985), 1567-1570.

12 Bennett, A. E., et al. "Sugar Consumption and Cigarette Smoking." *The Lancet* 1 (May 1970), 1011-1014.

13 Schroeder, K. L., and M. S. Chen, Jr. "Smokeless Tobacco and Blood Pressure." *New England Journal of Medicine* 312:14 (April 1985), 919; Hampson, N. B. "Smokeless is Not Saltless." *New England Journal of Medicine* 312:14 (April 1985), 919-920.

14 Pirkle, J. L., et al. "The Relationship Between Blood Lead Levels and its Cardiovascular Risk Implications." *American Journal of Epidemiology* 121:2 (February 1985), 246-258.

15 Glauser, S. C., et al. "Blood-Cadmium Levels in Normotensive and Untreated Hypertensive Humans." *The Lancet* 1 (April 1976), 717-718.

16 *Science News* 148 (October 21, 1995), 268.

17 Barnes, Broda O., M.D., and Lawrence Galton. *Hypothyroidism: The Unsuspected Illness* (New York: Harper & Row, 1976).

Chapter 9

Self-Care Options: How to Use Diet, Exercise, and Lifestyle Changes to Lower Your Blood Pressure

1 Resnick, L. M., R. K. Gupta, and J. H. Laragh. "Intracellular Free Magnesium in Erythrocytes of Essential Hypertension: Relationship to Blood Pressure and Serum Divalent Cations." *Proceedings of the National Academy of Sciences of the U.S.A.* 81:20 (October 1984), 6511-6515.

2 Foushee, D. B., J. Ruffin, and U. Banerjee. "Garlic as a Natural Agent for the Treatment of Hypertension: A Preliminary Report." *Cytobios* 34:135-136 (1982), 145-152.

3 "Reducing Hypertension: Is Diet Better Than Drugs?" *Alternative & Complementary Therapies* 3:1 (February 1997), 3. (Available from: Mary Ann Liebert, Inc., 2 Madison Avenue, Larchmont, NY 10538; tel: 914-834-3100; fax: 914-834-3582; 6 issues/$79).

4 *Hypertension* 22:3 (September 1993), 371-379.

5 Gordon, Laura. "Exercise and Salt Restriction May Be Enough for Mildly High Blood Pressure." *Medical Tribune* 8 (December 21, 1995).

6 Merlo, Juan, et al. "Incidence of Myocardial Infarction in Elderly Men Being Treated with Antihypertensive Drugs: Population Based Cohort Study." *British Medical Journal* 313

(August 24, 1996), 457-461.

7 Altman, Lawrence K. "Use of Heart Drug Is Found To Increase the Risk of Death." *The New York Times* (November 1, 1995).

8 He, Jiang, et al. "Oats and Buckwheat Intakes and Cardiovascular Disease Risk Factors in an Ethnic Minority of China." *American Journal of Clinical Nutrition* 61 (1995), 366-372.

9 Pietinen, P., et al. "Intake of Dietary Fiber and Risk of Coronary Heart Disease in a Cohort of Finnish Men." *Circulation* 94:11 (December 1996), 2720-2727.

10 Davidson, M. H., et al. "The Hypocholesterolemic Effects of Beta-Glucan in Oatmeal and Oat Bran." *Journal of the American Medical Association* 265:14 (April 10, 1991), 1833-1839.

11 Van Horn, L.V., et al. "Serum Lipid Response to Oat Product Intake with a Fat-Modified Diet." *Journal of the American Dietetic Association* 86:6 (June 1986), 759-764.

12 Pick, Mary E., et al. "Oat Bran Concentrate Bread Products Improve Long-Term Control of Diabetes: A Pilot Study." *Journal of the American Dietetic Association* 96:12 (1996), 1254-1261.

13 Goldstein, I. B., et al. "Home Relaxation Techniques for Essential Hypertension." *Psychosomatic Medicine* 46:5 (September/October 1984), 398-414; Brassard, C., and R. T. Couture. "Biofeedback and Relaxation for Patients with Hypertension." *Canadian Nurse* 89:1 (January 1993), 49-52; Whyte, H. M. "NHMRC Workshop on Non-Pharmacological Methods of Lowering Blood Pressure." *Medical Journal of Australia* 2:1 Suppl. (July 1983), S13-S16; Blanchard, E.B., et al. "Preliminary Results from a Controlled Evaluation of Thermal Biofeedback as a Treatment for Essential Hypertension." *Biofeedback and Self Regulation* 9:4 (December 1984), 471-495.

14 The Joint National Committee on Detection, Evaluation, and Treatment of High Blood Pressure. "The 1988 Report of the Joint National Committee of the American Medical Association." *Archives of Internal Medicine* 148 (1988), 1023-1038.

15 McGrady, A., et al. "Sustained Effects of Biofeedback-Assisted Relaxation Therapy in Essential Hypertension." *Biofeedback and Self-Regulation* 16:4 (December 1991), 399-411.

16 Aivazyan, T. A., et al. "Efficacy of Relaxation Techniques in Hypertensive Patients." *Health Psychology* 7 Suppl. (1988), 193-200.

17 Yen, Lee-Lan. "Comparison of Relaxation Techniques, Routine Blood Pressure Measurements, and Self-Learning Packages in Hypertension Control." *Preventive Medicine* 25:3 (May/June 1996), 339-345.

18 Gordon, N. F., and C. B. Scott. "Exercise and Mild Essential Hypertension." *Primary Care Clinics in Office Practice* 18:3 (September 1991), 683-694.

19 Grimm, Richard H., Jr., M.D., Ph.D., et al., *Journal of the American Medical Association* 275:20 (May 22/29, 1996), 1549-1556.

20 Hirofumi Tanaka, David R., et al., "Swimming Training Lowers the Resting Blood Pressure in Individuals with Hypertension," *Journal of Hypertension* 15:6, 0651-0657.

21 Murray, Michael T., N.D. *Natural Alternatives to Over-the-Counter and Prescription Drugs* (New York: William Morrow, 1994).

Chapter 11

Chinese Medicine: How It Can Help Reverse High Blood Pressure

1 *A Proposed Standard International Acupuncture Nomenclature: Report of a World Health Organization Scientific Group* (Geneva, Switzerland: World Health Organization, 1991).

2 Kaptchuk, T. J. *The Web that Has No Weaver* (Chicago: Congdon & Weed, 1983).

3 It would be impossible to cite every study from every journal around the world that might be relevant. A sampling of a few articles include: Tani, T. "Treatment of Type I Allergic Disease with Chinese Herbal formulas: Minor Blue Dragon Combination and Minor Bupleurum Combination." *International Journal of Oriental Medicine* 14:3 (September 1989), 155-166; Chen, A., M.D. "Effective Acupuncture Therapy for Migraine: Review and Comparison of Prescriptions with Recommendations for Improved Results." *American Journal of Acupuncture* 17:4 (1989), 305-316; Chen, G. S. "The Effect of Acupuncture Treatment on Carpal Tunnel Syndrome." *American Journal of Acupuncture* 18:1 (1990), 5-10; Chen, K., and H. Liang. "Progress of Geriatrics Research in Chinese Medicine." *International Journal of Oriental Medicine* 14:1 (March 1989), 49-56.

4 Zhuang, H., et al. "Effects of *Radix Salviae Miltiorrhizae* Extract Injection on Survival of Allogenic Heart Transplantation." *Journal of Traditional Chinese Medicine* 10:4 (December 1990), 276-281; Lu, W. "Treatment of AIDS by TCM and Materia Medica."

Journal of Traditional Chinese Medicine 11:4 (December 1991), 249-252; Di Concetto, G., M.D., and L. Sotte. "Treatment of Headaches by Acupuncture and Chinese Herbal Therapy: Conclusive Data Concerning 1,000 Patients." *Journal of Traditional Chinese Medicine* 2:3 (September 1991), 174-176.

Chapter 12
Lower Your Blood Pressure With Herbs

1 ESCOP, European Scientific Cooperative for Phytotherapy. (Meppel, The Netherlands: European Scientific Cooperative for Phytotherapy, 1992).

2 German Ministry of Health. Commission E. *Monographs for Phytomedicines* (Bonn, Germany: German Ministry of Health, 1989).

3 Lau, Benjamin H.S., M.D., Ph.D. "Effects of an Odor-Modified Garlic Preparation on Blood Lipids." *Nutrition Research* 7 (1987), 131-149.

4 Mindell, Earl L., R.Ph., Ph.D. *Garlic: The Miracle Nutrient* (New Canaan, CT: Keats Publishing, 1996).

5 Foster, S. *Garlic*. Botanical Series 311 (Austin, TX: American Botanical Council, 1991); Kleijnen, J., et al. "Garlic, Onions and Cardiovascular Risk Factors: A Review of the Evidence from Human Experiments with Emphasis on Commercially Available Preparations." *British Journal of Clinical Pharmacology* 28:5 (November 1989), 535-544.

6 Shibata, S., et al. " Chemistry and Pharmacology of Panax." *Economic and Medicinal Plant Research* 1 (1985), 217-284.

7 Brekhman, I. I., and I. V. Dardymov. "Pharmacological Investigation of Glycosides From Ginseng and Eleutherococcus." *Lloydia* 32 (1969), 46-51.

8 Bombardelli, E., et al. "The Effect of Acute and Chronic (Panax) Ginseng Saponins Treatment on Adrenal Function, Biochemical and Pharmacological." *Proceedings of the 3rd International Ginseng Symposium* 1 (1980), 9-16; Fulder, S. J. "Ginseng and the Hypothalamic-Pituitary Control of Stress." *American Journal of Chinese Medicine* 9 (1981), 112-118.

9 Joo, C. N. "The Preventative Effect of Korean (P. Ginseng) Saponins on Aortic Atheroma Formation in Prolonged Cholesterol-Fed Rabbits." *Proceedings of the 3rd International Ginseng Symposium* (1980), 27-36.

10 Hobbs, C. "Hawthorn: A Literature Review." *HerbalGram* 21 (1990), 19-33.

11 German Ministry of Health. Commission E.
Monographs for Phytomedicines (Bonn, Germany: German Ministry of Health, 1989).

12 Reuter, H.D. "Crataegus Hawthorn: A Botanical Cardiac Agent." *Quarterly Review of Natural Medicine* (Summer 1995), 107-117. (Available from Natural Product Research Consultants, Inc., 600 First Avenue, Suite 205, Seattle, WA 98104; tel: 206-623-2520; fax: 206-623-6340; $79/4 issues).

13 Berdyshev, V. V. "Effect of the Long-Term Intake of Eleutherococcus on the Adaptation of Sailors in the Tropics." *Voenno Meditsinskii Zhurnal* 5 (May 1981), 57-58. (Published in Russian).

14 German Ministry of Health. Commission E. *Valerian. Monographs for Phytomedicines* (Bonn, Germany: German Ministry of Health, 1985).

15 ESCOP, European Scientific Cooperative for Phytotherapy. *Valerian Root* (Meppel, The Netherlands: European Scientific Cooperative for Phytotherapy, 1990).

16 Hobbs, C. "Valerian: A Literature Review." *HerbalGram* 21 (1989), 19-34.

17 *Townsend Letter for Doctors* (May 1994), 432-434; *Explore! for the Professional* 4:5 (1993), 17-19.

18 Jin, H. et al. "Treatment of Hypertension by *Ling zhi* Combined with Hypotensor and Its Effects on Arterial, Arteriolar, and Capillary Pressure and Microcirculation." *Microcirculatory Approach to Asian Traditional Medicine*, edited by Nimmi, H., et al. (New York: Elsevier Science, 1996), 131-138.

Chapter 13
Alternative Medicine Options for Lowering High Blood Pressure

1 Wagner, H., and L. Sprinkmeier. "Uber die pharmakologischen Wirkungen von Melissengeist." *Deutsche Apotheker Zeitung* 113 (1973), 1159.

2 Franchomme, P., and D. Penoel. *Aromatherapie Exactement* (Limoges: Roger Jollois, 1990).

3 Tisserand, R. B. *The Art of Aromatherapy* (Rochester, VT: Healing Arts Press, 1977).

4 Czygan, F. C. "Essential Oils: Aspects of History of Civilization." *Atherische åle, Analytik, Physiologie, Zusammensetzung*, edited by K. H. Kubeczka, (Stuttgart, New York: Georg Thieme Verlag, 1982).

5 Dodd, G. H. "Receptor Events in Perfumery." *Perfumery: The Psychology and Biology of Fragrance* edited by van Toller, S., and G. H. Dodd (London: Chapman and Hall, 1988).

6 Steele, J. "Brain Research and Essential Oils."

Aromatherapy Quarterly 3 (Spring 1984), 5.

7 Lorig, T. S., et al. "The Effects of Low Concentration Odors on EEG Activity and Behavior." Journal of Psychophysiology 5 (1991), 69-77.

8 Belaiche, P. Traite de Phytotherapie et d'aromatherapie Tome I: L'aromatogramme (Paris: Maloine S.A., 1979).

9 Woolfson, A. "Intensive Aromacare." International Journal of Aromatherapy 4:2 (1992), 12-13.

10 Keller, W., and W. Kober. "Moglickeiten der Verwendung atherischer åle zur Raundesinfektion I." Arzneimittelforschung 5 (1955), 224; Keller, W., and W. Kober. "Moglickeiten der Verwendung atherischer åle zur Raundesinfektion II." Arzneimittelforschung 6 (1955), 768.

11 "Aromatherapy on the Wards: Lavendar Beats Benzodiazepines." International Journal of Aromatherapy 1:2 (1988), 1.

12 Tisserand, R. B. The Art of Aromatherapy (Rochester, VT: Healing Arts Press, 1977).

13 Fahrion, S. L. "Hypertension and Biofeedback." Primary Care Clinics in Office Practice 3 (September 1991), 663-682.

14 Namba, K., et al. "Effect of Taurine Concentration on Platelet Aggregation in Gestosis Patients with Edema, Proteinuria, and Hypertension." Acta Medica Okayama 46:4 (August 1992), 241-247; Ceriello, A., et al. "Anti-Oxidants Show an Anti-Hypertensive Effect in Diabetic and Hypertensive Subjects." Clinical Science 81:6 (December 1991), 739-742; Maxwell, S. R. "Can Anti-Oxidants Prevent Ischemic Heart Disease?" Journal of Clinical Pharmacy and Therapeutics 18:2 (April 1993), 85-95.

15 Galley, H.F., et al. "Regulation of Nitric Oxide Synthase Activity in Cultured Human Endothelial Cells: Effect of Antioxidants." Free Radical Biology and Medicine 21 (1996), 97-101.

16 Galley, H.F., et al. "Combination Oral Antioxidant Supplementation Reduces Blood Pressure." Clinical Science 92 (1997), 361-365.

17 Henry, H. J., et al. "Increasing Calcium Intake Lowers Blood Pressure: The Literature Reviewed." Journal of the American Dietetic Association 85:2 (February 1985), 182-185; Belizam, J. M., et al. "Reduction of Blood Pressure with Calcium Supplementation in Young Adults." Journal of the American Medical Association 249:9 (March 1983), 1161-1165.

18 Wimaladwansa, S., et al. "Mechanisms of Antihypertensive Effects of Dietary Calcium and Role of Calcitonin-Gene-Related Peptide in Hypertension." Canadian Journal of Physiology and Pharmacology 73:7 (1995), 981-985.

19 McCarron, D. A., et al. "Dietary Calcium in Human Hypertension." Science 217:4556 (1982), 267-269.

20 Dyckner, T., and P. O. Wester. "Effect of Magnesium on Blood Pressure." British Medical Journal 286:6381 (January 1983), 1847-1849.

21 Northeast Center for Environmental Medicine Health Letter (Fall 1992).

22 Skrabal, F., et al. "Low Sodium/High Potassium Diet for Prevention of Hypertension: Probable Mechanisms of Action." The Lancet 2:8252 (October 1981), 895-900.

23 Armstrong, B., et al. "Urinary Sodium and Blood Pressure in Vegetarians." American Journal of Clinical Nutrition 32:12 (December 1979), 2472-2476; Rouse, I. L., et al. "Vegetarian Diet and Blood Pressure." The Lancet 2:8352 (1983), 742-743.

24 Ivanov, S. G., et al. "The Magnetotherapy of Hypertension Patients." Terapevticheskii Arkhiv 62:9 (1990), 71-74.

Chapter 14

What Causes Stroke?

1 "Stroke Statistics." National Stroke Association Internet web site: http://www.stroke.org/.

2 American Heart Association Internet web site: http://www.amhrt.org/hs96/strokes.html.

3 "Stroke Statistics." National Stroke Association Internet web site: http://www.stroke.org/.

4 Ibid.

5 U. S. Department of Health and Human Services. Public Health Service, National Institutes of Health. Stroke: Hope Through Research (Pub. No. 83-2222, August 1983).

6 Levine, Jeff. "Study: Some People Risk a Stroke by Overusing Decongestants." Internet: CNN Interactive Heath Page (April 16, 1997).

7 "Study: Overweight Women at Greater Risk of Stroke." Internet: CNN Interactive Heath Page (May 20, 1997).

8 Kindenstrom, Ewa, et al. "Influence of Total Cholesterol, High Density Lipoprotein Cholesterol, and Triglycerides on Risk of Cerebrovascular Disease: The Copenhagen City Heart Study." British Medical Journal 433:309 (1994), 11-15.

9 Nagayama, Masao, M.D., Ph.D., et al. "Lipoprotein (a) and Ischemic Cerebrovascular Disease in

Young Adults." *Stroke* 25 (1994), 74-78.

Young Adults." *Stroke* 25 (1994), 74-78.

10 Peck, Peggy. "Elevated Lipoprotein (a) May Be the Strongest Predictor of Cerebrovascular Disease." *Family Practice News* (April 15, 1994), 2.

11 Davalos, Antonio, M.D., et al. "Iron-Related Damage in Acute Ischemic Stroke." *Stroke* 25:8 (1994), 1543-1546.

12 Perry, I.J., et al. "Prospective Study of Serum Total Homocysteine Concentration and Risk of Stroke in Middle-Aged British Men." *The Lancet* 346 (November 25, 1995), 1395-1398.

13 den Heijer, M., et al. "Is Hyperhomocysteinaemia a Risk Factor for Recurrent Venous Thrombosis?" *The Lancet* 345 (1995), 882-885.

14 Lalouschek, W., et al. "Hyperhomocysteinemia: An Independent Risk Factor for Stroke." *Fortschritte der Neurologie Psychiatic* 64 (1996), 271-277.

15 "Bypass Surgery Some Risk to the Brain." Internet: CNN Interactive Heath Page (December 18, 1996).

16 Phillips, Pat. "Fibrinogen Linked to Carotid Stenosis, Stroke." *Medical Tribune* (March 11, 1993), 3.

17 Ibid.

18 Resch, Karl L., M.D., et al. "Fibrinogen and Viscosity as Risk Factors for Subsequent Cardiovascular Events in Stroke Survivors." *Annals of Internal Medicine* 117:5 (September 1, 1992), 371-375.

19 Petitti, Diana B., M.D., et al. "Stroke in Users of Low-Dose Oral Contraceptives." *New England Journal of Medicine* 335:1 (July 1996), 8-15.

20 Jeppesen, Lise Leth, et al. "Decreased Serum Testosterone in Men with Acute Ischemic Stroke." *Arteriosclerosis, Thrombosis and Vascular Disease* 16:6 (June 1996), 749-754.

Chapter 15
Self-Care Essentials for Stroke

1 Orencia, Anthony J., M.D., Ph.D., et al. "Fish Consumption and Stroke in Men: 30-Year Findings of the Chicago Western Electric Study." *Stroke* 27:2 (February 1996), 204-209.

2 Gillum, R.F., et al. "The Relationship Between Fish Consumption and Stroke Incidence." *Archives of Internal Medicine* 156 (1996), 537-542.

3 Gillman, Matthew W., M.D., et al. "A Protective Effect of Fruits and Vegetables on Development of Stroke in Men." *Journal of the American Medical Association* 273:14 (April 12, 1995), 1113-1117.

4 "Carrots, Spinach and Diet Tied to Lower Stroke Risk." *Medical Tribune* (April 8, 1993), 7.

5 Keli, Sirving O., M.D., Ph.D., et al. "Dietary Flavonoids, Antioxidant Vitamins, and Incidence of Stroke: The Zupthen Study." *Archives of Internal Medicine* 157 (March 25, 1996), 637-642.

6 Mann, Denise. "Any Exercise at All Decreases Stroke Risk in Elderly." *Medical Tribune* (May 2, 1996).

7 Kiely, Dan K., et al. "Physical Activity and Stroke Risk: The Framingham Study." *American Journal of Epidemiology* 149:7 (1994), 608-620.

8 "Moderate Exercise Cuts Vessel Disease." *Medical Tribune* (March 26, 1992), 10.

9 Laino, Charlene. "Exercise from 25 On Guards Against Stroke." *Family Practice News* (August 26, 1993), 20.

10 Potempa, Kathleen, et al. "Benefits of Aerobic Exercise after Stroke." *Sports Medicine* 21:5 (May 1996), 337-346; Potempa, Kathleen, et al. "Physiological Outcomes of Aerobic Exercise Training in Hemiparetic Stroke Patients." *Stroke* 26:1 (January 1995), 101-105.

11 Wannamethee, S. Goya, Ph.D., et al. *Journal of the American Medical Association* 274:12 (July 12, 1995), 155-160.

Chapter 16
Oxygen Therapy: How It Can Help Stroke Recovery

1 Perrin, D. 1993 study in Great Britain (unpublished).

2 Warburg, O. "The Prime Cause and Prevention of Cancer." Revised lecture at the Meeting of the Nobel-laureates on June 30, 1966 (Bethesda, MD: National Cancer Institute, 1967).

3 Farr, C. H. Presented at the Fourth International Conference on Bio-Oxidative Medicine. Reston, VA (April 1-4, 1993).

4 Farr, C. H. "Workbook on Free Radical Chemistry and Hydrogen Peroxide Metabolism Including Protocol for the Intravenous Administration of Hydrogen Peroxide." Contains 32 citations with references in the workbook, and 123 in the protocol (1992). (Available from: International Bio-Oxidative Medicine Foundation. P.O. Box 13205, Oklahoma City, OK, 73113).

5 Farr, C. H. *The Therapeutic Use of Intravenous Hydrogen Peroxide* Monograph. (Oklahoma City, OK: Genesis Medical Center, 1987).

6 Farr, C. H. "Workbook on Free Radical Chemistry and Hydrogen Peroxide Metabolism Including Protocol for the Intravenous Administration of Hydrogen Peroxide." Contains 32 citations with references in

the workbook, and 123 in the protocol (1992).
(Available from: International Bio-Oxidative
Medicine Foundation. P.O. Box 13205, Oklahoma
City, OK, 73113).

7 Farr, C. H. *The Therapeutic Use of Intravenous
Hydrogen Peroxide* Monograph. (Oklahoma City,
OK: Genesis Medical Center, 1987); Baker, E. *The
Unmedical Miracle—Oxygen* (Indianola, WA:
Drelwood Communications, 1991).

Chapter 17
More Options for Treating Stroke

1 Ayers, Margaret E., M.A. "EEG Neurofeedback to Bring
Individuals Out of Level-Two Coma." *Biofeedback
and Self-Regulation* 20:3 (September 1995);
Ayers, Margaret E., M.A. "Electroencephalic
Neurofeedback and Closed Head Injury of 250
Individuals." *Head Injury Frontiers* (1987), 380.

2 Gey, K.F., et al. "Poor Plasma Status of Carotene and
Vitamin C is Associated with Higher Mortality from
Ischemic Heart Disease and Stroke: Basal
Prospective Study." *Clinical Investigator* 71 (1993),
3-6.

3 Clark, Wayne M., M.D., et al. "Need for Treatment of
Elevated Plasma Fibrinogen Levels in
Cerebrovascular Disease." *Heart Disease and
Stroke* (Available from Dr. Wayne M. Clark,
Department of Neurology L226, Oregon Health
Sciences University, 3181 SW Sam Jackson Park
Road, Portland, OR 97201).

Index

THIS BOOK COULD...

LEARN WAYS TO REVERSE AND PREVENT CANCER

Some of the Doctors in *An Alternative Medicine Definitive Guide to Cancer*:

Robert Atkins, M.D.
New York, NY
Learn about Dr. Atkins' multifaceted program to help the body overcome cancer.

Keith Block, M.D.
Chicago, IL
Dr. Block combines conventional therapy with immune-enhancing, detoxifying treatments to maximize cancer survival.

James W. Forsythe, M.D., H.M.D.
Reno, NV
An oncologist explains his use of immune-stimulating therapies.

Robert A. Nagourney, M.D.
Long Beach, CA
For those who are thinking of using chemotherapy, this oncologist can test for drug effectiveness first.

Jesse Stoff, M.D.
Tucson, AZ
All aspects of a patient's life—body, mind, and emotions—must receive therapeutic attention. Learn how.

Vincent Speckhart, M.D., M.D.H. Norfolk, VA
An oncologist for 22 years, Dr. Speckhart explains how he reverses cancer by removing toxins and repairing the immune system.

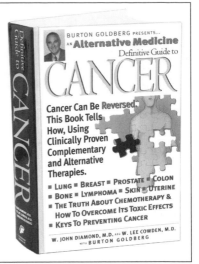

BURTON GOLDBERG PRESENTS...
AN **Alternative Medicine** Definitive Guide to
CANCER

Cancer Can Be Reversed. This Book Tells How, Using Clinically Proven Complementary and Alternative Therapies.

- LUNG ■ BREAST ■ PROSTATE ■ COLON
- BONE ■ LYMPHOMA ■ SKIN ■ UTERINE
- THE TRUTH ABOUT CHEMOTHERAPY & HOW TO OVERCOME ITS TOXIC EFFECTS
- KEYS TO PREVENTING CANCER

W. JOHN DIAMOND, M.D. AND W. LEE COWDEN, M.D. WITH BURTON GOLDBERG

©1997 by Future Medicine Publishing, Inc.
Publishers of *Alternative Medicine: The Definitive Guide* and the bimonthly magazine *Alternative Medicine Digest*

THIS 1,116-PAGE BOOK ILLUSTRATES MANY SUCCESSFUL ALTERNATIVES TO CONVENTIONAL CARE THAT CAN REMOVE THE ROOT CAUSES OF CANCER AND RESTORE YOU TO HEALTH WITHOUT FURTHER POISONING OR DAMAGING YOUR BODY.

CALL FOR YOUR COPY TODAY.
BUY A COPY FOR YOUR ONCOLOGIST AND INSIST THAT IT BE READ.

CALL 800-333-HEAL

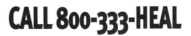

Valuable Information Featured in
An Alternative Medicine Definitive Guide to Cancer:

- Cancer patients treated with nontoxic botanicals had twice the survival rate after 1 year, and 4 times the survival rate after 2 years, compared to chemotherapy patients. Readers are unlikely ever to see such results published in American medical journals, which receive their primary financial support from the pharmaceutical industry.

- The medical director of a prestigious clinic reports that in 90% of his breast cancer patients there is a dental factor.

SAVE YOUR LIFE

The single most important, lifesaving book on cancer ever published—37 top physicians explain their proven, safe, nontoxic, and successful treatments for reversing cancer.

From W. John Diamond, M.D., director of the Triad Medical Center in Reno, Nevada, and W. Lee Cowden, M.D., cardiologist and consultant to the Conservative Medicine Institute in Richardson, Texas, comes the book that finally tells you how to be cancer free for life.

The book guides you through the safest and most effective treatment alternatives known today. Learn how leading practitioners use herbs, nutrition and diet, supplements, oxygen, enzymes, glandular extracts, homeopathic remedies, plus specialized substances such as Ukrain, Essiac, Carnivora, Iscador, 714X, shark cartilage, and many others to prevent and reverse cancers. Learn why the mammoth U.S. cancer industry does not want you to know about these successful alternatives. See the proof of treatment success in 55 documented patient case histories demonstrating how alternative approaches to cancer can make the difference between life and death—as these people found out:

It was a marvelous feeling. I was blossoming like a flower. After a short time, I regained my appetite, went on shopping sprees with my daughter, even went to shows. I began to live again! Can I ever repay Dr. Atkins for giving me the gift of life? Perhaps not. But if I stay well and healthy, I think that will be his greatest reward.

CLAUDETTE, 52—Metastatic ovarian cancer reversed

I'm well aware of what eating a proper diet has done for me. It not only cured me of cancer, but controlled my weight and relieved my hypertension, for which I had been on medication for 42 years.

ETHAN, 66—14 years after metastatic prostate cancer diagnosis

TO ORDER, CALL 800-333-HEAL

CURE YOUR HEADACHES...

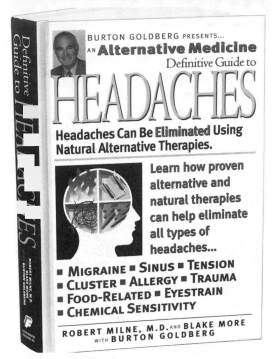

BURTON GOLDBERG PRESENTS...
AN **Alternative Medicine**
Definitive Guide to
HEADACHES

Headaches Can Be Eliminated Using Natural Alternative Therapies.

Learn how proven alternative and natural therapies can help eliminate all types of headaches...

- **MIGRAINE ■ SINUS ■ TENSION**
- **CLUSTER ■ ALLERGY ■ TRAUMA**
- **FOOD-RELATED ■ EYESTRAIN**
- **CHEMICAL SENSITIVITY**

ROBERT MILNE, M.D. AND BLAKE MORE
WITH BURTON GOLDBERG

If you suffer from headaches, this book could change your life. It is entirely possible that with this invaluable practical information, you may well put headaches behind you as something you once suffered from, but no more.

Robert Milne, M.D., and Blake More expertly guide you through the root causes and multiple treatment options for 11 major types of headaches, from sinus to migraine, cluster to tension.

We have made every effort possible to make this book practical and user-friendly for you. For a quick reference to headache types, symptoms, treatment options, use our Master Symptom Chart. If you suffer from tension headaches, turn directly to Chapter 6; if migraines are your millstone, see Chapter 7; and if you're not sure what type of headache you have, study the symptoms list in the Master Symptom Chart until you find the clinical term that best matches your condition.

No matter what kind of headache you used to have, after reading this book your head may never pain you again.

Hardcover ■ ISBN 1-887299-03-3
■ 6" x 9" ■ 525 pages

TO ORDER, CALL 800-333-HEAL

USING NATURAL THERAPIES

Say goodbye to headaches for the rest of your life. No matter what kind of headache you suffer from, thanks to the proven and effective health information in this book, your head may never pain you again. Your headaches, whether migraine, tension, sinus, cluster, or any of the 11 different types covered in this book, can be eliminated for good. Drawing on the entire field of alternative medicine, Robert Milne, M.D., Blake More, and Burton Goldberg tell you how, using chiropractic, herbalism, acupuncture, homeopathy, nutrition, bodywork, biofeedback, aromatherapy, and more, plus extensive self-care suggestions—all from leading experts in the field. In dozens of real-life success stories, learn how headache sufferers used these techniques and are now headache free.

Unlike any other headache book, *An Alternative Medicine Definitive Guide to Headaches* gives you the cutting-edge, practical, and easy-to-understand medical advice you need to make your headaches a pain of the past. Here's how the invaluable advice in this book helped these people become headache free:

It was so easy. To think of all those years I spent in pain, bouncing from one prescription to another, when all I had to do was stop eating sugar and dairy products for my headaches to go away.
—SUSAN, A FORMER MIGRAINER

I had thousands of dollars' worth of tests—CAT scans, MRIs, all kinds of things—but they didn't cure anything. Then with a nutritional supplement called essential fatty acids, I was handed the key to ending my headaches. —ROBERT, A REAL ESTATE BROKER

Decongestants only offered temporary relief of my sinus headaches. A naturopath gently massaged my face, neck, and stomach, then gave me homeopathy, herbs, and nutritional supplements. Within a week, I began to feel myself again, and now, 8 months later, my sinus headaches are completely gone.
—KATHERINE, A MASSAGE THERAPIST

TO ORDER, CALL 800-333-HEAL

ALTERNATIVE MEDICINE DIGEST

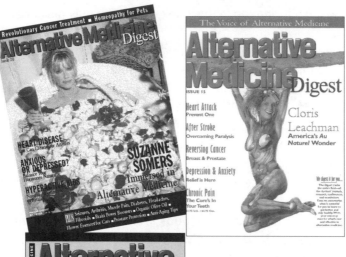

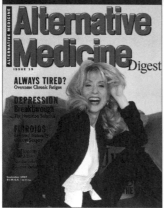

ORDER A SUBSCRIPTION TO THE BIMONTHLY *ALTERNATIVE MEDICINE DIGEST* TODAY.

TO ORDER, CALL 800-333-HEAL

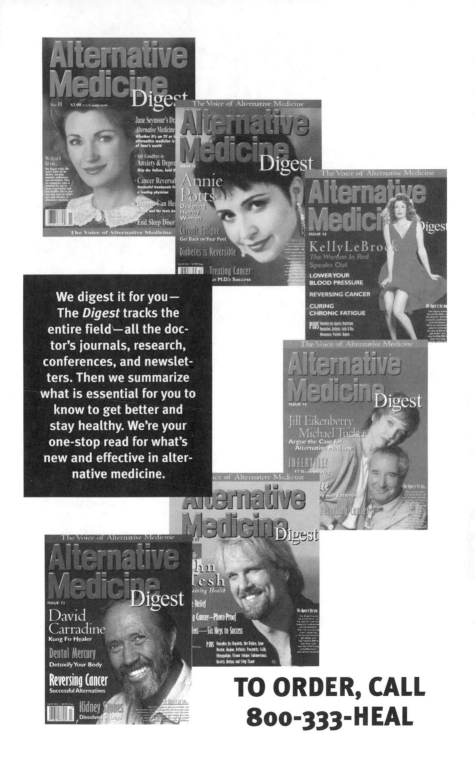

ALSO AVAILABLE FROM FUTURE MEDICINE

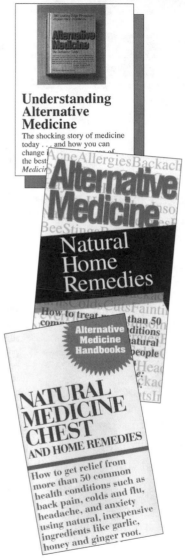

Understanding Alternative Medicine
The shocking story of medicine today . . . and how you can change

Alternative Medicine
Natural Home Remedies

Alternative Medicine Handbooks

NATURAL MEDICINE CHEST AND HOME REMEDIES

How to get relief from more than 50 common health conditions such as back pain, colds and flu, headache, and anxiety using natural, inexpensive ingredients like garlic, honey and ginger root.

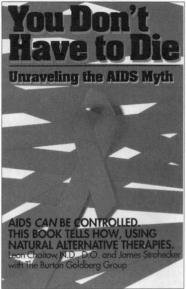

AIDS CAN BE CONTROLLED. THIS BOOK TELLS HOW, USING NATURAL ALTERNATIVE THERAPIES.
Leon Chaitow, N.D., D.O. and James Strohecker with The Burton Goldberg Group

- **You Don't Have to Die—Unraveling the AIDS Myth**
  319 pages, 5 1/4" x 8 1/4"
  ISBN 0-9636334-4-9

- **Understanding Alternative Medicine**
  Audio tape
  ISBN 0-9636334-6-5

- **Natural Home Remedies and Medicine Chest**
  72 pages, 4" x 7 1/2"
  ISBN 0-9636334-8-1

- **Natural Home Remedies**
  Video
  ISBN 0-9636334-7-3

TO ORDER, CALL 800-333-HEAL

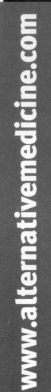
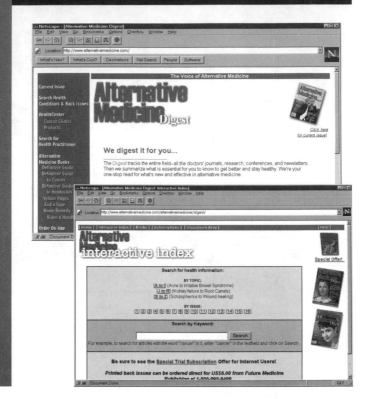

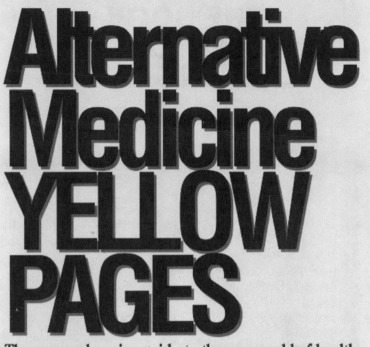

Alternative Medicine YELLOW PAGES

The comprehensive guide to the new world of health.

Become an active participant in your own well-being with the most complete directory of alternative therapies, health practitioners and products conveniently listed by type of therapy and location.

The perfect companion to the best-selling
Alternative Medicine: The Definitive Guide.

Put a one-stop telephone directory of 17,000 practitioners of alternative medicine around the U.S. at your fingertips. Find the alternative specialist by state and city, type of therapy, and health problem. Listings span back pain to weight management, arthritis to thyroid disorders. Learn even more about how alternative medicine can help end your health problem by browsing the hundreds of informative display ads throughout the book.

TO ORDER, CALL 800-333-HEAL

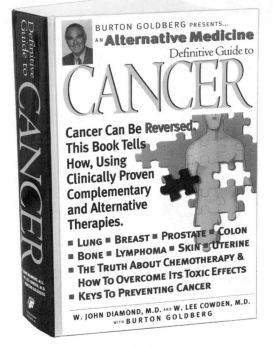